Judith S. Palfrey

Child Health in America

Making a Difference through Advocacy

The Johns Hopkins University Press
BALTIMORE

© 2006 The Johns Hopkins University Press
All rights reserved. Published 2006
Printed in the United States of America on acid-free paper
1 2 3 4 5 6 7 8 9

The Johns Hopkins University Press
2715 North Charles Street
Baltimore, Maryland 21218-4363
www.press.jhu.edu

Library of Congress Cataloging-in-Publication Data

Palfrey, Judith S.
Child health in America : making a difference through advocacy / Judith S. Palfrey.
p. ; cm.
Includes bibliographical references and index.
ISBN 0-8018-8452-7 (hardcover : alk. paper) — ISBN 0-8018-8453-5 (pbk. : alk. paper)
1. Child health services—United States.
[DNLM: 1. Child Advocacy—United States. 2. Adolescent Health Services—United States.
3. Child Health Services—United States. 4. Child Welfare—United States.
5. Infant Welfare—United States. WA 320 P159c 2006] I. Title.
RJ102.P348 2006
362.198′9200973—dc22   2006005263

A catalog record for this book is available from the British Library.

IN MEMORIAM
Anne E. Dyson

Contents

Acknowledgments

NEARLY TEN YEARS AGO, my friend Anne Dyson and I took a long walk through the streets of San Francisco. Up one hill, we talked about our families. Down another, we talked about children. Huffing a bit, we mused about how unfair life can be. Easing up on a level street, we wondered about how child health professionals could attack the big problems confronting American children. Annie wanted to do something to make a difference. She had a vision that she wanted to share. We talked and walked and thought about all sorts of things. One of them was writing a book like this. We talked of the fun it would be to do together.

Anne Dyson was an extraordinary person—a pediatrician, a businesswoman, and a philanthropist. She was convinced that pediatrics needed a fundamental realignment to address child health problems in the community. She believed that child health professionals could do a great deal of good through advocacy and that many of the young child health professionals were just waiting for the chance to speak and to act on behalf of children. As president of the Dyson Foundation, she worked to design a large experiment in pediatric resident education. Unfortunately, in October 1999, just as the national solicitation for proposals for the program was going out, she learned that she had an advanced, aggressive form of breast cancer. Even so, Anne never stopped plowing forward, positive in her beliefs and ardent in her efforts to improve the life chances and the health of children. She died almost exactly one year after the solicitation and one month after we celebrated the launch of the program: the Anne E. Dyson Community Pediatrics Training Initiative.

After Annie died, I decided that, to honor her and to fulfill her vision, I must write the book we had planned. I began work on the manuscript in the summer of 2003, drawing on the child health literature and the wealth of data available as a result of the 2000 census from government agencies and foundation projects.

Although I was working hard on the book, it was not until January 2005, listening to a student rendition of the song "Smile Though Your Heart Is Aching," that I understood that writing this book was my attempt to do just that—to smile with an aching heart, to capture what it means to fight with the odds against you and continue to laugh and love.

These days there is so much to make the heart ache. The pain of seeing child after child denied what they deserve, the sadness of losing friends and young patients to death in automobile crashes and by gunfire, the sorrow of lives crushed in natural disaster, lives burdened, harassed, and confused. And most especially the ache of all the uncaring by people who should know better, people in high places who owe children a fair chance.

But wallowing in sadness gets nobody anywhere—not Charlie Chaplin, not the little boy with cerebral palsy, not the little girl whose mother has bipolar disease. Annie Dyson knew that, and children know that. Children rebound. They run and play through the rubble of war and disaster. They dance in their wheelchairs, and they break the silence of the most solemn moments with a little coo, an outrageous giggle. When that happens, how is it possible not to smile? And where children are concerned, how is it possible not to care?

Fortunately, there are wonderful people who do care about children and children's health. I have been enormously fortunate to learn directly from many of them. First and foremost is Julius Richmond, whose wisdom, wit, and optimism have guided physicians, psychologists, child development practitioners, early childhood educators, public health professionals, public policymakers, and many others. His ability to keep the destination in his sights, never deviating from his original principles, is the essence of advocacy. It is not by accident that stories about Julius Richmond appear frequently in the pages of this book. He is a dear friend, and I am enormously grateful for his ongoing support and encouragement.

I have also been blessed by the guidance and friendship of such mentors and colleagues as Joel Alpert, Bron Anders, Betsy Anderson, Barbara Barlow, Richard Behrman, Steven Berman, Bill Bithoney, Joseph Carrillo, Tom Chapman, Bill Coleman, Morris Green, Robert Haggerty, Margaret Heagerty, Karen Hein, Renee Jenkins, Mel Levine, Phil Porter, Allan Rosenfeld, Ed Rushton, Steven Shelov, Cal Sia, Tom Tonniges, Debbie Walker, and Barry Zuckerman. I am particularly grateful to the principal investigators of the Dyson Initiative for their dedication to the ideals of community pediatrics and advocacy: Andy Aligne, Danny Armstrong, Gregory Blaschke, Arturo Brito, Chris Derauf, Steven Downs, Jeffrey Goldhagen, Matilde Irigoyen, Louise Iwaishi, Jeffrey Kascorowski, Stephen Ludwig, Dodi Meyer, Phillip Nader, Stephen Nicholas, Richard Pan, Vivian Resnick, Donald Schwartz, Laura Jean Shipley, Sarah Stelzner,

Nancy Swigonski, Daniel West, Earnestine Willis, Elisa Zenni, and the faculty and residents of their programs.

My colleagues and I have received generous support for our work from a number of individual donors, foundations, and federal agencies. Thanks go to Chris Degraw, Ann Drum, Rob Dyson, Barbara Finberg, Diana Gurieva, Ruby Hearn, Vince Hutchins, Paul Jellinek, Woodie Kessel, Margaret Mahoney, Merle McPherson, Ed Schor, and Chuck Yeager; my colleagues at Children's Hospital in Boston and Harvard Medical School, especially Lisa Albers, Hank Bernstein, Berry Brazelton, Laurie Cammisa, Mary Clark, Emily Davidson, Gary Fleisher, Fred Lovejoy, Bill Kiernan, David Nathan, Wanessa Risko, Emily Roth, Ron Samuels, Kate Weldon, Kim Wilson, and Alan Woolf; the associate chiefs of the Division of General Pediatrics, Joanne Cox and Leonard Rappaport; Karen Van Unen, Sarah Benioff, Brenda Brooks, Kusum Mathews, and Grace Chi of the National Program Office for the Dyson Initiative; Lisa "Sof" Sofis of the Pediatric Alliance for Coordinated Care. And in the Division of General Pediatrics, I thank Mindy Haake and Joan Lowcock for everything they do, day in and day out.

I am also grateful to Caitjin Gainty for her research help and to Naomi Sacks for keeping me moving forward. I also thank Jacqueline Wehmueller and Erin Cosyn at the Johns Hopkins University Press for making this book materialize.

For the past six years, my husband Sean and I have served as masters of Adams House at Harvard College. Talk about smiling and singing and looking forward: despite the terror of September 11, the personal trials of a number of the students, and the depth of tragedy for members of our staff, the 450 young people who surround us put life into perspective in their own full-of-wonder fashion. I have had the tremendous pleasure of writing this book in a place where life is all about promise. Just as Anne Dyson saw the promise in medical students and residents in training, I am convinced, by my time at Adams House, of the interest in and the excitement about child health advocacy among students just beginning their careers. Special thanks go to Michael Rodriquez and David Fithian, the current and former senior tutors; to Vicki Macy and Otto Coontz; and to the tutors Jorge Teixeira and David Seley.

Loving appreciation goes to so many dear people: my brothers and their families; the Rourke family—Mary, Carol, David, Ana, Caitlin, and Conor; to Antonia and David Isabel; and to Anna Tabor.

My fondest thanks are to my wonderful family: Katy and Quentin, John and Catherine, Jack and Emeline, and especially, Sean.

Introduction

SOMETHING IS WRONG IN AMERICA. We have the finest medical capability in the world and spend over $1,800,000,000,000 on health care each year, but our children still confront serious physical and mental health concerns. Families of children with disabilities go without comprehensive support. There are unconscionable disparities in child health status between white and nonwhite, rich and poor, educated and less educated families. As a nation we are not getting our money's worth. This paradox leads to the call for advocacy to fix the problem.

Frustrated and worried by the lack of accountability for children's health in Washington, in state capitals, and in city hall, child health professionals have become convinced that child health issues must be raised higher on everyone's agenda. The word *advocacy* has been increasingly prominent in the titles of pediatric journal articles, in the programs of national and regional meetings, and in the daily conversations of doctors, nurses, and social workers. Although child health professionals have always been concerned with the state of children's health, they have not always been as active in the campaign for children's rights as many other professional groups have been. Lately, however, child health providers have begun to question the status quo, suggesting changes in practice, reforms in policy, and a fundamental reassessment of professional attitudes. National ad hoc health groups, professional organizations, and multidisciplinary commissions have proposed directly engaging the social, environmental, and legislative factors that determine children's health in the United States.

I offer this book to affirm the urgent need for child health advocacy, to present a conceptual framework for child health advocacy, and to provide examples of best practices in advocacy as guidance for child health practitioners, teachers, and learners. I endeavor to illustrate why, where, and how advocacy is needed to improve the quality of clinical care delivery, enhance planning for children's health, and encourage a collective responsibility for children's health, growth, and development.

The Need for Advocacy

Socially determined health concerns. Children and youth face persistent and ever-changing health challenges. The roots of some of the most intractable problems (such as low birth weight, failure to thrive, substance abuse, depression, child abuse, teen pregnancy) lie deep in the community and the society. Isolated families and embattled communities often lack the resources that could protect the health of their children. By contrast, healthy families and communities promote the health of children. Child health advocacy builds on those strengths and works to spread community resources to all children and families.

Millennial morbidity. Scientific discoveries and the technologic evolution have created a new set of conditions full of both promise and peril for children and society. While many countries in the world still struggle with inadequate resources for children, it is just dawning on Americans that some of our most pressing child health problems grow from a surfeit of goods and distractions: too much food, too much TV, too many cars, and too much busyness. Many child health problems (obesity, Type 2 diabetes, asthma, injuries, anorexia, and bulimia) are caused or exacerbated by this surfeit. Child health advocacy works to understand how societal gain is best balanced with the promotion of children's health and development.

Chronic illness and disability. The child health conditions that consume the greatest medical and family resources are often the consequence of medical and surgical success. Children and youth with severe chronic illness (cystic fibrosis, sickle cell anemia, cancer, neurological disorders) who have survived well beyond former life expectancy for their conditions face enormous challenges in dealing with day-to-day life. Modern medicine has done a wonderful job preserving the lives of such children, but many of them now live between home and hospital, some in pain, many uncertain of their futures. Child health advocacy is needed to ensure that these children and youth have the best quality of life society can afford them.

Mental health concerns. Increasing numbers of children and adolescents manifest mental health disorders (depression, anxiety, thoughts of suicide). The cause behind this increase is far from certain, but the complex and changing patterns of family life, the stresses of a competitive society that is forever testing and measuring the merits of individuals, and the tensions children experience as they move back and forth between their culture of origin and the mainstream American culture all threaten the mental health of children and adolescents. Child health advocacy is needed to understand these relationships and to generate preventive strategies that address these mental health concerns.

Health care and health outcome disparities. The unfair distribution of health care resources has led to wide disparities in child health care outcomes. Minority and poor children are at significantly higher risk of death, illness, and mental and behavioral concerns than children who are white and have greater fiscal resources.

The Framework of the Discussion

In the child health professions, there is general agreement that it is time for increased activity in child health advocacy. But what exactly is child health advocacy? How do we define *advocacy?* What are the dimensions of child health? Is child health advocacy confined to certain problems, certain venues? Who does it? Who doesn't do it? How is it best done? How often does it succeed? When and why does it fail? This book draws on the child health literature and the experience of child health providers from a variety of backgrounds to tackle these and other questions.

"To advocate" means different things to different people. When groups of child health professionals gather to discuss advocacy at national workshops, their conversation can sound like the confusion of Babel. Each person draws definitions from experience. While one person considers advocacy a loud, public cry for national reform at the legislative and policy level, another maintains that getting a child with HIV infection into a summer camp is also advocacy. When these two people talk to each other, it is often in a confused cross talk. This book attempts to promote a fuller, more informed national conversation about children's health by systematically delineating the components of child health advocacy.

The framework offered here defines four types of advocacy: clinical, group, legislative, and professional. Each of these types of advocacy requires that the child health advocate base action on a deep understanding of the biologic, social, community, and political realities that attend the child or the problem. Each type of advocacy requires coordination among professionals, parents, agencies, and public officials. And each type of advocacy reaps its own rewards in terms of success, whether for one patient or for all children in the United States.

This framework is presented for discussion and elaboration. Others may suggest different or more theoretical constructs to explain child advocacy more fully. Such expansion will be welcome.

The Practice of Child Health Advocacy

This book includes lessons and cautions about child health advocacy. Doctors, nurses, parents, and others who wish to change the approach to child health now have models and tools at their disposal that were not available ten or twenty years ago. The past quarter century has witnessed serious exploration of the complex influences on child health. The development of comprehensive national and local databases has confirmed many hypotheses about social-health interactions. Pioneers in child health have tried new approaches to close in on the source of problems. Program planners have emphasized the quality of care delivery and have employed population-based methodology to ensure the widest possible distribution of child health knowledge and services. Many of these interventions have now been subjected to rigorous evaluation, and the results are encouraging.

Examples from the contemporary pediatric, public health, and nursing literature are presented throughout this book to give texture and meaning to the more theoretical constructs. I also tell the stories of some of the pediatric advocates whose lives and work contributed to the stunning child health improvements of the nineteenth and twentieth centuries. In the chapters on clinical, group, legislative, and professional advocacy, I describe the work of colleagues from around the United States. Many of the stories are from Baltimore, Boston, and New York, the cities I am most familiar with. Others are from the experiences of child health advocates around the country, including the twelve pediatric programs involved in the Dyson Initiative. What ties the practices together is the recognition that success in advocacy depends on strong partnerships among child health professionals, parents, community-based organizations, and policymakers. In the absence of these partnerships, the efforts of any one group are severely compromised. When the partnerships flourish, it is possible to address the serious problems of access to care, disparities in health outcomes, and lack of coordination of care for children with complex medical conditions. Grounding the models in a cultural context allows the very best care for children from all socioeconomic, ethnic, and racial backgrounds.

Recognizing that new comprehensive approaches are available, this book examines questions about how and why the approaches may or may not be adopted. What are the benefits of redesigning clinical systems to include parental and community input? Are there extra costs associated? Who pays? Who cares? How could a quality-focused agenda improve the outcomes for children and families? Why would an interweaving of private and public health goals and objectives lead to better health care delivery for both individuals and groups of children and youth? This book also explores how inertia may impede the child health advocates' agenda for change. Will there be ambivalence, uncertainty, and resistance among practitioners, parents, educators, and policymakers? What are the particular fiscal constraints that keep physicians and nurses locked into tight, traditionally defined service structures? What are the role definition barriers that obviate against professionals entering into partnerships with parents and representatives of community-based organizations? What are the psychological and sociopolitical impediments that restrict child health professionals in their attempts to improve the health and well-being of children? What are the warning signals that help advocates avoid false promises and dashed hopes?

For the most part, the practices described in this book are confined to the project stage. They have not been fully implemented at a scale that can have the general impact required for fundamental change. Charismatic leaders and early adopters can launch fabulous projects and keep them afloat over the short haul. For those in mainstream practice, a basic shift is required for long-term sustainability. Nurses, physicians, and families must want the change, and professional and public policies must allow the change. Much of advocacy is about anticipating a future when what now appears new or radical is accepted, common practice. The emphasis that many educators are now placing on the incorporation of advocacy into the training of future child health care providers is the attempt to make such attitudes and behaviors integral to being a child health care professional.

About This Book

Who is this book for? While the overall aim of the book is to discuss advocacy for children's health, the focus is on encouraging child health professionals to use the powerful tools of advocacy more explicitly than they have in the past. Drawing on examples primarily from pediatrics, the field I know best, I have tried to make the ideas in this book useful to practicing physicians, nurses, social workers, and other child health professionals, as well as to residents, medical and nursing students, public health providers and students, and college students considering a health care career. Many of the principles outlined in the book may be relevant for those in adult health as well. For those involved in clinical endeavors, the book aims to serve as a celebration of the victories of the past, a conversation with those who are currently active in advocacy, a point of discussion with those who have chosen to stay on the sidelines, and a road map for those who wish to live the advocate's life in the future.

The practice of child health advocacy is certainly not confined to professionals in child health. In fact it could easily be argued that the impact of parent advocacy groups, lawyers, schoolteachers, political scientists, journalists, and novelists have been as large as—or larger than—those of child health professionals themselves. If anything, child health professionals have been slow in joining the fray, despite the invitation from parents, community-based organizations, and other professional groups. Child health advocacy will only be effective when a wide range of professionals, community leaders, and families band together to identify crippling inefficiencies and silly bureaucratic barriers, to attack basic injustices, and to dream of the best for all children no matter how young, how vulnerable, or how ill they are.

It is my sincere hope to use this book to engage a conversation that addresses the questions, What are the most effective and successful approaches to ensure the health of all our children? and How do professionals, communities, and parents create partnerships that pull together powerful constituencies for change? To that end, I have endeavored to make this book accessible for families, health policymakers, child advocates, and child-focused professionals. One of my favorite expressions is, It takes two to tango and eight to do the Virginia reel. Child health advocacy is about doing the Virginia reel: getting into step with the other dancers, from varied backgrounds and with different experiences, beliefs, talents, and resources.

This book is written from the perspective of an observer whose lenses are heavily tinted by experiences in pediatric clinical and academic life. I beg the forbearance of readers who are not pediatricians when my own experience and vision delimit the discussion.

Why America? A few words about the domestic focus of this book are in order. With 10 million children dying annually from preventable causes around the world, the question can reasonably be posed, Why concentrate on child health in the United States? I have chosen to do so for several reasons. First, very practically, my own experience has been in the urban centers of the American northeast. The problems I have personally struggled with have resided in the row houses of East Baltimore; they have turned up at 1 a.m. in the emergency rooms in Washington Heights and the Bronx; they have been mired in controversy in the statehouse on Beacon Hill, and they have been buried in conference in the halls of Congress in Washington, D.C.

First-hand encounters with injustice drove me to write this book. I have wanted to come to grips with the juxtaposition of wealth and need, know-how and ineptitude, painful outcry and straggled response that is particular to America. In the United States, even in the face of abundant resources, children's issues are set to the side. They are considered inconsequential. Those who care about little children are accorded relatively little respect.

I have also felt a sense of urgency to speak up about what is happening in the United States as we have entered the millennium, a time of promise, a time of change, and a time of enormous risk for our children. The current highly political decisionmaking at the federal, state, and local levels jeopardize children's health. If the new policies that neglect the poor and threaten to dismantle the public health infrastructure are not reversed soon, children's health will be harmed substantially. Children's health and life chances in the United States have improved steadily over the past century. But the Katrina tragedy showed starkly that not all people share the same protections in the United States. It will be tragic if children's health suffers because of lack of advocacy.

If we have learned anything about successful advocacy, it is that it grows from a deep understanding of the sociopolitical factors that dictate local conditions. To address the horrible, mind-boggling health problems that children face around the world, we need advocacy at many levels—in the elementary schools of Durban, the colleges of Bangkok, and the medical schools of Calcutta; in the clinics of Belarus and the law offices of Jakarta and Kyoto; in the women's collectives in southern China and on the streets of Santiago. I hope that some of the work presented here will serve as encouragement to those engaged in child health to move more directly and visibly into the advocacy arena both here and around the world. Already, the forces bringing people closer together—the ease of transportation and communication—are opening up new opportunities for an international dialogue about children's health.

As American child health professionals engage increasingly in advocacy, the natural movement will be toward an inflected consideration of the roles they can and should play on the global stage. Some will find themselves providing direct clinical care; some will consult on group programs; some will fight political battles to free up dollars and euros and yen for children's health needs; and others will argue for a living wage for health professionals to curb the brain drain out of needy areas around the world. How the advocates work, whom they work with, where and when they have an impact will vary with the geopolitical conditions in each town, each country, and each region.

As long as the United States is as powerful as it is, what happens in the board rooms of New York and Detroit and Los Angeles and what happens in Congress can have significant behind-the-scenes impact on global child advocacy efforts. Even for those engaged on the world stage, it will be wise for some of their advocacy to be directed at those in power in the United States. Such action is necessary to counteract the arrogance of a nation that will not honor its debts to other nations, hoards its medical resources, and refuses to sign an international convention on the rights of the child.

What terms are used? A book about child health advocacy is fundamentally about children, and so from the start it is the important to define what is meant by *child health.* For the discussions presented here, that scope is long and wide. Childhood begins at least at birth (with child health care and issues related to child biology and development occurring from conception on). With the advent of adolescent medicine as a subspecialty of pediatrics, child health encompasses the portion of the life span until at least 21 or 22 years of age. Since young women become young mothers, many advocates urge that the preconceptual age be particularly emphasized. The word *children* generally connotes only a small segment of the population under discussion in this book, but the phrase "newborns, infants, children, adolescents, and young adults" is unwieldy. Therefore, I employ *child health* as all-encompassing and ask the reader to envision the entire group, from infancy to young adulthood, when they encounter this term.

Since many of the examples in the book are from specific age periods, I use the term *infancy* for newborns to age 1, *toddlers and preschoolers* for ages 2 to 5, *school-age children* or *children* for ages 6 to 12, *adolescents* for ages 13 to 17, and *young adults* for ages 18 to 22. For gender, the convention in this book is to alternate between *he* and *she* in examples unless there is a pertinent clinical or social reason to designate a specific gender. The terms *white, black,* and *Hispanic* are used in text, while the U.S. census delineation of *non-Hispanic white, non-Hispanic black, Hispanic black,* and *Hispanic white* are used in the tables.

How is the book organized? Throughout, I attempt to weave together the argument that child health advocacy is vastly underutilized in addressing the persistent concerns of children and youth, and I ask why this is so. I draw attention to the ways advocacy has been used effectively and suggest opportunities for amplifying the power of advocacy.

Chapter 1 sets the stage with a discussion of the need for child health advocacy and presents a typology for considering four interrelated components of child health advocacy. Chapter 2 tells the adventures of child health leaders whose advocacy over the past century has helped to improve the health of children and families. Chapter 3 details the current state of children's health in the United States, drawing on the 2000 census and other large databases. Chapters 4, 5, 6, and 7 discuss in detail the components of child health advocacy: clinical advocacy, group advocacy, legislative advocacy, and professional advocacy. In each of these chapters there are examples of successful approaches as well as a delineation of the tensions and concerns that can get in the way of full success. Finally, chapter 8 puts children's health issues into the larger social context. An appendix lists the websites that were helpful in the preparation of the book.

The hypotheses offered and the questions asked are invitations to readers to bring their own experiences and questions to bear on an examination of the issues. Advocacy for children depends on active engagement and the airing of all of our ideas and questions.

.

Child Health in America

Child Health Advocacy   1

HEALTH CARE IN THE UNITED STATES is second to none, and the available technology is advanced beyond anything that Jules Verne or H. G. Wells could have imagined. The tools for the prompt medical diagnosis, surgical management, and rehabilitative care of the child with an inflamed appendix are readily available. The same cannot be claimed for concerns such as child abuse, mental health problems, eating disorders, obesity, asthma, childhood aggression, and substance abuse, which are deeply rooted in social conditions. Although the tools for addressing these health concerns do exist, they are not in widespread use. Rather, child health professionals are constrained to practice medicine like a surgeon treating an abdominal catastrophe without the benefit of ultrasound, anesthesia, scalpels, or Kelly clamps. America spends over 15 percent of its gross domestic product on health care.[1] But something is missing.

Ten years ago a group of physicians, nurses, parents, and social workers met for an afternoon and asked a very simple question: What would the picture look like if children and adolescents in the United States were actually healthy? The group found that it was much easier to talk about disease than about health. They knew how to define HIV and AIDS; they could create lists of multiple congenital anomalies; they discussed autism and depression. There was no question about the black and blue face of domestic violence or about the lifelong toll of posttraumatic stress disorder. They agreed that health is the absence of these. And health is more.[2]

Health is a state of wholeness in body, emotion, and spirit. Healthy children participate actively in their communities and contribute to society. Attaining health requires the concerted effort of families and communities. More and more, the linkage between children's health and that of the community around them is being established.[3] Aware of the persuasive data that document the social determinants of child health outcomes, the group that gathered that day drafted the Bright Futures Children's Health Charter.[4] The charter calls for a preventive strategy that actively engages children and families but that also acknowledges the capacity of external forces (such as income, housing, schooling, and child care) to impact children's health. It is also mindful that factors such as race, ethnicity, and language are powerful predictors of inequity in health care and health outcome.

The Bright Futures Charter paints not a utopian vision but rather a practical hope for decent health services for all children. A short review of how the United States measures up on the charter's principles provides some insights into what's missing. Let's take a brief look at the items. The charter proposes that every child deserves:

To be born well. Being born well includes being born physically healthy and into an environment that nurtures a child's growth and development. Prematurity and low birth weight continue to threaten high numbers of children despite advances in obstetrics and newborn care. The causes behind early birth remain elusive, though a variety of prenatal predisposing factors are now known (smoking, malnutrition, high blood pressure). Data from the CDC's National Survey on Family Growth indicate that 50 percent of American children are born either unplanned or unwanted.[5] Forming families under those conditions certainly puts children at risk and could not be considered being born well.

To be physically fit. The United States is confronting an epidemic of child obesity. Since the 1970s, serious obesity among children ages 6 through 11 has increased from a rate of 3–4 percent to 14–16 percent, and the rate for adolescents (12–19 years old) has risen from 6 percent to more than 15 percent.[6] The level of fitness of the nation's youth is far from optimal and may be deteriorating. Only 8 percent of elementary schools, 6 percent of middle schools, and 6 percent of high schools offer daily physical activity or the equivalent. Shockingly, 30 percent of elementary schools do not even have regularly scheduled recess periods for children in kindergarten through grade 5.[7]

To achieve self-responsibility for good health habits. This goal presupposes a sophisticated approach to health education. Although the majority of the nation's schools report that they offer health education, the delivery of these services is highly variable, and monitoring requirements can be met by the report of minimal activities.[8]

To have ready access to coordinated, comprehensive, health-promoting, therapeutic, and rehabilitative medical, mental health, and dental care. There are serious problems when more than 8 million children lack basic health insurance, when only 20 percent of children who need to see a mental health professional receive even one visit, and less than 40 percent of children on Medicaid receive dental care.[9] The nation is far from meeting the aspiration of a health care system in which each child has an ongoing relationship with a primary care provider and access to consultative and hospital care.

To have a nurturing family and supportive relationships. A child's health begins with the health of his parents. In 2001, 542,000 children were living in foster care. Despite considerable hard work to obtain permanent placements for these children, that number remains unchanged since at least 1998. Approximately 50,000 children were adopted from the foster care program in 2001 (up from 37,000 in 1998), but more than 5,000 children in foster care ran away and 525 died, indicating the extreme vulnerability of these children and families.[10]

To grow up in a physically and psychologically safe home and school environment, free of injury, abuse, violence, and exposure to environmental toxins. Many children's environments pose direct health threats. School hazing, unwanted sexual advances, weapon carrying, and violence are prevalent in the nation's public schools.[11] Additionally, some schools are actually "sick buildings." Rising rates of asthma signal the compromised air quality of many urban environments. Many children live in old houses where rodents, roaches, and other antigens trigger bronchospasm and wheezing.[12]

To have satisfactory housing, good nutrition, a quality education, an adequate family income, a supportive social network, and access to community resources. Every night, more than 1 million children are homeless. For each homeless child, there are many others who live in crowded conditions in substandard settings. A third of homeless children have major mental illness, and up to half suffer from anxiety, depression, or withdrawal.[13] The wages of many working families are not adequate to pay for rent, food, and day care: 16 percent of American families have a less-than-poverty-level income.[14] Nearly 40 percent of the nation's 4th graders do not read at the basic level, and 12 percent of high school students drop out before graduating.[15] Many neighborhoods lack the necessary social service infrastructure to support families.

To have quality child care when her parents are working outside the home. A safe and stimulating environment is essential for children's health, growth, and development. The quality of day care environments varies greatly with major differences in long-term outcomes for children depending on the quality of the program. Child care costs on average from $4,000 to $10,000 a year. Families on the economic edge often must sacrifice greatly to ensure that their children are at least in a safe environment during the day.[16] Even if quality and cost were not issues, there are too few affordable child care slots for the more than 12 million babies, toddlers, and preschoolers who need them.

The opportunity to develop ways to cope with stressful life experiences. Stress is a part of every child and family's life. The charter's authors added this item to highlight the importance of young people learning to engage seriously with the world around them—the good, the bad, and the ugly parts of it. By stretching toward high goals and high standards and by being challenged (appropriately to their age and stage of development), children acquire the necessary cognitive, emotional, and social equipment for resilience in a complex and ever-changing world.[17]

To develop positive values and become a responsible citizen in his community. Even though the topics of moral development and social awareness can engender complex and frequently politicized discussion, experts in child health and youth development are increasingly engaging these topics. New evidence shows that young people who have developed a positive value base and have become involved in their communities have measurably better health and developmental outcomes than young people who have not.[18]

To experience joy, have high self-esteem, have friends, acquire a sense of efficacy, and believe that she can succeed in life. The pursuit of happiness is a fundamental American value. The authors of the Bright Futures Charter chose to close with a set of positive aspirations as the overall measure of children's health. That is what it would look like if children and youth were truly healthy.

The Call for Advocacy

The principles of the Bright Futures Charter shed light on the national failure to meet the basic health needs of all our children. We too rarely address the root causes of children's health concerns, and we have not met the goals our country has set for the health and well-being of children. Hence the uncomfortable backroom mutterings by some and the loud cries for child health advocacy by others. The call comes from all quarters—parents, students, philanthropy, and increasingly health care providers and other child-helping professional groups.

Families are not completely satisfied with the health care available for their children.[19] In June 1996 on the National Mall in Washington, D.C., an estimated 300,000 mothers, fathers, grandmothers, grandfathers, foster mothers, and foster fathers met together with clergy and social workers, police officers and doctors in one of the largest public gatherings ever to focus on children. The STAND for Children, organized by the Children's Defense Fund, tapped into a deep-seated unease among American families. The theme of the day was that children were not viewed as a priority by local, state, or federal policymakers. Celebrities, parents, and professionals all delivered the same message: until and unless there was a change in emphasis, there would continue to be serious gaps in services for all children and adolescents and disastrous problems for some.

Families of children with special health care needs have been particularly effective in advocacy and in sending a wake-up alarm to others about speaking up for children. A group of parents has organized Family Voices. With outreach to parents in every state, the group is calling for a fundamentally new kind of health care, one that focuses on a partnership between doctors and parents. The partnership when properly constituted affords both groups a strong leverage for change.[20]

College students recognize the need for advocacy for child health. As they engage in community service, they encounter situations that do not make sense. They meet families who cannot afford glasses for their children. They learn of newcomers to the United States whose children do not have a doctor to go to. They learn that the immigrant families are wary of signing up for health insurance coverage because they fear deportation. When the college freshmen go to volunteer in schools and after-school centers, they watch educators struggle to teach children who come from a wide range of history and experience. They marvel at the skill of the teacher who can explain advanced math to one of her fifth grade students while tenderly dealing with the outbursts of a mentally troubled youngster. As college students learn the intricate interweaving of the environment and health, they put together their own interventions. Some college students are leading the way in health service, advocating for new child health program development. In chapter 4, there is a discussion of Project Health, a sophisticated and effective college program with chapters at Harvard, Columbia, Brown, and George Washington Universities.[21]

When medical school applicants are asked to write their personal statements about why they want to go to medical school, they invariably say something like, "I want to make a difference. I want to change the way things are for families and children. What I see in the world needs changing if children and families are going to have the best we can offer. There are better ways, and I think that by getting trained as a diagnostician and an intervener, I can be part of making that difference." Increasingly, medical schools are reviewing their missions and modes of operation to react to these assertions.[22]

In response to the inequities they see during their clinical rotations in continuity clinics, emergency departments, and hospital wards, medical students and residents have organized committees on advocacy. They know what they can do in the health care environment, but they are frustrated by what they cannot do. Some medical students and residents respond by becoming angry or discouraged—turning off and turning away from their original intent to make a difference.[23] Others become creative and join together to form resident grassroots initiatives. They push the medical organizations and involve themselves directly in advocacy for children and families.[24]

Several philanthropic groups provide formal financial support for health care advocacy and leadership development. The Soros Foundation sponsors a fellowship under the rubric, Medicine as a Profession. The idea is to engage physicians in community service and to teach them to advocate for public health. The Soros fellowship was started in response to the commercialization of medicine. Early and midcareer physicians spend one to two years working with an advocacy organization.[25] The Dyson Foundation sponsored a pediatric advocacy fellowship from the early 1990s through 2002 to develop a cadre of young physician leaders who addressed health care problems simultaneously from a biomedical and an advocacy perspective.[26] In 2000, the Dyson Foundation launched a major national effort, the Anne E. Dyson Community Pediatrics Training Initiative (CPTI), to integrate advocacy skills into pediatric house officer training. In 2005, the CPTI was incorporated into the activities of the American Academy of Pediatrics. The purpose of the initiative is "to develop a new generation of pediatricians with skills and knowledge of community-based medicine advocacy, and the capacity to improve the health of all children in their communities." Among others, the Robert Wood Johnson Foundation, the Joseph P. Kennedy Foundation, and the Annie E. Casey Foundation sponsor fellowships in health policy and systems change. Several of the training programs of the Maternal and Child Health Bureau have modules on child health advocacy as core elements.[27]

Professional pediatric organizations are also involved in advocacy for children. The American Academy of Pediatrics has been particularly vocal in the call for health care insurance and access for all children. The vision of the academy's Community Access to Child Health (CATCH) program is that every child in every community should have a "medical home" and all necessary services to reach optimal health and well-being.[28] Academic organizations such as the Ambulatory Pediatric Association and the Society for Pediatric Research have also found that advocacy is an important complement to the work their members do in the office, at the bedside. and at the bench.[29]

So what is child health advocacy, anyway? When child health providers decide that it is time to heed the call for advocacy, how do they do it? What do they find themselves getting into? Who is there to give them a hand? How do they know if they are aiding the efforts for children or just adding to the confusion? Let us delineate some principles that describe advocacy and consider the implications for child health practice.

What Advocacy Is

Advocacy is expressed in many ways. Daumier's proper Parisian *advocat* stands tall in court pleading his case. Speaking out, speaking up, speaking for. Jane Addams and Upton Sinclair venture into the dark corners of society to shed light on the abuses of child labor, poverty, and urban blight. Sticking their necks out, taking risks, uncovering abuse. Rosa Parks and Martin Luther King Jr. confront the wrong that has cheated them and their loved ones. Fighting back, combating the enemy. Wilbur Cohen reforms the way things are done, remakes the broken systems. Building, creating, making something new and whole. *To advocate* comes from the Latin for *to speak to* or *to voice*. The advocate sees and hears and then speaks up.

Because children cannot speak for themselves, it is natural for health care providers to stand as witnesses for their rights and causes. An emergency room doctor notices that child traffic victims seem to be struck crossing the same intersection, and it is time to call city hall. A managed care company refuses for the third time to pay for a prosthesis for a little cancer patient, and it is time for the nurse clinician to speak to the insurance company. The primary care physician learns that a quarter of his families have no health insurance, and it is time to question the system.

Advocacy is rewarding, even fun. There is nothing like the excitement of a CATCH meeting, with child health providers from around the country swapping success stories—a CATCH physician, for example, relating that she and her colleagues convinced the state legislature to expand health insurance coverage to children at 1.5 times the poverty level. Capturing and channeling the exhilaration of such advocates is the purpose of the learning collaboratives sponsored by the National Initiative for Child Health Quality.

Advocacy is creative. If we are stuck in the mud, what tools and resources are available to dig ourselves out of a bad place? Creativity often involves shifting the frame of reference. There is huge benefit in engaging people with different perspectives. They look at the same old intractable problem from a novel angle, one that might just work.

Advocacy is practical. While the image of the advocate evokes a sense of drama, there is a lot less of Joan of Arc under her flying standard and a lot more of Rosie the Riveter securing bolt after bolt into place. It is down-to-earth, day-to-day work. Yes, passion, rhetoric and a sense of righting wrongs fuel the efforts; but in the end the essence of advocacy is in the little details, the letter writing, the faxing, the actual fingers doing the dialing to get a child that urgent orthopedic appointment, the car driving out to the hazardous waste site, the turning up at 7:30 a.m. at an Individualized Education Plan meeting, the chasing down of the newly arrived Cambodian child who didn't return for a tuberculosis skin test reading.

Advocacy frequently takes place behind the scenes. Often the beneficiaries of tremendous efforts of advocacy have no idea what has transpired on their behalf. The family of a child who is able to receive free care for a cardiac operation does not need to know how long and hard the surgeon worked, how many calls he made, and who was opposing his bid for funding for such care. For those who work in large institutions, advocacy is for outsiders and insiders. Advocates often need to decide whether they can effect change best by working within the current system, making adjustments and incremental modifications, or by removing themselves to an outside vantage point, where the institution becomes "they," not "we." Creativity, practicality, and keeping the concerns of the children in mind help with the choice of that path.

What Advocacy Is Not

Advocacy is not (or should not be) self-aggrandizement. Some people avoid playing the advocate's role because they dread the limelight. They recognize a potential advocacy pitfall in the messenger becoming the message. Effective advocates learn to walk the delicate balance that allows them to use the force of their personality and authority while maintaining humility and objectivity. They know that a cause is often best championed by an individual, identifiable leader—someone who can articulate a coherent and concise message. On the other hand, they know that the personal qualities of the leader must not overwhelm and subsume the essence of the campaign.

Advocacy is not partisan. It is not the role of child health advocates to further the careers of individual candidates, and there are negative consequences for aligning with one political party or another. Nonetheless, there is every reason for advocates to hold political figures accountable for child health and to engage them at opportune times. Elected officials should be challenged about where they stand on child health policy, and they should be willing to receive information about the current status of child health and health care delivery. These officials cannot be at all places at all times. It never hurts for child health advocates to bring news from the front lines and to suggest initiatives and interventions.

Advocacy is not starry-eyed dreaming. Empty rhetoric gets us nowhere. With the tools now available for systematic planning, such as those spelled out in Healthy People 2000 and 2010, and with the enormous emphasis throughout health care on evidence-based medicine and outcomes orientation, advocates who do not have a well-articulated course of action with clear time lines and points of accountability will be doomed in their efforts.

Advocacy is not synonymous with community medicine or public health. Nor is child health advocacy reserved for problems facing the poor and underserved. Because the disenfranchised disproportionately encounter complex and deeply rooted health problems, advocacy is a common response. But this in no way precludes child health providers from speaking out about concerns that affect middle-class children and youth. Moreover, advocacy is not exclusively a tool for the generalist. Pediatric medical and surgical specialists and nurse clinicians benefit equally from having advocacy skills as part of their armamentarium.

Advocacy is not always about medical people taking the lead. Often professionals other than nurses and physicians lead the way, open the issue to outside scrutiny, and then ask for child health assistance to provide critical evidence or technical assistance. Such was the case in South Africa when, in the early 2000s, a group of lawyers took on the African National Congress and the Mbeki government about their failure to provide antiretroviral therapy to patients with HIV/AIDS.[30] The lawyers created the Treatment Action campaign and brought the case to court. Realizing that their case would be much strengthened by focusing on children, they asked a group of pediatricians to join them in their Save Our Babies campaign. The doctors were able to frame the debate around prenatal treatment and to provide data that significantly weakened the government's case. Advocacy is not all about leadership. It is a lot about skilful teamwork.

Those who champion the cause of the young, the poor, and the down-trodden find that it is not easy work. They must endeavor continually to understand the champion's relationship with those being advocated for. Clearly, infants and small children will always depend on adults to articulate their needs and concerns. In fact the advocate's assessment of personal success is that children are able to depend on him or her over the long haul for improvements in life chances. For advocates working with adolescents, families, and communities, a nuanced response involves discovering and then reinforcing the strengths of those being advocated for. Success comes on the day when the advocate no longer speaks "for" but rather speaks "with" the adolescents, families, and communities.

Above all, advocacy is not boring. Advocacy is an antidote to the routine of the daily grind. It provides a vantage for periodic assessment of what is working and what is not. It is a compass to be sure that all the work is going toward some greater purpose.

The Barriers to Child Health Professionals Getting into Advocacy

Even though a number of effective advocates have been child health providers (some of whose stories appear in chapter 2), advocacy itself has not been considered a core activity of child health provision until recently. Most child health providers, in fact, do identify advocacy as something they do: they participate in their town councils, they volunteer a night a month at the homeless shelter, they testify before the legislature on the importance of newborn screening. But this advocacy is usually an extra, something to be done at the end of the day or at the end of one's career.

If we are to make progress in answering the call for clinician's involvement in advocacy, it is helpful to understand what keeps advocacy from being an integral piece of child health provision. At least four reasons underlie the resistance and the maintenance of the status quo: (1) the basic structure of medical practice, (2) risk avoidance, (3) an inherent tension between advocacy and science, and (4) confusion on the part of child health providers about what advocacy is and how it should be practiced. Let us explore each of these barriers.

Medical practice is traditionally reactive, not proactive. Emergency rooms and operating theaters exist to respond to critical events. Primary care doctors are on call to assist families of children who are sick in the night. Medical practice focuses on one patient at a time. This means that the underlying patterns of ill health within a community are easy to miss.

American child health providers are not held accountable to any community or to the general public. Health care providers tend to think of themselves as professionals who are primed and ready for those who seek their services; they are not directly responsible for those who cannot access or afford those services. They are busy enough with the patient who is right there right now. They sincerely hope that the needs of others will be taken care of by somebody else. The daunting problem in child health is that it is not always clear who that "somebody else" is.

Some child health providers are conflict-averse or do not want to sacrifice their hard-earned position and prestigious job. There is a kind of drama to advocacy that may make it seem dangerous: Do I really want to stick my neck out? Taking a stand rarely comes naturally and generally necessitates a great deal of soul searching.

For physicians and nurses, coming down unequivocally on one side of an argument flies in the face of much of the academic training and scientific rigor that goes into making them medical professionals. Medical and nursing education teaches clinicians to look at all possible explanations for a problem. The process of going through a differential diagnosis allows for posing a series of hypotheses: It could be this, but maybe it is that. An advocacy stance involves digging in the heels, so advocates want to be certain that their mission is the right one.

Finally, the biggest barrier is the confusion about what advocacy encompasses. Child health professionals and trainees who wish to be advocates are often unable to gauge what they are accomplishing. The absence of a common language about child health advocacy frequently compromises their effectiveness.

Framework for Child Health Advocacy

It may be time to struggle with defining the components of child health advocacy, if for nothing else than to allow people working together to converse about what they are about. It may be helpful to define subtypes of child health advocacy: clinical advocacy, group advocacy, legislative (or systems level) advocacy, and professional advocacy.

Clinical Advocacy

Clinical care for individual children seen every day is more effective if the child health provider has a broad view of health, is versed in family-centered care, and has a finger on the pulse of the community. Health care providers do not always consider how much better their day-to-day care could be if they thought in advocacy terms and incorporated advocacy attitudes. Wanting to ensure that the children who come to the office or clinic receive the very best care available is an advocate's stance. Building one's practice as a medical home and using quality improvement tools are clinical advocacy. Reaching out to other agencies in the community to ensure that individual children and families have their needs addressed reflects a full understanding of the social determinants of health problems and shows that the clinician wants to be part of the larger solution.

Group Advocacy

Often the same problem confronts classes of children (for example, children with disabilities, children in foster care, or gay and lesbian youth). In these situations, a specialized group program augments clinical care. Any child's problem that is similar to that of other children may find its solution in the group. Child health providers can design effective interventions for a group of children who share the same risks, concerns, and life circumstances. One of the most practical aspects of group advocacy is the fact that policymakers and philanthropists often respond positively to appeals for financial support to resolve a particular, well-defined, categorical problem. Outcome measurement and monitoring are reasonably straightforward in group work.

Legislative Advocacy

Advocacy to improve systems involves high-level policy change and high-cost intervention. Often child health providers find that no matter what they do, no how matter how creative and persistent they are, their patients do not receive the services they need. The problems are at the systems level; the solutions must be there too. To fix health insurance problems, state and federal funds must be identified. To house children, the tax base must change and lower-rate mortgages must be created. To meet the increasing demand for home-duty nurses, new nurses must be trained and their salaries be covered. These issues demand legislative advocacy. Now the placards come out and the letter-writing skills are honed. Effective systems-level advocacy grows out of partnerships and an understanding of how power is accrued and how it is best wielded.

Professional Advocacy

The fourth type of advocacy looks at the question, What is getting in my way of doing my own day-to-day work and how can I remove those barriers? Occasionally there is need for change in the way the profession of medicine is practiced. A number of national reports codifying child health needs indicate that it would be timely to modify professional responsibilities, placing more emphasis on community medicine and child health advocacy. To effect this change requires taking a hard look at preconceived ideas about practice, followed by advocacy within the profession to adjust to the new demands.

Paths to Success

For the past fifty years, Julius Richmond has stood out as one of the most effective child health advocates. His story appears in chapter 2, but for now let us focus on his model for ensuring success in health efforts for children and families. Figure 1.1 is the graphic rendition of his multidimensional thesis. He argues that if advocates wish to accomplish long-lasting, meaningful change they must attend simultaneously to three key domains: knowledge base, social strategy, and political will. These components are in a dynamic equilibrium, continually interacting with and reinforcing one another.

Knowledge Base

The knowledge base in the basic science and clinical areas of pediatrics exploded over the course of the twentieth century, with major discoveries in biochemistry, metabolism, fluid and electrolyte balance, microbiology, and many other areas. By contrast, until very recently, the knowledge base in the larger arena of child health has suffered from little attention, investment, or creativity. The science of epidemiology has been vastly underutilized. For example, until the adoption of E-codes for designating the external cause of the injury a child had sustained, the pediatric nurse practitioner who wanted to do a study of trauma in her catchment area could learn how many children died of this cause, but she could not get detailed information about cases in which the child had not died, even those left with serious disability. The data simply were not collected, and there were no systems for doing so.

One of the most important and least heralded accomplishments of the late twentieth century was the advance in the quantity, quality, and accessibility of child health data. Since the late 1980s, leaders in child health policy have insisted on the collection of a standardized set of child health indicators. Moreover, several funders (the Agency for Health Policy Research and the Maternal and Child Health Bureau at the federal level and the Annie E. Casey Foundation in the private sector) have concentrated much of their effort on the creation of large data sets. As a result, the pe-

Figure 1.1. Schema for Successful Advocacy

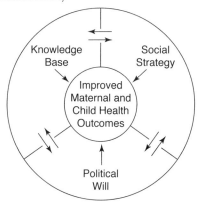

Source: Richmond JB and Kotelchuck M, The Effects of Political Process on the Delivery of Health Services, in McGuire C, Foley R, Gorr D, and Richard R, eds., *Handbook of Health Professions Education* (San Francisco: Jossey-Bass, 1983), p. 386.

diatric child health world can now find extensive, well-tabulated, trended data sets that they can access with relative ease.

Since Julius Richmond first began discussing the knowledge base, the technical capability for display of information has soared. In 1985, when an investigator wanted to spice up an article with a pie chart or bar graph, it would literally cost her several weeks of work and up to $100 per camera-ready figure. Now, using a computer graphic package, all she needs to do is click her mouse ten or twenty times to create a figure. Moreover, a large amount of beautifully collected, validated information is available for display to everyone on the Internet. (The appendix lists the data sets found to be most comprehensive and user friendly during the preparation of this book.)

There are two big caveats about the new data availability. First, while most of the information is well collected and standardized, there is a tremendous amount of it, which can be quite overwhelming. Second, Mark Twain knew a thing or two when he said, "There are three kinds of lies: lies, damned lies, and statistics." He was expressing the caution that goes with the use of any powerful tool. Just as one would carefully bone up on the use any new piece of equipment to avoid accidental harm, child health providers who wish to use data effectively must invest time in acquiring a basic understanding of epidemiology, statistics, and demography.

The knowledge base in child health comprises not only these new big population-based data sets but also a deep understanding of child growth and development and a familiarity with the interventions and best practices that are showing promise for children and youth. As child health advocates analyze potential approaches to child health problems, an understanding of the different considerations for the several stages of childhood—fetal, newborn, infant, toddlerhood, early childhood, school age, adolescent, and young adult—improves the chances for their success.

Social Strategy

Social strategy answers the questions, How do I get this good idea from here to there? What is the first step, the second? How do we know we are on our way? Do we have a clear idea of where "there" is? As Richmond says, "You cannot get very far if you don't know where you are going." The recognition of the importance of precise social strategy defines the real advocate.

As a result of poorly articulated social strategies, many projects fail despite great potential. Social strategy is the driver for each of the four types of advocacy described in this book. The essential components of the social strategy are the delineation of feasible objectives, the description of the target population, the garnering of help from key individuals and groups, and the involvement of stakeholders along with the shared celebration in the case of success as well as the refusal to blame in the case of failure. A social strategy to tackle a daunting issue such as youth violence might be to break the large problem into several smaller, manageable problems and resolve them step by step. A first step may be, for example, getting thirty new after-school slots in the east section of town by next April.

Richmond often uses the campaign for the worldwide eradication of smallpox as an example of social strategy. After a careful needs assessment, the world public health bodies targeted their resources on the areas where the rates of smallpox were the highest. They then fanned out to contiguous areas to address the remaining pockets of infection.

A critical element of social strategy is communication. The social strategy chosen for each type of advocacy varies depending on the problem, the group affected by the problem, and the players chosen to address the problem, but what does not vary is the need for all players to be kept abreast of progress and dilemmas. One particularly effective social strategist remarked that she keeps a note over her computer that says, "Have you told absolutely everyone who needs to know?"

Social strategy also depends on relationships. Not periodic formal meetings of people from different agencies but long-standing, deeply rooted relationships—I trust you, you trust me—born of hard experience working shoulder to shoulder over time and against odds. The social strategist who understands relationships has a pretty thick address book and remembers special days and occasions with a card, a note, or an email. She might turn up unexpectedly one day just to have a cup of coffee, drop off a new interesting book, and see what's up in the neighborhood. You never know what great plans might arise from that fifteen-minute chat.

While social strategy is aimed at accomplishing an objective for children and keeping them in the center, the wise strategist is always aware of the competing agendas of all those involved. It is human nature for people to want to know what benefit they or their agency will derive from getting involved. The savvy social strategist continually reminds his partner about all the great things that are in it for him. There is nothing wrong with appealing to enlightened self-interest.

Political Will

When Julius Richmond talks about political will, he is referring to politics at both governmental and street levels. Senators and congressmen, aldermen and the town meeting all evince political will, and they can generate the fiscal resources to get the job done. But just as important, the opinion and vote of the veterinarian and the middle-school teacher sway the direction of what happens for children and youth. There can be successful pilot projects, child health demonstration models, and an accepted best practice, but nothing will change permanently until the larger society wants that change. If advocates do not engage all the powers that be, the work they have done will rest in a spiral-bound notebook on a library shelf.

The skills required to garner political will are rarely taught in medical school, and child health providers generally do not have the time to spend learning which senator and which community leader to touch base with first and whose name to mention to whom. Child health professionals who are serious about wanting to effect change find partners who have walked the halls of the statehouse for years and who know the ins and outs, the procedures, and the absolute no-nos. In the chapter on legislative advocacy (chapter 6), we discuss the practical issues relating to such teamwork in establishing political will at the government level.

The larger issue of political will brings us back to the question posed at the beginning of this chapter. We might well ask the question with a slight twist: What does it take for society to ensure that children and youth are as healthy as they possibly can be? The elementary question is whether anybody cares, and if they do care how do they show their com- mitment to and support for children's issues? To get to the bottom of this issue, it is worthwhile for us to explore children's place in American so- ciety and then to elaborate what changes the public would have to want in order for children and youth to be as healthy as they possibly can be. This analysis is featured in the last chapter. For now, let us turn our at- tention to the stories of child health advocates who have been successful in making a difference for children and youth over the past 150 years.

2   A History of Child Health Advocacy

THROUGHOUT AMERICAN HISTORY, advocacy has been a natural component of the child health enterprise. As a backdrop to the present, let's revisit the experiences of some of the many men and women who have made a difference by speaking up. These stories show not only how child health advocates witnessed problems but also how they documented what they saw in their efforts to understand the social and environmental underpinnings to child health. They described the problems and demonstrated the ways to correct them.

Abraham Jacobi and Job Lewis Smith: Founders of American Pediatrics

Considered by most historians as the fathers of modern American pediatrics, Abraham Jacobi and Job Lewis Smith created a field that combined the principles of medicine, public health, and advocacy. They recognized the need for each of these components as they worked with children and families in New York City in the latter half of the nineteenth century. At the time, there were few accurate data to inform child health action, but the problems were apparent at every turn and these physicians battled the problems head on.

Abraham Jacobi came to New York from Germany in the 1850s, bringing with him the method of systematic observation that was then emerging in Europe.[1] His writings, which established the science of children's growth, health, and development, argued that children's anatomy and physiology were substantially different from that of adults and that unique processes moved an individual from fetal existence, through infancy, childhood, and adolescence. He speculated that children and youth might also respond to illnesses in a distinct fashion. He had little sympathy for practitioners who attributed all childhood illness to proximal events like teething. He is said to have coined the term *paediatrics* to define the new field of medical study.

Jacobi was struck by the large disparities in deaths between poor children and the children of privileged families. Like him, many of the poor were immigrants. Personally motivated by issues of social injustice, he joined others in calling attention to high infant and childhood mortality as markers of political corruption. Jacobi believed that a government that plays by the rules will see itself as the protector of its most vulnerable citizens.[2] He would continually admonish his newly adopted country to respect those rules.

Job Lewis Smith came from a distinctly American background, complete with Puritan forebears.[3] His education was less grounded in the emerging scientific method than was Jacobi's. Nonetheless, his first mentor, Austin Flint at the University of Buffalo, had inculcated in him the clinical values of close observation and meticulous documentation.[4] Smith followed his brother Stephen in setting up practice in New York City. Coincidentally, he arrived in that city the same year as Jacobi. While Jacobi lived and worked in the Bowery neighborhoods of southern Manhattan, Smith took up residence and began seeing patients at the northernmost edge of the city, at 49th Street, where Rockefeller Center would later be built. He described the deplorable living conditions of the shanties the poor laborers called home: "The streets were not sewered, and refuse matter from the shanties and the stables, the two often built together, was dumped upon the open spaces. . . . In one small room are found the family, chairs usually dirty and broken, cooking utensils, stove, often a bed, a dog or cat, sometimes more or less poultry. . . . The water used is sometimes the Croton, which is brought to the shanties in pails, usually from one of the avenues. In other places, where the Croton hydrants are too far away, and the ground is marshy, the water is obtained from holes dug a little below the surface. This water has a roiled appearance and unpleasant flavor."[5]

With such an unclean water supply, it was no wonder that large numbers of children succumbed to infectious diseases. Smith documented that, each summer, 3,000 children in New York City died of diarrhea. Both Smith and Jacobi devoted themselves to upgrading hygiene and nutrition for infants and young children. Smith also worked with the Asylums and Foundling Homes to improve the cleanliness of the milk supply. When it became clear that infants were dying because midwives were feeding them watered-down cow's milk, Smith advocated for the increased reliance on wet nurses and breast-feeding. His interventions slowly began to save lives.

Jacobi created one of the first American child public health campaigns with the pamphlet "Nine Rules to Avoid Summer Diarrhea."[6] In simple, direct language, he urged mothers to breast-feed if at all possible. He suggested alternating the breast-feeding with cow's milk, loaf sugar, and brandy. If water had to be given, it should be laced with a little whiskey. One wonders whether the alcohol might have worked as a disinfectant. He urged mothers to stop milk once diarrhea had started. He also advised going to the doctor. In language that says a good deal about the times, he wrote, "When you see the doctor, trust in him and not in the women. They do not know better than you do yourself."

The problem with Jacobi's advice was that there were very few doctors for the families to "go to." In 1888 the inaugural gathering of the American Pediatric Society attracted fewer than fifty people.[7] Even if every doctor knew the latest in the care of an infant suffering from summer diarrhea, the ratio of pediatricians to children was one for every 400,000 children. Few of these child-oriented physicians were available to care for the poor immigrant families that Jacobi worried so much about. One solution to the problem was to affiliate health dispensaries with training institutions. Doctors in training needed patients to learn from. This alliance of convenience exists to this very day and has both good and bad features.

From different backgrounds, Abraham Jacobi and Job Lewis Smith held worldviews shaped by totally different experiences. Their personalities, too, were different, Jacobi being so outspoken that he was forced to leave his native country, and Smith being quiet, often speaking more with his expressive eyes than with words. But both men recognized the need for a new field to address issues unique to children, and their parallel and combined efforts began to define pediatrics as a specialty that based action on scientific evidence. They concurred that social determinants were key factors in children's health status. As the first and second presidents of the American Pediatric Society, these two early pediatricians founded a professional discipline that included speaking up and acting on one's convictions as explicit parts of the job description.[8]

Jane Addams and Alice Hamilton: Hull House and Beyond

The 1889 opening of Hull House in Chicago was a watershed in the history of American child advocacy.[9] Jane Addams, an Illinois miller's daughter, established Hull House as a community center for the many families who were pouring into Chicago from Italy, Syria, Greece, Russia, and Poland. Some came to flee oppression and pogroms, some came for work, some for adventure. Addams modeled Hull House on Toynbee Hall in East London, where young university students "settled" to engage in the real problems of the real world. The large, rambling mansion on Halstead Street became the residence, or settlement house, for a dynamic group of women and men. Under Jane Addams's leadership, their collective work literally changed the face of America's social response to the needs of children.

Early on, Addams observed how harsh social conditions contributed to dreadful child health outcomes. "We learned to know the children of hard-driven mothers who went out to work all day, sometimes leaving the little things in the casual care of a neighbor, but often locking them into their tenement rooms. The first three crippled children we encountered in the neighborhood had all been injured while their mothers were at work: one had fallen out of a third-story window, another had been burned, and the third has a curved spine due to the fact that he had been tied all day long to the leg of the kitchen table, only released at noon by his older brother, who hastily ran in from a neighboring factory to share his lunch with him."[10]

Hull House welcomed more and more of these "little mites," who found their way to this place of safety, where the residents provided shelter, food, comfort, and fun. One of these residents was Alice Hamilton, a physician and bacteriologist teaching at the Women's Medical School of Northwestern University.[11] At Hull House she began a baby clinic and parent education programs. A keen observer, well trained in epidemiology, Hamilton kept careful records. Her study of childbearing was one of the first systematic analyses to correlate high infant mortality rates with frequent pregnancies.

In the early 1900s druggists legally dispensed cocaine to anyone who could pay the few cents it cost. Distressed by the drug's effects on children, Addams described "a young Italian boy who died, a victim to the drug at the age of seventeen. He had been in our kindergarten as a handsome merry child, in our clubs as a vivacious boy, and then gradually there was an eclipse of all that was animated and joyous and promising, and when I last saw him in his coffin, it was impossible to connect the haggard, shriveled body with what I had known before."[12] Alice Hamilton documented the extent and chemical effects of cocaine addiction among boys in the Chicago neighborhoods, and in 1907, her epidemiological and laboratory data were instrumental in the passage of a state law banning the sale of cocaine to minors. She was to continue to combine the triple methods of epidemiology, laboratory research, and legal advocacy throughout her lifetime of battling disease.[13]

Hamilton noticed that many of the workers who visited Hull House suffered from ailments such as stomach cramps, "lead palsy," and wrist drop. Employing what she called her "shoe leather epidemiology," she made it her business to explore the working conditions of the factories that employed large numbers of immigrant men, women, and children. Using the precise scientific method she had learned at the Universities of Leipzig and Munich and at the Pasteur Institute, she correlated working conditions, specific industrial practices, and illness symptoms. Overnight, her 1908 paper on occupational causes of illness and disability established her as the expert in the state of Illinois on industrial disease.[14] In 1910 she conducted an extensive statewide survey of manufacturing practices, documenting 578 cases of lead poisoning among workers in a number of industries, including enamellers of bathtubs. Hamilton's conservative approach served her well (she would not diagnose lead poisoning until she could identify a "lead line" on the patient's gums), so that her data were incontrovertible. Now that we have the benefit of blood lead tests, we know that gingival deposits do not appear until the blood lead level is in the dangerous fifty-to-seventy micrograms per deciliter range for several months.[15] Her work convinced the state of Illinois to increase industrial safety regulations. In 1911 the U.S. Department of Labor appointed Hamilton to oversee the national program on industrial hazards and occupational health.

Hamilton's move to Washington was part of a larger pattern. Hull House had become a springboard from neighborhood advocacy to state and national advocacy. Julia Lathrop and Grace Abbott moved from Chicago to the Children's Bureau, Florence Kelley served on the Illinois Bureau of Labor Statistics, and Frances Perkins became the U.S. Secretary of Labor.[16] The brilliance of the Hull House group was their ability to move from the specific to the general. They recognized what the children and families in Chicago needed and took advantage of that experience to advocate for all American children and families. They realized, too, that the federal government was more likely than state governments to take on the role of advocate. Fortunately, most of the Hull House women were from generous and supportive families, because it was common for government appointments to come without pay.

In 1919, in recognition of her pioneering the field of occupational health, Hamilton was recruited by Harvard University to be the first woman ever appointed to the faculty. She had proved herself to be a scholar, a scientific expert in an emerging field, and a creative advocate. Despite personal reticence, she had learned to speak up in the fight for fundamental change in the workplace. When she came to Harvard, though her intellect fit the mold of the other faculty, her gender did not. Her assistant professorship was contingent on her agreeing that she would not sully the faculty club with her presence, that she would not attempt to join the academic procession at graduation, and most of all, that she would not lay claim to the free football tickets that were a favorite perk of those with faculty rank.[17]

Hamilton's advocacy on the part of lead-exposed workers was to have a profound influence on child health. Although lead had been recognized since the time of the Roman Empire as potentially poisonous, each human epoch seemed to forget the lessons of previous era. The tell-tale signs—high infant mortality, intellectual impairment, neurological disability, and untimely, gruesome deaths—have reappeared repeatedly among children because they drank juice from lead-glazed cups or played in lead-laced soil or nibbled lead-filled paint chips.[18] It was not until Hamilton opened her industrial laboratory at Harvard that conclusive scientific evidence defined the pathophysiology and the dose-related effects on human cellular biology. Typical of the soft-spoken Hamilton, she had convinced the lead industry to fund her research. These businessmen were not entirely pleased with the upshot of her work, which caused them to submit to regulations and to pay substantial workmen's compensation claims.

Hamilton often found herself engaged directly with the power elite, whether at an international peace conference, in the halls of Congress, or at the Department of Labor. In 1925 she was asked to join a number of the nation's industrial tycoons on a commission charged with deciding about the addition of lead to stabilize automotive gasoline. Her intuition was that lead in any form was probably a health hazard, but as a scientist she had to agree with the majority opinion that there were no data on the direct effects of lead in gasoline. Maybe there would be no ill effects. Who knew? Truthfully, no one knew. Not Alice Hamilton, not anyone. There was not enough evidence to stop progress, to hold back the economy, and to deny jobs. It would not be for another fifty years until the lead vapors spewed from the millions of Fords and Chevrolets that crisscrossed the U.S. highways that the nation woke up to the fact that almost every American baby was born with lead ions in their body. The blood lead level of 88 percent of the children in 1976–80 was more than ten micrograms per deciliter.[19]

Although Alice Hamilton could not stop the wheels of progress of the automobile industry, her very presence at the meetings where major industrial decisions were made represented the kind of progress that the residents at Hull House were trying to achieve. They were determined to give a voice to the voiceless and power to the powerless. They were asserting that macroeconomic forces filter down into the world of families, that what may be good for General Bullmoose may not always be good for little girls and little boys. Like the other women and men of Hull House, Hamilton elevated child and family concerns so that they had to be taken seriously. It was hard for opponents to argue either with the well-researched, well-documented facts she produced or with the political coalitions she built.

The residents of Hull House knew the power of the published word. Their observations on the relationship between educational levels and poverty got the nation thinking about schooling in new ways. Their documentation that high fertility rates translated into high infant mortality stimulated new understanding of population dynamics. They got people thinking about the role that birth control measures might play in the alleviation of poverty. With the other Progressives, they documented the health hazards in air and water. They provided information on the need for regulation of foods and drugs. Over time, their ideas would be translated at the federal and state levels into formal oversight and responsibility for programs that serve vulnerable populations.

The environment of Hull House itself provided the incubation for the ideas, the methodologies, and the strategies of activists like Alice Hamilton. When Jane Addams created the settlement house, she designed an environment where young dynamic women and men could try out new ideas, debate, caucus, and support one another in their schemes. Far from settling down, they branched out and literally changed the odds, especially for families and children who were doing their own settling in their newly adopted country.

Helen Taussig on Broadway

Photographs of Helen Taussig always feature her hands, hands that touched and softened pain, hands that listened, and hands that learned.[20] Because she often approached life problems from a different angle from other people, she felt, saw, and deduced different things.

Born in Cambridge, Massachusetts, in 1898, Helen Taussig experienced a childhood filled with adversity.[21] She suffered whooping cough and deafness and lost her mother to tuberculosis. Further, she was a girl. But for all that, she ultimately made some of the most groundbreaking discoveries in the history of pediatrics, helped establish the subspecialty of pediatric cardiology, and set off a cascade of activity in cardiac surgery whose full impact is only being appreciated now, more than a half century later.

Following in her mother's footsteps, she attended Radcliffe College for two years and then completed undergraduate studies at Berkeley. Always interested in science, she considered studying public health at Harvard, but Harvard would not grant degrees to women. So she followed the advice of an anatomy professor at Boston University and enrolled at the Johns Hopkins School of Medicine in Baltimore.[22]

After graduation, Taussig joined the Hopkins Pediatrics Department. There, the department chair Edwards Park was creating specialty services to focus on the physiology and pathology of specific organ systems. Because of Taussig's interest in heart disease, in 1930 Park assigned her to direct the new Children's Heart Clinic at the Harriet Lane Home. By this time, Taussig had lost most of her hearing and depended on lip reading. How would a deaf woman be able to direct a clinic for children with heart disease? Until the 1920s and 1930s cardiologists relied almost exclusively on the stethoscope. Listening to the heart sounds, they intuited the child's anatomy and pathology.

Perhaps it was precisely because Taussig could not hear well that she advanced the field of cardiology. She used the new technologies of X-ray and fluoroscopy to watch the heart. And she used her hands. Her fingers felt for the heart's point of maximal impact. Her palm gently stretched on the babies' chest to feel for heart murmurs, pericardial rubs, and the galloping beat of a failing heart. She was a marvelous diagnostician, and she never let a question go unanswered.

Especially interested in questions about congenital heart disease, Taussig delved into some problems that had stumped scientists for centuries. Why were blue babies blue? What was the course of their circulation? Why was their heart not sending blood to the lungs to pick up oxygen? Why did so many new babies die? To answer these questions she went to the pathology lab. Whenever a baby with a congenital heart condition died, she would work with the pathologists to delineate the distorted anatomy of a malfunctioning heart. With medical artists, she drew the details of the heart chambers, the valves, and the vessels: some were too big, some were too small, and many were heading in the wrong direction. There was a mixed-up twist during embryonic life that would cut off life out of the womb. She catalogued her findings in her classic book *Congenital Malformations of the Heart.*[23]

Taussig asked a further question: she wondered not so much why babies with congenital anomalies and cyanotic heart disease died as why some of them lived. What was protecting them? They struggled, they didn't grow well, they grunted and gasped, but they did survive. Placing her hand on their little chests, she felt the reason why. The ductus arteriosis (the connection between the aorta and the pulmonary arteries) that allows babies' blood to be oxygenated in fetal life generally closes shortly after birth. In babies with normal hearts, having an open ductus arteriosis is unnecessary. In fact, it is a hazard. In the normal course of the first few days of life, the ductus arteriosis shuts down.

For babies whose pulmonary arteries are blocked so that they cannot get blood to and from their lungs, an open ductus arteriosis provides that hidden back route that every knowing commuter cuts over to when the main highway is tied up. Helen Taussig discovered that the blue babies who survived did so by relying on that special back road. She asked the next question: Why can't we make a permanent detour for these children? If we could construct a permanent shunt between the aorta and the pulmonary artery, then maybe we could keep these children alive a lot longer. Taussig's ideas hit home with Alfred Blalock, the new hotshot surgeon recruited to Hopkins from Nashville to head the cardiac surgery program.[24]

Blalock's surgical success was a team affair. That story has now received nationwide acclaim through the PBS series *Partners of the Heart.*[25] A brilliant surgeon, diagnostician, and thinker, Blalock had as brilliant a partner in Vivian Thomas, whose background as a black man without a college education excluded him from the medical profession, especially on the midcentury Johns Hopkins medical campus. Taussig, Blalock, and Thomas are now credited with the stunning success of the first blue baby operation, carried out on November 9, 1944, on a 9-month-old girl with tetralogy of Fallot. She weighed just nine pounds and was so frail that Blalock wrote in his postoperative note, "The patient stood the procedure better then I anticipated."[26] At the end of the operation, Taussig exclaimed from the head of the operating room table, "The baby is a lovely color now!"

The Children's Heart Clinic was a busy place. Children with heart disease came from all over the country. With an epidemic of acute rheumatic fever under way, hospital clinics and wards throughout the country were filled with children and youth with rheumatic fever's characteristic symptoms of arthritis, carditis, and skin problems. Children also suffered another poststreptococcal disorder, acute glomerulonephritis; their bodies were swollen, and their lungs were so filled with edematous fluid that they could not breathe. Other children suffered from Saint Vitus's dance and Syndenham's chorea.

Rheumatic fever is a prime example of a disease that is caused by the coalescence of biologic and environmental factors.[27] The three factors most implicated are (1) specific strains of beta hemolytic Streptococcus A, (2) immunological systems that cannot distinguish a bacterial antigen from the protein that makes up the delicate leaflets of a child's heart valves, and (3) overcrowded living situations and lack of proper nourishment. Because of her experience with rheumatic heart disease, Taussig was one of the first physicians to pinpoint the biologic-environmental interface of disease etiology. She understood why the doctor's black bag and sturdy walking shoes are valuable equipment for child health professionals.

In just the same way that Helen Taussig followed the path of congenital heart disease to the anatomy table, she followed the rheumatic fever story to the streets. It bothered her that so many of her patients were poor, that they seemed burdened by multiple problems. She employed a social worker to visit the homes of her patients, to climb the famous white steps of the Baltimore row houses, to walk up and down the now dilapidated real estate of the once posh Broadway, to see what else she and the clinic could do for the children. Taussig did not send her social worker out to report back in a month or two; she went with her. She sat down at the kitchen table, listened to the children babble and yell and squabble. Seeing four or five children sharing a bed, she became convinced that the social conditions of the children were a big part of the children's health problem. The answer to a rheumatic fever cure was here just as much as it was in the clinic.

Over her life Helen Taussig made enormous contributions to children, to child health, and to the advancement of child health science. She perceived things that others did not perceive. She knew that many of the secrets lay right in front of her and that if she asked the right question she would be able to follow the right path to the answer. And the answers she found changed the life chances for untold numbers of children and families.

Roland Scott and 350 Years of White Brainwashing

In 1950 Roland B. Scott applied for membership to the medical staff of the National Children's Hospital in Washington. While many doctors had to wait four or five months to hear about their appointments, for Scott it would be five years.[28] This was in spite of the fact that he was a graduate of a fine medical school, had received his pediatric training in a top-flight residency program, and was currently the chief of pediatrics at a sister institution. But that neighboring institution was Howard University, and Roland Scott was black, so the problem lay not in Roland Scott's qualifications but in white resistance to equality among the races. Throughout his career, even into his late years, Scott, "the father of sickle cell disease," had to contend with racism.[29]

Born in Texas, the son of a small businessman and a supportive mother, Roland Scott was a natural scholar. He fell in love with chemistry and excelled in his studies. In 1927 he chose the historically black Howard University over the University of Chicago, his mother having counseled him that a young black man might find himself isolated in a predominantly white social environment. At Howard he found encouragement from mentors that included Ralph Bunche, Alan Locke, and Percy Julian.[30] He stayed on at Howard for a productive medical school career. The chief of pediatrics, Alonzo Smith, recognized his talent and encouraged his budding interest in childhood illness.

Scott chose the University of Chicago for his pediatric training. Life has its coincidences: Scott, who would become the world's most distinguished scholar in the field of sickle cell anemia, happened to take his residency at the same university where in 1910 James B. Herrick first described a case of sickle cell anemia, in a medical student.[31] Perhaps the greatest lesson Scott learned during residency was the precise art of physical diagnosis. Throughout his career he would perfect his skill as he carefully documented every aspect of sickle cell disease.

At the end of Scott's training, Alonzo Smith recruited him back to Washington, D.C. This recognition by the faculty at Howard did not prevent Roland Scott's suffering the stings of racism from other quarters: despite passing the examinations of the American Board of Pediatrics, he was initially rejected by the American Academy of Pediatrics because of race; and although he had joined the Chicago Medical Society, an affiliate of the American Medical Association, when he applied for membership in the comparable association in the nation's capital, his request was denied.

Roland Scott's personal brushes with racism made him keenly aware of how social factors intertwine with health and social outcomes. Tactful and politically astute, he focused his advocacy on clinical action. Every day, in the emergency room and on the wards of the Howard Hospital, he diagnosed and treated seriously ill children with the painful, swollen hands and feet, the invasive infectious complications, and the long-term consequences of sickle cell anemia. He documented everything he saw. During his career, Scott wrote more than 250 articles, many of which form the classical description of sickle cell anemia.[32]

In the 1940s and 1950s there was little sophistication in the epidemiology of pediatric illness. Scott's careful depictions of sickle cell disease woke the rest of the pediatric community to the differential in childhood morbidity based on race. His studies showed that sickle cell anemia accounted for much of the excess mortality and shortened life expectancy among black children.

In 1945 Scott became the chairman of pediatrics at Howard. In his leadership position, he pushed for laboratory space and research dollars to probe for better scientific understanding of the cause of sickle cell disease. Early on he had difficulty tapping traditional funding sources. Fortunately, several black sororities and fraternities supported his efforts. Somewhat unexpectedly, a radio station in Connecticut also took up the cause.[33] These gifts helped Scott gather the data he needed to advocate for large-scale federal support. His testimony before Congress was critical to the passage of the Sickle Cell Control Act of 1971, which provided funding for ten sickle cell centers, including one at Howard.[34]

Scott's advocacy laid the foundation for scientists at the centers to elucidate the specific pathophysiology of sickle cell disease. Their findings added to the basic understanding of how genetic abnormalities translate into disease. Scientists working at the centers learned how the change in one nucleic acid in one gene on one chromosome calls the body to manufacture an amino acid, whose aberrant physical structure causes a cascade of abnormal hematologic and systemic outcomes. Here was Watson and Crick's 1953 model played out in human physiology.[35]

Despite the fundamental laboratory breakthroughs, Scott found that he had to keep reminding government funding agencies that bench research was only one step in a long process. Children continued to suffer from crises and strokes and to die from sickle cell disease. In the late 1970s, when sickle cell research funding was in decline, Scott knew that he had to up the tempo in his call for action. "Interest in sickle cell, like many other diseases is like the latest hairstyles, fashions, and dances—it goes in cycles."[36]

It vexed Scott that few of the children's parents understood the signs and symptoms of sickle cell disease, let alone its complex genetic basis. He ached when children came to the hospital late in the course of a crisis or an infection. He worried about the distrust on parents' faces and wondered whether they were receiving adequate information and support when clinicians tried to explain the disease's recessive inheritance pattern. Scott saw racism at work in the poor communication to black families about the basic facts. He spoke of "350 years of white brainwashing." To a *Washington Post* reporter in 1972, he said, "Black people were taught to look down on everything that was part of their heritage."[37]

In the 1970s and 1980s, as the genetic origin of illness was first being made clear to the lay public, the major conditions considered to have a genetic base were insanity and mental retardation. Many black communities, bitterly hurt by the horrible Tuskegee experiments, were leery of a further conflation of race and disease. The white medical community had ignored the illnesses of black people and literally had abused their black brothers and sisters in the name of science. Scott anticipated a difficult battle in communicating how the crucial new information explained some racial disparities in health. When sickle cell disease was discovered among people in Mediterranean, South American, and Arabian countries, Scott was able to disentangle race from genetics and believed that these epidemiologic findings were a huge contribution to moving toward a solution.

Roland Scott was an effective advocate because he knew how to use science to influence decisions. He always presented his own personal experience. He understood the importance of biding his time until the propitious moment. He also knew that his own passionate journey held an undeniable poignancy. His forcefulness came from knitting these elements together and never giving up in the face of adversity or discouragement.

Robert Haggerty, Joel Alpert, and Barry Zuckerman: Primary Health Care

In the late 1950s and early 1960s, many department chairmen began to reexamine general pediatric care. In Boston, Charles Janeway tapped his chief resident, Robert Haggerty, to scrutinize problems in child health and community medicine.[38] Haggerty had always contended that house officers did not treat enough common problems. As the grandson of a general practitioner, tagging along in the summers on house calls, he knew that medicine's purview was a lot wider than the wards at 300 Longwood Avenue.

Haggerty designed the Family Health Care Program as a model health delivery system. It soon became the site for residents' clinics and medical student teaching. Trainees learned to care for pregnant women, attend the birth of the child, and follow up with the new baby and his siblings. Young faculty began to clamor for opportunities to work with the children and families. Something special was going on. The doctors and nurses who flocked to the little building on Francis Street found like-minded professionals, including other health clinicians, sociologists, and social workers. Here were colleagues who wanted to get a handle on why, in some families, children were sick all the time, while in others the children flew through the early years with little more than an occasional cold.

Haggerty built in a comprehensive research component to follow co-horts of patients and their families through diary recordings of the details of everyday life. These data would allow the research team to study the complex interactions of community events, family factors, and children's health. Would a move, the death of a grandparent, the birth of a sister, or a parent's job loss have an impact on Danny's tendency to asthma or to stomachaches? If so, how did those stresses operate?

In a classic study, Haggerty and his team showed the relationship between stress and infection. Within the two weeks after a significant household stress, children were at four times increased risk of infection by Streptococcus A, the bacteria that caused rheumatic fever.[39] Here was a big link in the chain of observations that colleagues like Taussig and Scott were making. Clearly, children's immunological systems had more than one master. Bacteria and virus might be calling many of the shots, but poverty, overcrowding, and stress were getting their orders in too.

In 1964 Haggerty was recruited to Rochester, New York, as chief of pe-diatrics at Strong Memorial Hospital, where he continued to wed medical care with research. He and the sociologist Klaus Roghmann conducted a groundbreaking community health study of children and families in six distinct neighborhoods. Their book, *Child Health and the Community,* established the tight interaction of community factors with child health outcomes.[40] They also brought into play the notion of the "new morbid-ity," conditions such as developmental and behavioral problems, sub-stance use, interpersonal violence, and child abuse. These health prob-lems were plaguing families and needed addressing.

Haggerty and Roghmann demonstrated that they could affect health outcomes area by area. Two neighborhoods alike on the surface and sim-ilar with regard to ethnicity and poverty status (the factors most people thought accounted for health-related effects) could have quite different health outcomes, depending on whether one of the neighborhoods had a health clinic that supported and educated families. The community itself was such a living, breathing, powerful force that Haggerty coined another phrase, *community pediatrics* and developed partnership models of health care that incorporated families and communities.

When Haggerty left Boston, Joel Alpert took on the leadership of the

Family Health Care Program. He received a grant that gave him the opportunity of defining *primary health care*. At the time the concept was open to many interpretations and some confusion. In 1974 Alpert and his colleague Evan Charney published their work in a government monograph.[41] They defined four anchoring points for primary care. Primary care should be (1) continuous, (2) longitudinal, (3) the first contact, and (4) family focused. In 1976 Alpert and the Family Health Care Program published a critically important article entitled "Delivery of Health Care for Children: Report of an Experiment."[42] Using a randomized controlled trial, Alpert and his team showed that primary care met the needs of the children and cut down on inappropriate emergency room use and preventable hospitalizations.

Alpert was encouraged by Janeway to consider the position of the department chair at Boston City Hospital and to use his skills to build a systematic and equitable health care delivery system for a large, generally underserved population of children. At the time, Boston City Hospital suffered from the worst that city bureaucracy has to offer: poor facilities, poor pay, poor attitudes, and enough under-the-table dealings to make Boss Tweed blush. Alpert knew the horror stories of offices without desks, telephones without dial tones, and clinic rooms without examining tables. But Alpert did not get things done by being nice. He had an edge, a presence, and a persistence that had earned him the reputation of being a bulldog. When the fact that Alpert was going to become chair of pediatrics at Boston City Hospital became public knowledge, it was common to hear, "If Joel can't do it, nobody can."[43]

With little to lose and lots to win, Alpert would be one of a small number of pediatric department chairs around the United States who began to see primary care and community pediatrics as their principal academic commitment. He recruited a strong faculty: men and women who had practical ideas for how to make primary care delivery a rich solution for the health care problems of the children they saw day to day. One of these faculty members was the developmental pediatrician Barry Zuckerman. He was most interested in what it meant to deliver comprehensive services as part of primary care. As Alpert designed and refined the primary care model, Zuckerman worked at how best to meet the needs that patients brought to the clinic door—needs for housing, for food, for green cards, for drug treatment, and even for extrication from an abusive situation.

In the late 1970s and early 1980s the escalation of national health care costs drove a reassessment of health care delivery and health manpower. Government-sponsored studies showed a high ratio of special- ists to generalists (especially in adult medicine), and Alpert's studies and those of others documented that an emphasis on primary care and gen- eralism might be cost saving. Given these facts, the government decided to establish new training programs and incentives for physicians to enter primary care careers, passing Title VII of the Public Health Service Act. The Alpert-Charney definition of *primary care* was incorporated into the legislation and its regulations.

Most of the push for an academic focus on primary care has been positive and has succeeded in shifting the specialist-to-generalist ratios. The manpower shortages in pediatrics now are among the subspecialties. On the negative side, however, the wedding of academics with primary care for the poor has the potential to perpetuate two systems of care, a private one for those with health insurance and a public one—the uni- versity training programs—for the poor. Poor families often turn to uni- versity training programs as their default health center, and universities respond by setting up continuity clinics that serve the dual function of responding to community need and preparing the future child health workforce. By definition, these combined clinical-teaching settings fight an uphill battle to be as efficient and to provide as dependable care as a private doctor's office or a neighborhood health center. On the other hand, these settings do serve as incubators for important innovations. Barry Zuckerman, who succeeded Alpert as chair at the Boston Medical Center, has introduced highly successful programs like Reach Out and Read, Pathways to Health, Healthy Steps, Project Health, and Family Ad- vocacy Program into the clinical mix.[44]

Haggerty, Alpert, and Zuckerman have defined generalism, primary care, and community pediatrics. They have lifted the sights of academic institutions and federal funding agencies about what the practice of high-quality primary care and community pediatrics can accomplish. They have also opened the door to combining the best of primary care and the best of public health into an approach that all child health prac- titioners can embrace.

Julius B. Richmond: Head Start, Healthy People, and the Tobacco Wars

Julius Richmond is the consummate advocate.[45] Never satisfied, he looks, he sees, he questions, and when he gets an answer, he uses his enormous political know-how and strategic acumen to change things. He also never works alone and never seeks personal aggrandizement or credit.

Born in Chicago in 1916 Richmond was raised partly in the city and partly in rural Illinois in a boy's private boarding school, where as the only Jewish student he learned the minority perspective. He began his residency in pediatrics at Cook County Hospital. After the attack on Pearl Harbor, he joined the Air Force, serving from 1942 until 1945 and the end of the war.

On his return, he received funding as a Markle Scholar, and from 1948 to 1953, he conducted basic research on the autonomic nervous system to document individual differences in infants and young children.[46] He was one of the first people to point out how infant brain growth depends on organized input from the external world. Before the advent of sophisticated brain imaging, he and his research colleagues documented the elaboration of synaptic connections in infants. He would demonstrate the intricate and vulnerable interactions of the newly forming brain, and he would take the next logical step to argue the importance of early cognitive stimulation.

In 1953 Richmond moved to the State University of New York in Syracuse, where he teamed up with Bettye Caldwell, a child psychologist and perfect collaborator for Richmond. Finding such a like-minded partner as Caldwell was just the kind of "incidence of coincidence" Richmond loves to talk about: the right colleague at the right time in the right place asking the right questions.

Richmond and Caldwell worked with infants and toddlers in the poorer neighborhoods of the city. At first they simply assessed and described the development of the children, but what they found disturbed them greatly. Although the children sat up on time, walked on time, began to speak on time, at about 18 months of age, their learning curves and development eventually slowed down. Developmental test scores of some of the toddlers actually fell into the abnormal range. These were not ill or retarded children. What was going on?

Richmond and Caldwell began to visit the children's homes. What they found disturbed them even more. There were the bare essentials: food, shelter, and minimally acceptable clothing. But there were no toys, no books, no crayons or paints. There were no blocks and puzzles; no cow jumping over the moon, nor were there reminders of the families' heritage in Africa or the Caribbean or South America. They hypothesized that the families' sheer poverty left them with little energy to supply developmental stimulation to the children.

The two investigators' response was to write an early childhood curriculum and to enroll children in a preschool at the Syracuse campus. After all, that was what college-educated women had been doing for years. A comparison of children who attended Richmond and Caldwell's preschool to a group that had not had that advantage showed the familiar pattern of developmental loss, beginning at eighteen months, among the children denied the preschool experience. The youngsters who had attended the enrichment program had normal developmental trajectories. with no missed milestones. The early childhood curriculum had made an enormous difference, and word spread that poverty's effects on children could be overturned.

As it turned out, the new head of the Office of Economic Opportunity (OEO), Sargent Shriver, was on the lookout for programs that could help families climb their way out of persistent poverty.[47] In his 1964 State of the Union address, President Lyndon Johnson had declared a war on poverty and charged his administrative aides to come up with the weaponry to attack the root causes of social devastation.[48] Shriver called Richmond to Washington and asked him to put a full-scale program into place—tomorrow. Few people could have mounted the kind of response that Richmond did, implementing a nationally directed program for 500,000 children at nearly 3,000 sites. As the first national director of Head Start, Richmond traveled to small towns, rural villages, and big city neighborhoods throughout America. Over and over, he witnessed the same deprivation that he and Bettye Caldwell had encountered when they visited homes in New York State. He found children denied nurturing, children taken for granted, and children whose potential was being wasted.

He also found allies in the towns and cities, men and women who knew that the situation for young families could change. They recognized in Head Start a practical mechanism to turn things around but also knew that Head Start should invest in the community itself, should take advantage of the talents of local people. Under the umbrella of Head Start, these community leaders could introduce young children to language and song, pictures and stories about their heritage and their future. Years later Richmond would say that Head Start has succeeded so well because it rests on "contracts between the federal government and local communities, which have proved to be remarkably effective in giving people in local communities—and particularly parents—ownership and commitment for the health, education, and welfare of their young children."[49]

As Richmond learned more about the needs and the strengths of communities, he identified gaps in the delivery of health care to young children. In the bayous and the backwaters, out where the tall wheat blew and in the swelter of the inner cities, Richmond recognized the dearth of easily accessible health care clinics for children. He was impressed by the ideas that community members brought to him. Richmond listened and responded with the kind of idea that Shriver could run with. How about a new type of community-organized, community-run health clinic? The OEO wanted to ensure the "maximum feasible participation of the poor." What better way to create participation, ownership, jobs, and community health than to build and run these clinics? And so the neighborhood health center movement was born.

In 1967, with the change of presidential administrations, Richmond made his way back into the academic world, with leadership roles at the State University of New York in Syracuse and then at Harvard. But Richmond was not to stay away from Washington for long. In 1977 President Carter appointed him assistant secretary for health and surgeon general of the United States.[50] With his new authority, he turned his attention to some unfinished business: long-term federal commitment to the neighborhood health centers. He worked with Congress to pass the Health Services and Centers Act of 1978. Nearly $3 billion was authorized to fund services in community health centers, migrant centers, and primary care programs and to offer grants-in-aid for community-generated public health initiatives.[51]

Julius Richmond has the rare ability of moving easily from the specific to the general, from the smallest detail to the integrated whole, from one child stacking green and purple blocks to a nation of youngsters preparing for life. He sees in the individual and in the moment what can be in all people in the future. He lives in two time zones: now and thirty years from now. Although Head Start will always be heralded as his great gift to the children of the United States, and neighborhood health centers as a stunning contribution to health care delivery, the Healthy People concept and methodology was his gift to the nation as a whole.[52] For the first time someone asserted that a nation could be well, that its people could be not only free from disease but also truly healthy. *Healthy People,* Richmond's 1979 report, threw down the gauntlet to every agency in the government, every member of Congress, every person working in the private health sector, including academics, to meet 226 health goals by the year 1990. The document elevated the notion of health and at the same time it put health attainment in the hands of all citizens. The brilliance of the report was in breaking the task of creating a healthy nation into manageable parts, each with concrete, measurable end points.

As surgeon general, Julius Richmond inherited the ongoing tobacco wars from his predecessors. In the 1960s the publication of studies linking tobacco smoking to lung cancer had drawn the battle lines between the public health establishment and the tobacco companies. With his belief in the power of documentation and data, Richmond decided that the most valuable and strategic thing he could do as surgeon general was to collate the scientific evidence implicating tobacco's disease potential. He was subjected to name-calling, abuse, and personal attack by the big tobacco companies, but he persisted. His foresight has paid off in billions and billions of dollars of legal settlements against the tobacco industry (most of which are being appealed by the tobacco companies). Because Richmond made sure that the scientific facts about the hazards of smoking were in a publicly available government-published form (in the 1979 anniversary report on smoking), the tobacco companies had to explain their continued promotion of a known harmful substance. They have had a particularly difficult time claiming ignorance of the cumulative effects of tobacco smoke—so much so that the Food and Drug Administration proposes to regulate tobacco as a drug.[53]

Throughout his career, Richmond has straddled the two worlds of politics and academics. In his roles as professor of pediatrics and psychiatry and the dean of a medical school, he was interested in preparing the social strategists of the future. Just as he has made groundbreaking contributions in the policy arena, he has also effected significant change in how child health is viewed, practiced, and taught in universities, medical schools, and academic health centers. Together with thought leaders in pediatrics like Milton Senn, he was convinced that child health professionals needed to be deeply versed in child development. He has championed research into the causes of mental retardation and has chaired numerous panels and advisory councils on the epidemiology of child developmental and mental health disorders. He has been the major adviser to national studies on special education and on the long-term consequences of prematurity. He was one of the first pediatric leaders to call for recognition of child development as a critical discipline. He helped launch the campaign that culminated in 2000 in the board certification of developmental-behavioral pediatrics as a subspecialty.

Julius Richmond has always had his eye on the future. With a grand optimism, he envisions a world that is just and kind and that cares about children and families. But with a feet-on-the-ground realism, he plans every step of every action and crafts every political maneuver. Because he sees advocacy as a gift one generation gives to another, he cultivates the careers of young colleagues, helping them to see as he sees, to dream as he dreams, and to act as he acts—for communities, families, and children.

Margaret Heagarty and Barbara Barlow: Pocket Parks, Gardens, and Community

When Margaret Heagarty was the chief of pediatrics at Harlem Hospital, visitors to her seventeenth-floor office were invariably treated to her Irish storyteller's depiction of the creation of the Harlem Injury Prevention project.[54] Sitting behind a cluttered desk, surrounded by gifts from pediatric residents from Nigeria and Egypt and India, she would lean back and with a gleeful little smile tell how she and pediatric surgeon Barbara Barlow decided to tackle the problem of injuries and violence in Harlem. "One day, my chief of pediatric surgery marched in here and said, 'I just won't do it again! I will not stitch up another child with a knife or glass wound until we start finding out what is happening on the streets and in the playgrounds.'" That day in the mid-1980s the Harlem Injury Prevention program took off. From it has grown a nationally replicated system, the Injury-Free Coalition for Kids, which is saving countless child lives and improving basic living conditions in neighborhoods all over America.[55]

To get to the bottom of the injury and violence problem in Harlem, Heagarty and Barlow knew that they needed facts. What better place to gather them than the routine morning report? Every day at 8 a.m. the interns and residents would shuffle into Heagarty's office to recite the histories and physicals of the children who had been admitted to the hospital the night before. They would describe the falls, the scrapes, and all too often the knife or bullet wounds. They would talk about the 911 calls, the screaming ambulance siren, the workup in the emergency ward, and the sewing and patching in the operating theater. All the information for investigation was there, but no one had ever taken a systematic approach to assembling it.

Heagarty supplied the residents with three-by-five index cards and asked them to log the names, addresses, and ages of the children they treated; to describe the nature of the injuries and the pertinent medical details; and radically, to record where the incident happened and how the injury was sustained. Pretty soon, she and Barlow began to discern a pattern. Certain streets and certain playgrounds were breeding grounds for hospital admissions.

Armed with this information, their creativity, and the resolution to make a difference for the children in Harlem, Heagarty and Barlow set out to find partners who could help them clean up the playgrounds and improve the street environment. These partners included epidemiologists from the Columbia School of Public Health, political leaders from the councilman's office, the police, urban planners, and philanthropists. Margaret Heagarty also relies a fair amount on Saint Anthony. With the data on injuries, the behind the scenes politicking and a patron saint in the mix, dollars and help began to flow to the project, with particularly strong support from the Robert Wood Johnson Foundation. Then step-by-step, Heagarty's group renovated parks, established a baseball program (which some years later would send a team to the World Series of Little League), and inaugurated a dance program and arts studio right in the Harlem Hospital. Within a few years, injuries had decreased by 60 percent, and the Harlem area was distinctly safer than sections of the city with comparable sociodemographic characteristics.[56]

The success in Harlem spurred Heagarty and Barlow to try to replicate the program in other communities, using the recipe, one part community leadership, one part motivation for change, one part ingenuity. Heagarty and Barlow found community leaders all over: in police stations, beauty parlors, schools, churches. Like Barlow and Heagarty, these citizens were interested in improving their neighborhood; in teaching neighborhood children some basics, like how to cross the street safely; and in turning vacant lots into garden plots and playgrounds. Surely, there were people like this all over America.

When the project officers at the Robert Wood Johnson Foundation saw the program's positive results, they urged Barlow to consider a dissemination strategy. Together, they formed the Injury-Free Coalition for Kids (IFCK), which by 2004 was operating forty sites in thirty-seven cities.[57] Although the programs share one common element—their administrative home in a pediatric trauma center—the philosophy of the program is that local conditions cause particular injury patterns. Fixing those conditions depends on local response. In Providence, Rhode Island, the Buckle-Up Faithfully program is sponsored primarily by rectors of the African American churches, who deliver car safety sermons. In Phoenix, where most backyards boast a family swimming pool, Oliver Otter advises young children that they "otter be water wise." In Seattle teenagers, in a program called Shot through Our Eyes, wield cameras and take thought-provoking pictures about community hazards.

Prevention works. Childhood injuries can be decreased by community engagement, beautification projects, good play and sports equipment. and antibullying and antiviolence interventions. Preventive activities even affect the health care bottom line, certainly for insurance companies. Perhaps one of Heagarty and Barlow's biggest triumphs occurred when Saint Anthony brought the All-State Insurance Company to the good doctors' door. The partnership with All State has allowed several of the IFCK groups to design and build new playgrounds for children. When even one five-year child does not end up with serious head trauma in the intensive care unit, insurance companies save hundreds of thousands of dollars, and a productive life goes forward.

Calvin Sia: The Medical Home

In 1958, on the day he opened his private pediatric practice in Honolulu, Cal Sia doodled on his newly printed prescription pad.[58] He looked expectantly out the window and peered at the phone. He paced and waited for patients. That was probably the last day he ever waited for anything. He determined that his would be a practice that was proactive, that planned ahead, and that avoided crises. He wanted to step in early enough to prevent ill health and injury. He believed that it was critical for his office to be efficiently connected to resources so that none of his patients would ever have to wait either. Years later, he would chair the American Academy of Pediatrics committee that drafted the medical home statement.[59] He would work tirelessly to promote the principles that (1) any child health team includes not only medical practitioners but also the family and the community, and (2) child health is an ongoing, dynamic process.

The roots of Sia's advocacy are in his family background. Born in Beijing, he was raised on the value of service. Sia recalls an event in the 1930s involving his father, who was an infectious diseases specialist. During the visit of a multimillionaire American industrialist to China, the businessman's young son began to display signs of paralytic polio, including severe respiratory compromise. The visitors turned for help to Cal Sia Sr. Sia had been working with opium addicts who had developed respiratory complications from their morphine addiction. To support these patients' breathing, he was using a newly developed apparatus, the iron lung. It occurred to him that the iron lung could get the young American through the acute phase of his infection. This bold approach saved the boy. Much moved at his father's courage, Cal Sia wanted to be like him, a different strain of physician, one who would take chances and practice bold medicine.

In 1939, because of Japanese rule, the Sia family left China and joined Cal Sia's grandparents in Hawaii. The grandparents, both physicians, cared for Chinese immigrants working on the island's vast farms and pineapple plantations. The grandfather, Dr. Li, and grandmother, Dr. Kong, were instrumental in founding Chinese cultural institutions in Hawaii, including the first Chinese church, a Chinese newspaper, and Chinese cultural clubs. An active practitioner throughout her life, Sia's grandmother delivered more than 6,000 babies. The Chinese church was the center of much of the activity in Sia's youth. Because of the emphasis his deacon parents placed on community service, young Cal made an early life decision to become a doctor. During medical school at Western Reserve, in Cleveland, Ohio, he worked on infectious diseases, including polio, and on pulmonary interventions through mechanical ventilation He was easily wooed into pediatrics and readily accepted the overtures of the child health faculty.

After medical school and internship on the mainland, Sia returned to Hawaii for residency. He stayed on to open his practice in the community, with close ties to the University of Hawaii Medical Center. He continued as chief of Newborn Services and subsequently became chief of staff of the Children's Hospital. As the newest and youngest pediatric practitioner in town, he found that when patients did start trickling in to him, he got all the difficult problems, those that had baffled or overwhelmed his fellow child health colleagues. Many of these complicated cases involved multiple organ systems, cognitive and emotional concerns, and the need for input from multiple community systems.

To design his clinical office, Sia sought help from colleagues throughout the community. He visited schools; he talked to the directors of social service agencies; he discovered who could be trusted to support children and families. He became involved with Easter Seals Hawaii, the United Cerebral Palsy association, the Salvation Army, and other philanthropic societies. In 1965 he helped found the Variety School for Learning Disabilities. He became active in the American Academy of Pediatrics and the Hawaii State Medical Association and served as president of both groups.

As he became active in organized medicine, Sia realized that he had a natural gift for advocacy and learned the advantage of getting to know influential people. Sia met Senator Hiram Fong at a dinner, for example, and later Senator Fong arranged for Sia to be appointed to the Advisory Council for the National Institute for Child Health and Human Development, the branch of the National Institutes of Health that sponsors pediatric research. On that council Cal Sia widened his circle of nationally influential colleagues to include leading health scientists like Samuel

Katz, Philip Dodge, and Norman Kretchmer. He also was able to learn about up-coming grants from the Children's Bureau and made sure that Hawaii responded to the request for proposal; millions of dollars were awarded to the state for an innovative child abuse prevention program, Hawaii Healthy Start. Working with Senator Daniel Inoye, whom he had met on a flight to Washington, D.C., Sia was able to help launch the national Pediatric Emergency Medical Services program.

Cal Sia's name is almost synonymous with the medical home concept: that children and youth deserve accessible, family-centered, comprehensive, continuous, and coordinated care from their medical providers. The term *medical home* was first used by the American Academy of Pediatrics in the 1970s to denote a formal medical record for gathering all of a child's health information into a central document. The problem of dispersed medical data has only gotten worse since that time, despite the advent of computer technology. The countervailing pressures of specialization and subspecialization and the burgeoning of laboratory and radiological testing have led to an explosion of medical information about individual children and youth. Data may be lodged in a surgeon's file cabinet, on a gastroenterologist's laptop, in a neurologist's handheld PDA (personal digital assistant), on a hospital laboratory server, or on the computer at the school-based clinic. All of this information actually belongs to the child and the family, but the chore of assembling it in one place can be difficult. The medical home is the common ground for coordinating these data into a comprehensive approach to a child's health and related needs.

Unlike Abraham Jacobi, who warned mothers to shun the folk wisdom of other women, Sia's concept of a medical home builds on the mutual respect of parent and professional: both have something consequential to offer. Moreover, the medical home can function only if parents are key actors. Family-centered care is the ideal. Mothers and fathers articulate their hopes and dreams for their children and work with doctors, teachers, and other to realize those aspirations.

While Cal Sia proposes a medical home for all children, the model is especially applicable to children with special health care needs. If a child is born with spina bifida, the medical home approach would call for the team of family and health care provider to compose a list of the specialists and therapists who will be caring for the child and a timeline of anticipated surgeries and interventions. The aim is as few emergencies and unanticipated events as possible.

Doggedly persistent, Sia has waged a sophisticated campaign to insert medical home language into government standards, federal request for proposals, the position statements of the American Academy of Pediatrics, the Future of Pediatric Education II blueprint, and the pronouncement of various state medical societies.[60] Through his national involvement in the American Medical Association, he has helped to introduce the notion into the care of adults as well as children. The term *medical home* now regularly shows up in the literature of parent groups such as Family Voices, in family practice journals, and on the websites of state public health and medical agencies. How did the term find its way to all these far-flung locations, newsletters, and press releases? Odds are high that one night the representative of the organization or agency had a lovely conversation over rubber chicken with a certain visionary doctor from Hawaii.

Phillip Porter, Ed Rushton, and Tom Tonniges: The CATCH Program

In Cambridge, Massachusetts, in the early 1970s, Phil Porter wore many hats.[61] He was a teacher of pediatrics and public health, chief of the Cambridge City Hospital's Pediatrics Department, director of Maternal and Child Health, and the head school doctor. And now somebody wanted him to take on Head Start! Having so many obligations in so many directions would frazzle most people, but Phil Porter embraced the chance to travel into uncharted waters and to try to pull together a coordinated health care scheme for children and families in Cambridge. He envisioned fashioning the component parts into to a larger whole, creating a truly seamless set of services for the children and youth of his city.[62]

The 1970s was a time of great opportunity for creative thinkers. The birth rate had dropped, and town and school administrators were open to ideas for making good use of empty space. If at all possible, they wanted to preserve the staff slots they had fought so hard to accrue—nobody likes to take a backward step. In Rochester, Bob Haggerty and Klaus Roghmann were describing the "new morbidity" in children and adolescents and urging pediatricians to go outside the clinic door to practice in and with the community to counter such problems among children and youth as pregnancy, substance abuse, violence, and school failure. Phil Porter was to galvanize national action around those problems.

For good reason Phil Porter earned the nickname "the Johnny Appleseed" of community pediatrics. With his slight slump, warm smile, disarming manner, he was a master storyteller. He kept audiences on the edge of their seats as he told of pediatricians in St. Paul, Minnesota, joining forces with Catholic parish priests because both groups were sickened by the high rates of abortions among the city's teenagers. Together, they founded one of the nation's first school-based clinics for adolescents—a place where nurses and doctors would not shy away from honest engagement with young people about sexuality and contraception. He described a pediatrics practice in Great Barrington, Massachusetts, joining early education providers to deliver comprehensive, integrated health and education interventions. He traveled the United States promoting the kind of multidimensional community pediatrics he had assembled in Cambridge. Before long, the Robert Wood Johnson Foundation began to fund his activities: the RWJ Healthy Children Program laid the groundwork for what would become the Community Access To Child Health (CATCH) program of the American Academy of Pediatrics.

One of Porter's stories featured the pediatrician Ed Rushton, who practiced in a small town in northern Florida. Rushton had seen too many poor families water down their stews to make ends meet. Florida's Medicaid program allotted health insurance benefits only to the most desperately impoverished families, and the amount that the state paid clinicians barely covered the time of the office assistant who had to fill out the reams of triplicate forms to justify the patient's visit. Ed Rushton took matters into his own hands, creating an innovative outreach program for poor families. Working with the health department and with the other private pediatricians in town, he crafted a comprehensive program for children that combined public health clinics (responsible during weekday hours) with a contracted on-call pediatrician service (for nights and weekends).

In the late 1980s Ruby Hearn, the vice president of the Robert Wood Johnson Foundation, approached the American Academy of Pediatrics with the question, Would the AAP be interested in taking on Porter's Healthy Children project as a new initiative? The project would empower child health providers in their towns and cities to try to resolve the problem of poor health care access for the children and youth, who somehow never made it to their offices. The AAP leadership decided to take on the project and recruited Ed Rushton to Chicago to be the first director of the CATCH program.[63]

In the beginning the AAP and others struggled to define CATCH. Was it a program, a call to action, a club, a philosophy? Somehow, the lack of definition didn't seem to matter. Maybe that was because CATCH was about defying definitions. People who were performing CATCH-like activities knew what it was. Before long, CATCH physicians were popping up all over. The AAP, the Robert Wood Johnson Foundation, and the Maternal and Child Health Bureau developed a mechanism to bring the can-do, action-oriented ideas of the practitioners monetary support and technical assistance to move ideas to action. In 1989 Healthy Tomorrows funding allowed CATCH to take off as a distinct mechanism for the local improvement of child health access. There would not be a definition, but there would be funds for action.

Ed Rushton knows pediatrics and he knows pediatricians. His "y'all come" personality made it easy to invite the pediatricians in Eastern Maine and in the Four Corners to get together in regional meetings to consider what would benefit the children in the area and what would actually make the pediatricians' lives a little easier. Avoiding nighttime phone calls is high on every pediatrician's list. Ed Rushton always argued that CATCH activities tied in to community-based prevention could be a win-win proposition.

When it was time for Rushton to pass on the baton of community pediatrics at the AAP, Tom Tonniges, a pediatrician from Nebraska, was chosen to succeed him.[64] Tonniges had practiced for eighteen years in Hastings. When he first arrived in the town, he was astonished by the high infant mortality rate and considered it his duty to recruit an obstetrician to the town. Within five years there was an active obstetric service in town, and infant mortality had been cut in half. The AAP knew that Tonniges would be an inspiring leader for community pediatrics and for CATCH. He had been an ardent campaigner for newborn hearing screening.[65] In practice, he had instituted OAE (otoacoustic emissions) screening in the local nursery and spoke up about the importance and feasibility of such screening. As a member of the AAP leadership, he kept both general community pediatrics issues and specific practices in the forefront. As director of community pediatrics at the AAP, Tonniges took the disparate ideas and components of the possible community outreach efforts of pediatricians, the beyond-the-boundaries work, and found ways to organize them into distinct programs: Healthy Child Care America, the Breast Feeding Initiative, the Medical Home Initiative, and Native American Health.[66]

Anne E. Dyson: A Different Kind of Doctor

Anne Dyson often described herself as a pediatrician who cared for children in the larger sense.[67] She supported innovation, new program development, and new ideas. She was a larger-than-life figure who was at the same time a pediatrician, a successful businesswoman, and a philanthropist. She knew from her medical practice what problems children and families confronted. She knew from her business life how to solve systems dilemmas. And she had the personal commitment to use the funds that were left in her care to address the inadequacies she perceived in pediatric health care.

Anne Dyson was the only daughter of Charles Dyson, a wealthy businessman who had made a fortune after World War II through mergers and acquisitions.[68] Dubbed by *Forbes Magazine* "the inventor of the leveraged buy-out," Charles Dyson began his work career as a bookkeeper and used his natural business sense and good timing to build a successful financial company. By the early 1990s he was regularly listed among the 150 richest people in the nation. Parallel to his private business career were Dyson's public contributions. During World War II, as a consultant to the secretary of war, he was one of the authors of lend-lease. He was a founder and financial supporter of Common Cause. His outspoken support for freedom of speech and his public stance against the Vietnam War earned him a spot on all three of Richard Nixon's enemies' lists. He said that being on those lists was "an endorsement of good standards."

Charles Dyson and his wife Margaret felt strongly that the money they had acquired brought with it the obligation of giving back in meaningful ways. His children grew up knowing that what mattered most to their parents was that they identify pressing needs and use the money and influence at their disposal to make a difference for the people around them. Annie Dyson considered these values her parents' most important legacy.

As a young woman, Anne Dyson was attracted both to business and to medicine. She surprised her family when she announced her intention to attend medical school, but her parents encouraged her to follow her own path. She initially thought that that path would lead her into psychiatry, but she became increasingly interested in pediatrics. After completing her training at Weill Children's Hospital at Cornell, Dyson became an instructor in the resident continuity clinic at the University of Illinois at Rockford. During those years, she became convinced that there was a serious deficiency in pediatrics and in pediatric training. She was deeply moved by her teaching encounters with the trainees. Intern after intern presented her with truly distressed patients. The young doctors felt frustrated by their inability to intervene for patients who suffered from ills that did not respond to the pills and potions in the traditional pharmacopoeia. It seemed to Dyson that the residents were swimming against the current. She became convinced that these inadequacies of the health care system were leading young doctors to lose confidence. She worried that the system was creating a sense of failure and ineptitude in the very people who were the hope of the future.

Juggling the multiple responsibilities of her life, Dyson moved between the financial world of Fifth Avenue to Union College, where her husband was president, to the boardrooms of the Dyson Foundation and multiple other groups. She spent days on end at the American Academy of Pediatrics, as one of the most stalwart members of the Friends of the Academy. With all the coming and going and meeting and greeting, managing money and deals and business matters, she maintained her practice skills by serving as the doctor at the Hole in the Wall Gang camp in Connecticut.[69] She loved coming back each summer, watching as the children with cancer, hematological disorders, and AIDS played and made friends and lived as full a life as they possibly could. She was a doctor in the larger sense, but she knew that the grounding for everything she did came from the care of individual children.

Like her father and mother, she was committed to using the family fortune to effect tangible change. Much of her work was behind the scenes. She and her mother made substantial contributions to the Dana Farber Cancer Institute to support basic science research on both childhood and adult cancers. She began the Big Apple Circus Clown Care Unit, which now has groups in children's hospitals all over the country. She saw to it that the CATCH program of the AAP was on firm footing. It was not unusual for her to hand an encouraging check to a young pediatrician who was caring for children in an innovative way.

In 1996 Marian Wright Edelman and her son Jonah Edelman asked Anne Dyson to help with the Stand for Children, an event to be held on the National Mall in Washington, D.C. Dyson arranged for medical care for the hundreds of thousands of people who would attend and asked her friend Paul Newman to donate enough lemonade and bottled water to avert heat stroke among attendees. At the end of that day, impressed by the energy and good will of the crowd, Anne Dyson felt that there must be something more that could be done. She also knew that she was in a position to be part of that something more. As president of the Dyson Foundation, she consulted with colleagues and experts around the United States, asking them all the same question: How can the foundation best use its resources to improve the stakes for children? She met with child advocates to discuss the possibility of launching a children's movement. She visited the AARP offices in Washington to explore setting up a membership organization for families. She considered creating extensive national programs to fight child abuse and teenage pregnancy. But always she came back to the same idea: the education of the pediatricians of the future. An education that would involve the community.

In her travels Anne Dyson had met a number of young people who took risks and defied the odds. She wanted to keep alive the spirit she saw in young medical students entering residency programs. What happened to crush their idealism? Where did the determination to make a difference fade into an acceptance of the status quo? Pediatric training programs do a great job of instilling competence and confidence in young physicians as they care for desperately ill neonates in the neonatal intensive care unit and for children with complex, multiorgan failure in the medical special care ward. How could pediatric training programs build that same sense of success and skill into the work of saving the lives of children threatened by poverty, hunger, violence, racism, and ethnic misunderstandings? Dyson decided to launch an initiative devoted to training the doctors of the future in community medicine and advocacy.

She gathered together pediatricians and educators to design an experiment in pediatric training. She would challenge medical schools and residency programs to prepare young physicians with the skills and attitudes they needed to take on the health concerns of the millennium and to lessen community health hazards. They would learn how to be effective advocates for their young patients and their families. They would not accept unfair community and societal conditions that bred poor health for children. They would use their talents and voices to improve conditions that promote the growth and development of children.

The novelty in Anne Dyson's idea of introducing advocacy into pediatric training was that most child health advocates of the past were physicians in the middle or latter parts of their careers. These experienced physicians came to advocacy because they were frustrated with the conditions that beat down children and families and because they wanted to devote time and energy to work toward change. Anne Dyson proposed to integrate advocacy into the fabric of pediatric preparation, to make it part of the breathing in and breathing out of everyone in the child health profession. Advocacy, she believed, should not be the responsibility of a few brave souls at the culmination of their careers. It should be the daily life's work of everyone who cares about children's health. That would be a sea change for pediatrics but one that she believed the field was prepared for. The young people were ready to dance. She would build them a dance floor.

Anne Dyson fought all her life against unfairness, only to suffer the ultimate unfairness in her own life. Shortly after she and the consultants at the New York Academy of Medicine had put the final touches on the request for proposal for the planned advocacy training initiative, she discovered that she had breast cancer. She lived for one year from the day the request for proposal was sent out in the mail to every medical school in the country. As the letters of intent and proposals poured back in to the foundation, she read each one with deep interest. She would even bring stacks of proposals with her to read during chemotherapy sessions. The idea of an advocacy training program had hit a nerve. Faculty members, deans, community leader, residents, and hospital administrators "got it." They could see the value of an organized approach to advocacy. They also understood there would be a benefit to young people in learning the culture, customs, mores, and resources of the communities where their patients lived. As she read the proposals, she knew that she had expressed concisely what was wrong with current training and was offering the mechanism for moving forward in the direction that many if not most residents were already poised to go.

Anne Dyson lived only long enough to welcome the first six residency sites in the Community Pediatrics Training Initiative.[70] With her mentor Fred Rogers and her great friend Bud Trillin, she encouraged the programs to be bold, to take risks, and to work hard to produce "a different kind of doctor."[71] Anne Dyson believed deeply in the ingenuity and creativity of individual people. She did not script what the sites should do or how they should do it. She trusted that each group would respond to local challenges. And they have. They have made strong partnerships with families and community-based organizations. They have improved the quality of the clinics and offices where they work. They have celebrated the rich cultural diversity and traditions among the patients they care for. They have identified barriers to care, documented health disparities, and uncovered impediments to health insurance coverage. They have devised interventions to address inequities; they have spoken up and spoken for. They have done all the things Anne Dyson knew they could do.

The child health advocates whose stories are told here have dealt with children in different parts of the country at different times in history, but they have had many similar experiences and held several observations in common. They recognized that the health of the children that they were responsible for depended on a complex array of factors including the community that the children lived in, the physical and emotional environment around the children, the exposures and risks that the children encounter in the course of everyday life, the assets and resources available to the children and their families. The advocates knew that keeping children healthy or alleviating the suffering imposed by chronic illness or disability meant nothing less than ensuring that health services were available and accessible, defining *health* broadly, and measuring accessibility in terms of not only language and culture but also structure.

The Current Status of   3
Child Health

WHEN LAUREN ELIZABETH MATTHEWS drew her first breath at 12:05 a.m. on January 1, 2000, she became a citizen of the wealthiest nation the world has ever known. She joined 71 million children and youth aged 0–18, representing a quarter of the total U.S. population.[1] By comparison, youth were more than 35 percent of the population in 1960 during the height of the baby boom.[2] Lauren's life expectancy is 80 years. Pete John San Nicholas, the first American boy born in the millennium, can expect to live 75 years. One hundred years ago, an infant girl could anticipate living only until age 48 and an infant boy until age 47.[3]

Changing Demographics

Lauren and Pete have become part of a wonderfully diverse and culturally rich country. As they grow and go to elementary and middle school, the children in their classes will be drawn from all races and ethnicities. Nationally, 58 percent of their age-mates will be white, 20 percent Hispanic, 15 percent black, and 7 percent other ethnicities.[4] As they make their way through school and on to college, they will have the chance to be friends and teammates with children who were born literally all over the world (figure 3.1).[5]

There is vast economic diversity as well. By contrast to the opportunity that racial and ethnic diversity affords, the huge income differentials among youth have created an ever-widening gap between those who have and those who do not have. Eighteen percent of the nation's children live in poverty, and that poverty is distributed unequally.[6] Thirty-four percent of black children and 30 percent of Hispanic children come from families whose total income is below poverty (less than $19,307 for a family of four).[7] In stark contrast, only 10 percent of white children are poor. At the other end of the income distribution, 29 percent of children live in families with incomes of more than $75,240 for a family of four, and 13 percent of young people enjoy very high annual incomes, of $112,860 or more for a family of four.[8]

Most American families reside in metropolitan areas: 30 percent in

Figure 3.1. Trends in U.S. Immigration, 1900–1990s

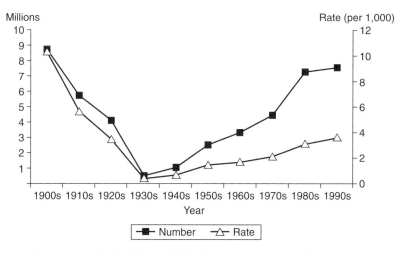

Source: U.S. Census Bureau. *Statistical Abstract of the United States: The National Data Book* (2000).

central cities and 50 percent in suburbs,[9] a profound change from 1900, when the majority of Americans lived in rural environments. In the first half of the twentieth century, families poured into the cities to search for employment; they made their homes in tightly knit, thickly settled neighborhoods. Since 1950 there has been a steady movement out of central cities, with a threefold decline in urban population density.[10] At the turn of the millennium, there seems to be a subtler population shift in the making. The original move out of the cities was typified by the flight of white affluent families. The exodus from inner cities now in- cludes families in general. Until a very short time ago, one could expect that poor children would be in inner-city and rural environments and wealthier children would live in suburban settings. In the early twenty- first century, many poor families with children are migrating into small towns and suburban areas.[11] States such as Nevada, Arizona, Colorado, Florida, and Georgia are also experiencing a high influx of families.[12]

Nearly 70 percent of American children live with two parents who are not necessarily their biologic mother and father.[13] Because of high rates of divorce,[14] many children move between households, often spending time in reconstituted families, bunking with their new stepbrothers and stepsisters. Twenty-six percent of white children, 33 percent of Hispanic children, and 61 percent of black children live in single-parent homes, mostly with their mother.[15] Children in single-parent Hispanic and black

Figure 3.2. Percentage of Children in Poverty by Family Type

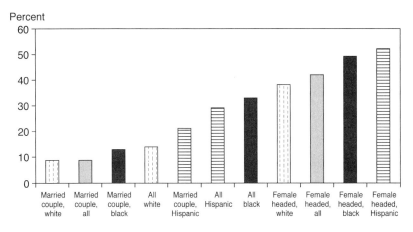

Percent

Source: ChildTrends Data Bank available at www.childtrendsdata.bank.org/pdf/4 (accessed October 1, 2005).

households are nearly five times as likely to be poor as children in two-parent white families (figure 3.2). Two newly emerging phenomena are father-only households and grandparents raising their grandchildren (1.5 million children are primarily cared for by grandparents).[16]

Some boys and girls live in single-child households, where the world revolves around them.[17] Other children share their living space with cousins and uncles and aunts in overcrowded apartments.[18] Some very unfortunate children do not have a home at all; they live in shelters, welfare motels, and even on the street. Each year, half a million youth are in the custody of the state in foster care arrangements.[19] Only 160,000 American children under 18 years of age are institutionalized, generally as a result of psychosocial difficulties, mental illness, or extremely severe disabilities.[20]

Access to technology is a major part of children's worlds: 99 percent of U.S. homes have a television set, and 66 percent have three or more.[21] Only 3 percent of American children live in families without a telephone; 48 percent of children and adolescents have access to the Internet at home.[22] The "neighborhood" that most American children live in is not bounded by Elm and Third. In fact, many children do not know their postman or the butcher at the Piggly-Wiggly. Their neighborhood includes the TV studios of Los Angeles and New York. They know the intimate details of the most recent relationship between nonactors on the show *The Real World*. They have seen in real time what real war is, and they are only a remote-control click away from the latest suicide bomber attack in the Middle East.

Americans spend a lot of time on the move, and their children come with them. Ninety-three percent of families have a car, van, or truck.[23] In their fast-paced lives, children move back and forth from before-school care, to school, to after-school care. They come into contact with adults who are their teachers, their bus drivers, their counselors, and their volunteer reading coaches. But many of those encounters are brief and largely uncoordinated with one another.

Children are less and less likely to experience the natural world in any but the most contrived fashion. They may watch an educational video on the Amazonian rain forest, but their direct encounters with the natural environment are becoming increasingly limited. Unless they are one of the 1–2 percent of children who live on a farm (or belong to 4H), they are unlikely to witness the birth of a lamb or spend time wandering in the woods, studying the habits of red squirrels. By the time they reach college age they will immediately and easily identify a thousand corporate logos but will be able to name no more than ten plants.[24]

Children and adolescents spend a large share of their time and energy in school. Unfortunately, the report card the educational establishment brings home each year is pretty disappointing.[25] Nationwide, only a third of public school 4th graders are at or above the proficient level in reading; in central city public schools, fully half of 4th grade students cannot read at the basic level. In large cities like Los Angeles, Chicago, and the District of Columbia, as many as two-thirds of the children are poor readers. Although there has been modest improvement in these rates in the early 2000s, there is a long way to go.

Thirteen percent of American students do not graduate from high school. The high school completion rate in 2003 was 92 percent for white youth, 85 percent for black youth, and 69 percent for Hispanic youth.[26] Such disparities play out in the life chances for the young people in the world of further education and employment.

The facts and figures that describe Lauren and Pete's world are now readily accessible to anyone with a questioning mind, a few hours to spare, and a computer with Internet access. The data form an increasingly valuable component of the knowledge base available to those who are interested in advocating for improvement in the health and well-being of children and youth. Let us now review what is known about

Table 3.1. Leading Causes of Death, by Age Group, 2000

Rank	< 1 year	1–4 years	5–14 years	15–24 years
1	Congenital anomalies	Unintentional injury	Unintentional injury	Unintentional injury
2	Short gestation and low birth rate	Congenital anomalies	Malignant neoplasms	Assault (homicide)
3	SIDS	Malignant neoplasms	Congenital anomalies	Suicide
4	Maternal complications	Assault (homicide)	Assault (homicide)	Malignant neoplasms
5	Placenta, cord, and membranes complications	Heart disease	Suicide	Heart disease
6	Respiratory distress	Influenza and pneumonia	Heart disease	Congenital anomalies
7	Unintentional injury	Septicemia	Chronic lower respiratory disease	Cerebrovascular diseases
8	Bacterial sepsis	Perinatal period	Benign neoplasms	Influenza and pneumonia

Source: Centers for Disease Control, table 7, Deaths and Death Rates for the 10 Leading Causes of Death in Specified Age Groups: United States, preliminary 2000, *National Vital Statistics Report,* 49 (2001): 25.

children's health status in general and then assess what impact socioeconomic, racial/ethnic, and health systems have on that status.

Causes of Child Death

Each year, the Centers for Disease Control in Atlanta report on the leading causes of death by age group. These mortality statistics keep a finger on the pulse of the nation's health. Table 3.1 shows the child and adolescent death report for the year 2000.

Under 1 Year

The infant mortality rate is a sensitive indicator of child and community health, reflecting the effectiveness of both the public and private health care sectors.[27] During the twentieth century, the U.S. infant mortality rate fell dramatically, from nearly 140 per thousand in 1900 to 7 per thousand in 2002.[28] Many factors contributed to the decline, including improved maternal and prenatal services, advances in obstetrics and neonatal intensive care, and improvements in standards of living (clean water, improved availability of nutritional foods, and so on).[29]

Questions about the effectiveness of the American system arise because, in international comparisons, the U.S. rate is twenty-seventh, just below that of Cuba.[30] Of greater concern, the rate for black Americans is

Figure 3.3. Infant Mortality by Race, 1940–2001

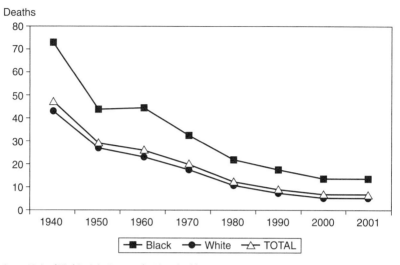

Source: *National Vital Statistics Reports,* vol. 52 (2003), table 31.
Note: Deaths under 1 year, per 1,000 births.

uncomfortably close to the rates for Barbados and Costa Rica, countries that spend half to two-thirds as much of their gross domestic product on health as the United States does.[31] Figure 3.3 shows the persistent black/white disparity in infant death rates.

The majority of infant deaths occur in the neonatal period, with much of the mortality related directly to birth complications from prematurity, low birth weight, respiratory distress syndrome, and high-risk pregnancies. Low birth weight is a problem in 7 percent of all births and 13 percent of births to black women.[32] In 2001 nearly a third of infant mortality could be attributed to birth-related issues. In addition, 5,513 infant deaths (20 percent) were the result of congenital anomalies. Sudden infant death syndrome (SIDS) accounted for 2,234 infant deaths (8%).[33]

Early Childhood

After the first year of life, mortality rates improve considerably. Infant mortality is measured as deaths per 1,000, whereas early childhood mortality is so infrequent that the figures are reported with denominators of 100,000. At the turn of the century the fear of life-threatening infectious diseases kept families and physicians on high alert at all times. Over the course of the twentieth century the advent of vaccines and the availability of antibiotics decreased the overall death rate and changed the shape of the mortality pattern. In 2000 injuries were the first cause of mortality among 1- to 5-year-olds.[34] Although injuries have always been a major hazard for little children, their prominence was not quite so apparent in the past, largely because other causes overshadowed them.

In the late 1980s and early 1990s, HIV infection was consistently one of the top ten causes of death for children aged 1–4.[35] That HIV/AIDS does not appear on the 2000 Centers for Disease Control chart as a cause of mortality for young children is a testament to the combined efforts of infectious disease investigators, academic health centers, public health agencies, the pharmaceutical industry, public policymakers, and hundreds of thousands of individual clinicians, community-based organizations, outreach workers, and families. HIV's absence from the list of childhood deaths is a direct result of this massive national collaborative effort, specifically the 076 prenatal AZT protocol, which prevents the transmission of HIV from mothers to infants.[36]

School-Age and Adolescence

School-age children experience the lowest levels of mortality of any age group. In 2000, 4.3 per 100,000 school-age children died in motor vehicle injuries, 0.9 per 100,000 in drowning accidents, and 0.9 per 100,000 as a result of firearm catastrophes.[37] The next most common cause of death among 5- to 14-year-olds was malignant neoplasms. While cancer rates for children under 20 years of age have been rising (a 16 percent increase from 1975 to 1995), death from cancer has shown a substantial 40 percent decrease over the same time period.[38] This change is due to the stunning improvements in oncology care and the availability and effectiveness of multidrug treatment. The five-year survival for children under 15 with acute lymphocytic leukemia has moved from 3–5 percent in 1964 to more than 85 percent in the late 1990s.[39]

During the adolescent and young adult years, the mortality rate pattern signals the perils that young people face. Teenagers must adapt to rapid biologic, environmental, and social change. As they create their own new world and try to mesh it with the competing expectations of their friends, family, and school, they take risks, try on new identities, and experiment with new life choices. Unfortunately, some of the risks they take are too great. Injuries account for nearly half of the deaths among 15- to 19-year-olds.[40] In 2002, automobile-related injuries accounted for half of these injury deaths. Homicide accounted for 14 percent of adolescent deaths and suicide for 11 percent. Nearly 5 percent were due to neoplasms and approximately 3 percent to diseases of the heart.

All is not bleak in teen health. In fact, the 28 percent decrease in teen deaths from 1990 to 2000 is cause for celebration. During just one decade the rate of deaths among 15- to 19-year-olds fell from 71 to 51 deaths per 100,000.[41] The vast majority of deaths among adolescents are from preventable causes, and this significant decline is a testament to the effectiveness of age-targeted interventions such as graduated licensing and substance abuse and violence prevention programs.[42]

Causes of Child Illness
Acute Illness

No child gets through the early years without his or her share of colds, tummy bugs, scrapes, cuts, and broken bones.[43] Miniepidemics of viral illness, streptococcal pharyngitis, and giardia are the norm in schools and day care centers. During the first five years of life, the average child will experience nearly thirty bouts of illness.[44] One in three children has at least one visit to the emergency room per year.[45] Antibiotics, vaccines, travel, and group experience affect the epidemiology of acute illness. The advent of vaccines has reduced the occurrence of many childhood illnesses. Table 3.2 shows the near elimination of certain diseases such as diphtheria, measles, rubella, and polio. Since the 1985 licensure of the HiB vaccine, cases of invasive disease due to hemophilus influenza Type B have decreased from 20,000 per year to fewer than 100 per year. The routine use of the pneumococcal vaccine has decreased the risk of sepsis and pneumonia.[46] The availability of powerful and effective antibiotics has improved the response to bacterial infections such as sepsis and meningitis.[47] Hospital stays for many common infectious diseases have decreased dramatically.[48]

Two acute childhood conditions, respiratory syncytial virus (RSV) and rotavirus infection currently account for a great deal of early childhood morbidity.[49] RSV is responsible for as many as 100,000 hospitalizations a year. It is estimated that 2–5 percent of patients hospitalized with RSV die annually. Rotavirus infection accounts for as many as 2.2 million annual infections and puts 55,000 children in the hospital each year. These two illnesses cause a tremendous number of missed day care, school, and work days. The molecular structure of both of these viruses is now well understood, and vaccines to prevent both illnesses are in the pipeline.[50]

Microbiologic agents evolve and emerge as pathogens without warn-

Table 3.2. Decrease in Nine Childhood Diseases by 1998 through Use of Vaccines

Disease	Baseline 20th-century annual morbidity	1998 provisional morbidity	Percent decrease
Smallpox	48,164[1]	0	100.0
Diphtheria	175,885[2]	1	100.0[3]
Pertussis	147,271[4]	6,279	95.7
Tetanus	1,314[5]	34	97.4
Polio (paralytic)	16,316[6]	0[7]	100.0
Measles	503,282[8]	89	100.0[3]
Mumps	152,209[9]	606	99.6
Rubella	47,745[10]	345	99.3
Congenital Rubella Syndrome	823[11]	5	99.4
Haemophilus influenzae type b	20,000[12]	54[13]	99.7

Source: Adapted from Impact of Vaccines Universally Recommended for Children, United States, 1990–1998, Morbidity and Mortality Weekly Report, April 2, 1999, pp. 243–48, available at www.cdc.gov/epo/mmwr/preview/ mmwrhtml/00056803.htm#00003753.htm (accessed October 13, 2005). See also www.childrensvaccine.org/html/ general_information.htm (accessed April 2, 2006).

Note: Baseline twentieth-century annual morbidity and 1998 provisional morbidity from nine diseases with vaccines recommended before 1990 for universal use in children (United States).

1. Average annual number of cases, 1900–1904.

2. Average annual number of reported cases, 1920–22, 3 years before vaccine development.

3. Rounded to nearest tenth.

4. Average annual number of reported cases, 1922–25, 4 years before vaccine development.

5. Estimated number of cases based on reported number of deaths, 1922–26, assuming a case fatality rate of 90%.

6. Average annual number of reported cases, 1951–54, 4 years before vaccine licensure.

7. Excludes one case of vaccine-associated polio reported in 1998.

8. Average annual number of reported cases, 1958–62, 5 years before vaccine licensure.

9. Number of reported cases in 1968, the year reporting began and the first year after vaccine licensure.

10. Average annual number of reported cases, 1966–68, 3 years before vaccine licensure.

11. Estimated number of cases based on seroprevalence data in the population and on the risk that women infected during a childbearing year would have a fetus with congenital rubella syndrome.

12. Estimated number of cases from population-based surveillance studies before vaccine licensure in 1985.

13. Excludes 71 cases of Haemophilus influenzae disease of unknown serotype.

ing and with varying levels of virulence. Experience with the AIDS epidemic demonstrates how life-threatening viral and bacterial agents can appear any time, anywhere, despite the best scientific understanding and available therapeutic responses. One of the biggest concerns regarding acute conditions is the emergence of bacteria that have developed resistance to everything in the powerful antibiotics armamentarium. Methicillin-resistant strains of staphylococcus aureas (MRSAs) are now isolated in hospital-acquired infections among infants, children, and youth.[51] Community-acquired MRSAs raise a new alarm.[52]

Organisms resistant to penicillin and its congeners are becoming more and more common in American communities.[53] Amoxicillin resistance among hemophilus influenza and strep pneumoniae has become a significant problem in many areas of the country. As a result, the national infectious disease experts have urged the "judicious" use of antibiotics.[54] Until the late 1990s pediatricians and nurse practitioners would treat children with even the earliest and mildest signs of otitis media (middle-ear infection) with antibiotics, despite the knowledge that 30–40 percent of such infections were caused by viruses, which do not respond to anti-microbial therapy. Because vaccinations protect most children from the most serious bacterial infections, watchful waiting in equivocal cases has been a reasonable replacement for the overtreatment caused by a low threshold for therapy. The campaign for the reduction of antibiotic use has led to a substantial decrease in both diagnosis and drug therapy for otitis media.[55]

The downside to the powerful effectiveness of immunizations is complacency. The absence of reminders of the serious threat that viruses and bacteria pose to children's health has led some parents to doubt the need for vaccines or antibiotics and to look to "natural cures" instead.[56] Several factors are driving this movement. There are legitimate concerns about unnatural additives in foods and medicines and the potential of these agents to cause harm. There is also some confusion about antibiotic resistance, with parents believing that it is their children rather than the bacteria that develop the resistance. Finally, some parents mistrust vaccines because of highly publicized, incorrect assertions that certain vaccines are associated with negative child health outcomes.[57] The unfortunate consequence is a group of parents who are now choosing not to immunize their children, placing their own and other youngsters at risk for diseases that, because of immunization, have come under some level of control.

Globalization has a continuously unfolding effect on infectious disease patterns and potential microbiologic exposures. One of these effects is certainly the need for biopreparedness in the wake of the 9/11 attacks and the realization that microbiologic agents have the potential for death, illness, and massive disruption.[58] Preparedness scenarios have to take into account the fact that young children are often in group care and away from home, that exposed children need to be isolated, that families need to be contacted, and that children unable to return home must be cared for. The ease of travel is another effect of globalization, with its possibility of child travelers encountering hepatitis A, cholera, and malaria.[59]

Chronic Illness

Every year, the Centers for Disease Control conduct a national telephone survey to monitor the U.S. immunization program. In 2001 the Maternal and Child Health Bureau arranged to add a special set of questions to the State and Local Area Integrated Telephone Survey to determine the number of American children with special health care needs. The bureau's definition of children with special health care needs is "children who have or are at risk for chronic physical, developmental, behavioral or emotional conditions and who also require health and related services of a type or amount beyond that required by children generally."[60] The survey indicates that 9.3 million American children (13 percent) meet this definition.[61] A variety of factors contribute to the existence of so large a group, especially cohort survivorship, epidemics, developmental and behavioral conditions, and the multigenerational perpetuation of disease and disability.

Cohort Survivorship

Advanced medical and surgical technologies have greatly improved the life chances of children with conditions such as heart disease, cystic fibrosis, sickle cell anemia, various cancers, and congenital anomalies.[62] For example, the mean age of death for children with cystic fibrosis was 6 months in 1960; in 1998 it was 32 years. Conditions considered incompatible with life a quarter century ago (such as hypoplastic left heart syndrome) are now regularly treated in state-of-the-art academic centers and have high survival rates. For some serious conditions, definitive treatments cure the children completely with no need for ongoing medication or therapy. More commonly, though, there is not a cure. Many children depend on medication or medical procedures (such as gastrostomy feeding or the use of oxygen) for their survival and function.[63] Once these medication regimens and procedures become routine, most children are able to live fairly normal lives. For some less fortunate youngsters, life is filled with ups and downs, good days and bad ones, and the price they and their parents pay for survival is high.[64]

Children with complex medical conditions present significant challenges both to medical care facilities and to the community as a whole. They have a close interaction with the medical care system because their very survival often depends on the availability of state-of-the-art medical care, highly specialized equipment, newly licensed or experimental medications, and such extraordinary measures as extracorporeal membrane oxygenation and bone marrow or organ transplantation. Hospitals who care for such children are experiencing sharp rises in the severity of illness in their case mix.[65] This is coming in the face of increasing costs and the introduction of the eighty-hour workweek for resident physicians. The complexity and chronic nature of health conditions among hospitalized children has catalyzed the creation of new systems of care. Physicians, nurses, pharmacists, and others now practice in teams. Because the stakes for these children are so high when they are in the hospital, inpatient teams generally use highly protocolized treatment plans (called clinical practice guidelines, or CPGs) to guarantee the highest standard of quality and to prevent systems-level errors.[66]

Children with chronic conditions can, in general, participate fully in community life. If families, health care providers, and service agencies plan ahead using an individualized health plan (IHP), children can attend school safely and productively. The community inclusion movement questions the long-held beliefs that people with disabilities are best served in segregated, specialized institutional settings. By definition, community placement of children with complex conditions depends on a larger group of people having in-depth understanding of the underlying conditions, emergency responsiveness, and general care of people with disabilities.[67]

Cohort survivorship has meant that clinicians and scientists have had the opportunity to follow the natural course of many chronic conditions to new levels. For instance, as children with cystic fibrosis are living into adulthood, the extent of their endocrine involvement of the pancreas with full-blown diabetes is becoming more manifest.[68] The early onset of Alzheimer's disease in Down syndrome patients has provided new insights into the aging process as well as some hints about the location of the Alzheimer genes.[69] The longer survival of young people with HIV disease has uncovered a variety of protective immunologic mechanisms.[70]

Youth who have been treated successfully for cancer show up disproportionately on the rosters of oncology clinics because of recurrent complications or because they confront new and different cancer growths.[71] Children may sustain organ failure secondary to cancer treatment, since many of the drugs are toxic to the liver, kidney, heart, and lungs. In the case of many survivors, the experience of a second cancer opens a window for research into the basic mechanisms of vulnerability to neoplastic illness. In some situations, the tumor may be the regrettable but unavoidable consequence of the previous cancer treatment regimen. Just when a family learns to cope with the basic illness, their child may be hit with a serious secondary problem. Some families sound as if they have attended medical school, because they learn from their child's course the pathophysiology of nearly every organ system as well as the side effects of the majority of the drugs in the pediatric pharmacopoeia.

Facing each of these problems is hard for even the most emotionally intact individuals and families and can cause mental health and behavioral breakdown. In situations where there are additional emotional risks, the presence of chronic illness may seriously compound the problem.[72] The siblings of children with chronic illness may also be susceptible to the emotional consequences.[73]

Epidemics

In 1980 HIV/AIDS hit the United States as it did many other nations. While many decried the U.S. response to the crisis as too slow,[74] the multipronged, team-level response demonstrated the capacity of the medical care system, public health, drug companies, and families to collaborate. The inverted U shape of figure 3.4 documents the stages of the epidemic among babies: increasing incidence until the early 1990s and then a slow decrease.[75] New evidence suggests that the HIV agent was probably in the environment as early as 1968 and did not emerge fully until the early in the 1980s.[76] The virus made a substantial attack on certain vulnerable populations: infants born to women engaging in drug use or prostitution were at high risk of becoming infected with HIV through vertical transmission from mother to baby during the perinatal period. Once an effective drug intervention (maternal AZT) was discovered, an all-out effort led to the dramatic reduction in HIV rates.[77] The babies born during the height of the HIV epidemic reached school age and adolescence in 2000. They are a small and unique segment of the population of children with chronic illness and depend on complex drug regimens for their survival. They experience developmental delay and school-related difficulty.[78] The social acceptance of people with HIV is increasing, yet these children are still stigmatized, and many families elect not to tell their children their diagnosis in order to protect them from the psychological impact.

Preventive efforts have tremendously reduced the incidence of new perinatal cases of HIV, and the United States has avoided the sharp rise in these cases that demographers and statisticians predicted early in the epidemic. Nonetheless, there continue to be young new recruits into the ranks of the infected, though from a different cohort: adolescent and adult young women ages 15–24. Initially, HIV was rarely seen in women,

Figure 3.4. Incidence of Perinatally Acquired AIDS, 1985–2000

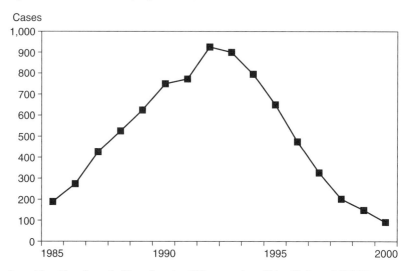

Cases

Source: Adapted from Centers for Disease Control, available at www.cdc.gov/hiv/graphics/images/L207/L207.ppt (accessed 10/11/2005).

and heterosexual spread was uncommon. In 2000, however, 47 percent of cases of HIV in 15- to 24-year-olds were female. Heterosexual contact and intravenous drug use caused the majority of these cases. These disturbing facts make it clear that the epidemic is wreaking havoc especially among young women of color.[79]

Several new chronic disease epidemics have recently caught the public's attention (see figure 3.5). Each of these conditions has substantial physical and functional impact as well as the predisposition to serious adult consequences.

Asthma. Nationally, asthma rates for those under 18 years of age have risen from 4 percent in 1982 to 6 percent in 1996.[80] Worldwide, the reasons behind this dramatic increase remain a mystery. Because asthma affects children in cities disproportionately, contenders for the cause are overcrowding, air quality, smoking, stress, and environmental triggers in the homes.[81] Despite new asthma drugs and treatments, morbidity and mortality from asthma are still unacceptably high for children and youth. Interns and residents speak of some children with asthma as "frequent fliers" because they are seen so often in the emergency room and admitted so many times to the hospital. In 1993 there were nearly 200,000 hospital admissions for asthma in people under age 25.[82] Children with

Figure 3.5. Prevalence of Child and Adolescent Health Conditions, Early 1980s and Mid-1990s

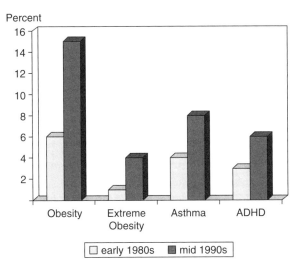

Source: James Perrin, Armstrong Award Lecture, 2004, with permission

asthma in the United States miss an estimated 10 million days of school per year.[83]

Obesity. Acknowledgment of the epidemic of childhood obesity came in the last years of the twentieth century, when the national growth charts for children and adolescents were being reissued. The charts were revised to reflect the heights and weights of the racially and ethnically diverse population of children in the United States.[84] The standards developed in the 1920s and 1930s using growth parameters of boys and girls living in Iowa or those developed by Stuart in the 1930s on Euro-American children in Boston were no longer representative. The new data gave unequivocal evidence of a general average increase in height and weight at every age as well as a growing number of children and adolescents who met the criteria for obesity. Monitoring by the Centers for Disease Control reveals an entire nation trending toward overweight. In 1991, no states reported adult obesity in more than 19 percent of their population, whereas in 2002 a rate of 15–19 percent obesity was reported by twenty states, twenty-nine reported 20–24 percent obesity, and one state a more than 25 percent obesity rate.[85] Among children, the increases are equally startling. In 1971–74, 4 percent of children ages 6–11 were considered overweight, whereas a 1999–2000 study reported that a full 15 percent of children in that age group were overweight—more than a tripling in the twenty-five-year period.[86]

Childhood obesity sets young people up for particularly pernicious physical and psychological ill effects. Children who are overweight are teased. They are excluded. When other children poke fun at them, adults often titter in tacit approval rather than reprimand the jokesters. Academic and job performance are affected by obesity, at least in part through the impact on self-esteem.[87] The long-term health consequences of childhood and adolescent obesity are staggering.[88] Children who are overweight have a significantly increased chance of developing Type 2 diabetes. It is predicted that if the current trends continue, a third of children in the United States will be diagnosed with Type 2 diabetes by the time they are adults.[89]

Diabetes. Type 2 diabetes used to be considered "adult onset," but the disease is no longer confined to adulthood. Although the numbers are not yet solid, it is clear that there is a precipitous rise in the number of childhood cases, likely as a consequence of the obesity epidemic. Type 2 diabetes does not respond to insulin but rather to diet. The behavioral and lifestyle changes that are recommended for obesity are also appropriate to treat this disease.

Developmental and Behavioral Conditions

Since 1975 the U.S. Department of Education has been keeping statistical tabs on educationally relevant disabilities in order to monitor and manage the Individuals with Disabilities Education Act (IDEA). Estimates from IDEA are that in 1999–2000 nearly 5.5 million children and youth ages 6–17 had disabilities that required special educational intervention. This is 11.4 percent of the estimated enrolled school population for these ages. Another 284,000 young adults ages 18–21 were also served through the special education program. The distribution of the children in special education was 2.9 million children and adolescents (50.5 percent) with learning disabilities, 1.1 million (19.2 percent) with speech or language problems, 614,000 (10.8 percent) with mental retardation, and 470,000 (8.3 percent) with serious emotional disorders. The other 12 percent are categorized as having hearing, vision, orthopedic conditions, autism, or developmental delay.[90]

Other developmental/behavioral disorders have been taking on particular prominence in the past two or three decades, especially autism and attention deficit hyperactivity disorder (ADHD). Controversy abounds about why (or even if) the incidence of these two conditions is increasing. Are there new toxic exposures? Have nutritional or lifestyle alterations caused the abrupt surge in the worldwide number of cases of autism? Is the epidemic of ADHD real? Or is there an epidemic of overidentification? In addition to these are problems such as mental health, substance abuse, and risky sexual behaviors.

Autism. The autism spectrum disorders (ASD) are serious conditions that affect children's ability to communicate with others both through language and through conventional social interaction.[91] Current estimates are that 4–6 per 1,000 children meet criteria for ASD. Both international and national studies document increases in the diagnosis of autism and pervasive developmental delay over the past twenty-five years, with some estimates as great as a tenfold increase.[92] Although there is some concern that this change may signal new environmental health hazards, no specific agent has been identified. Most specifically, no causal relationship has been documented between immunization for measles-mumps-rubella and the incidence of autism, despite a large-scale media campaign promoting this unproven theory.[93] At least part of the explanation for increased numbers of children with autism is better identification and diagnostic precision, especially after the 1994 revision of the *Diagnostic and Statistical Manual.*[94]

ADHD. Attention deficit hyperactivity disorder is a functional condition that affects children's ability to concentrate on meaningful tasks. Children with ADHD are inattentive, impulsive, distractible, and perseverative. They can be fidgety and overly active, and they often invade the space of other people without thoroughly appreciating the impact that their activity has on others. Children with ADHD often are in a hypersensitive state, where any outside stimulation is noxious to them. They sometimes cannot screen out irrelevant information and sensory detail. Children with full-blown ADD or ADHD can be severely compromised in their day-to-day abilities and functioning. Making the diagnosis of ADHD requires a careful assessment and confirmation that the child's symptoms occur in at least two settings (usually home and school). Since there is no human being alive who does not on occasion manifest one or another of the ADHD symptoms, it is easy to understand how the possibility of an ADHD diagnosis can be raised at one time or another for many children. In 2000, with estimates for the prevalence of ADHD ranging from 4 to 12 percent, the American Academy of Pediatrics promulgated guidelines to improve the rigor and consistency of diagnosis.[95]

Mental health disorders. Mental health disorders among children and youth are seriously disabling, resulting in increasing rates of emergency room visits and hospitalizations each year. The use of psychotropic drugs rose by 5 percent from 1997 to 2000.[96] Life-threatening disorders such as suicidal depression and severe anorexia nervosa are beginning at earlier and earlier ages.[97] One manifestation of the increase in mental health disorders has been an upward trend in the number of prescriptions for psychotropic drugs for children and youth. It is estimated that by the time a cohort of young people has graduated from high school one quarter of them will have been regularly taking a medication for a psychiatric condition at some point in their life.[98] In many regions of the country these mental health problems are causing considerable concern because there are not enough facilities and trained professionals to care for these children and youth.

Substance abuse. The 2003 Youth Risk Behavior Surveillance Systems report on high school students indicates high involvement with intoxicating substances among this age group.[99] Almost half of the teenagers drank alcohol during the past month, with 30 percent reporting that they engaged in episodic heavy drinking within the past month. A fifth of the students had used marijuana in the past month, nearly a tenth had "ever" used cocaine, and 12 percent had ever sniffed or inhaled intoxicating substances. This extensive drug use places many of these young people at risk for long-term dependence or addiction. In the short term, the dangers of drinking and driving are paramount, as are the increases in violence and promiscuous sexual behavior with intoxication.

Smoking is a prime contributor to cardiovascular and pulmonary ill health in adulthood, and people who begin smoking at or before the age of 15 have double the chance of dying from lung cancer than do people who begin smoking later in life.[100] Cigarette smoking begins for many people in the middle childhood and adolescent years. According to the 2003 report, 58 percent of high school students ever smoked cigarettes, 22 percent smoked cigarettes during the past month, with 10 percent smoking on twenty or more days of the past month. Favorable trend data indicate a decline in smoking among teenagers that began in 1996.[101]

Asset data are now being linked with information on health habits. The 2001 National Household Survey on Drug Abuse Report: Academic Performance and Youth Substance Use documents that young people ages 12–17 who had positive school experiences and found their schoolwork meaningful were less likely to use substances than students who viewed their educational experience negatively.[102] Investigators who study spirituality have found that young people who believe in forgiveness (for themselves and for others) are less likely to abuse drugs and alcohol than young people for whom the spiritual dimension is less prominent in their lives.[103]

Sexual behaviors. Youth sexual behavior is generally measured by assessing the age at first intercourse, birth control and condom use, teen pregnancy rates, and annual numbers of abortions. The Youth Risk Behavior Surveillance Systems report for 2001 indicates that 46 percent of high school students had ever had sexual intercourse. Among the 33 percent of students who had had intercourse in the past three months, 58 percent used condoms, but only 18 percent used birth control pills.[104] In 2001 the birth rate among 10- to 14-year-old mothers was 0.8 live births per 1,000 girls of this age; among 15- to 17-year-old mothers, the rate was 25.3; and among 18- to 19-year-olds, the rate was 75.8.[105] Girls under 18 years of age are much less likely to receive prenatal care in the first trimester than pregnant women in general (approximately 60 percent versus 80 percent).[106] Although the birth rate for young adolescents remains unacceptably high, with the U.S. rate at twice that of England and nine times that of the Netherlands and Japan, the good news is an appreciable and steady decrease in teen births over the past decade. Moreover, this decline appears related to better preventive intervention among teens, since the decrease in teen births has been paralleled by a significant decline in the number of abortions over the same period.[107]

Trends in the occurrence of sexually transmitted diseases reflect some aspects of teen sexual behavior. The 2000 rates of gonorrhea and chlamydia among 15- to 19-year-olds were 516 and 1,373 per 100,000, respectively. While far less common, cases of syphilis among adolescents are also reported routinely to state public health facilities.[108] As mentioned above, of greatest concern is the continued small but steady number of teenagers, both male and female, who are acquiring HIV infection. The distribution of AIDS cases has changed markedly since the beginning of the epidemic. The finding that 57 percent of the 13- to 19-year-olds with HIV infection were girls challenges the health care system to reassess practice with regard to prevention of sexually transmitted diseases.[109]

Multigenerational Cycle

Children with serious chronic conditions can now survive into adulthood and become parents, sometimes with an ensuing multigenerational cycle of illness. Their children may be at risk for the same disease, or the children may develop health problems as a result of the therapy their parent received. Women with "childhood onset" (Type 1) diabetes have a high rate of obstetrical complications and fetal loss and four times the rate of congenital anomalies.[110] Infants of diabetic mothers are often premature and suffer from serious lung disorders. The babies are physically large at birth, because their mothers' hypoinsulin state has left them bathed in a high sugar load. These newborns can be very hard to manage because of hypoglycemia and respiratory distress. As growing children, they are at increased risk of developing insulin-dependent diabetes.[111]

Success with metabolic screening has contributed a new level of complexity to the chronic illness picture. Whereas children with diseases such as phenylketonuria (PKU) used to die very early on or end up in institutional care because of severe retardation, adherence to a phenylalanine-free diet has changed the morbidity and mortality of the disease. The current concern is with "maternal PKU." When treated female children get to childbearing age, the cycle begins again.[112] Women with PKU must keep strictly to their diet so that their infants are not compromised. Because of careful monitoring and high levels of medical and nutritional input, children of mothers with PKU now rarely suffer complications from the condition. They, of course, must be put on the same elimination diet as their mothers.

It remains too early to predict the courses for children born to other cohorts of survivors, but there is every reason to expect that young people with various forms of chronic illness will be among the parents of the next generation. This means that obstetricians will be delivering babies of mothers with conditions that never before saw the inside of a labor and delivery suite. Gynecologists and internists will be caring for a new generation of people who have already endured many disease experiences.[113]

Disparities in Health and Health Care

Where a child lives, how much his parents make, and what his skin color is all have profound and additive effects on health and well-being. Acknowledgment of these effects and the disparities in health outcomes has taken some time in coming but is now a central element of public health surveillance and is beginning to be factored into clinical medicine.

At least three intertwined factors account for child health outcomes: (1) the child's basic biologic and genetic predisposition and vulnerabilities, (2) environmental exposures, and (3) the resources and responses of the health care system. Serious inequalities in the health care delivered to different subgroups of children are the subject of much recent scrutiny.[114] For some children and some conditions, these inequalities in care literally tip the scale, resulting in measurable differences in health outcomes. New large data sets—meticulously collected by geographic, socioeconomic, racial, and linguistic characteristics—demonstrate just how important these relationships are.

Geography and Health

Geography plays a considerable role in child health. Children who live in certain locations are more prone to particular health risks than children with the same characteristics who live in other areas. Children in California are at higher risk of earthquakes. Youth in the Gulf states may suffer from floods and hurricanes. Health conditions also vary by location. Worldwide studies show a twentyfold variation in asthma prevalence (from 1.6 percent to 36 percent) depending on geographic location.[115] Immigrant children who never wheezed in their native country may respond to environmental triggers in their new home by developing full-blown asthma. This experience has been documented for children from India and Malaysia who have moved to England and Australia, generally into more urbanized environments.[116] There is still controversy over what it is about the urban environment that predisposes a city child to illness, but asthma is an immunological disorder, and a variety of environmental agents—including air pollutants, cockroach antigen, and animal dander—have been implicated as the most likely suspects.[117]

Urban areas present increased risk for other child health problems as well. Childhood injury registers record a much higher rate of fatal falls for children living in urban areas (with high-rise apartment buildings) than for those living in suburbs and rural areas.[118] Moreover, lead poisoning is much more common in children living in central cities because much of the housing stock is old. Houses built before 1958 are far more likely to have been painted with lead-containing paint than those built after the paint companies voluntarily began to make lead-free paint. The 1978 federal ban on lead in paint ensured that newer houses would be far safer for children. Older houses may also be in poor repair, with peeling paint and plaster exposed to the exploring fingers and lips of toddling 1- to 2-year-olds.[119]

While life in the city elevates the risk for some conditions, suburban and rural environments present health hazards as well. Children living in the southern climates, where family and neighborhood swimming pools are common, are more likely than children in other parts of the country to drown or be injured in a pool accident.[120] Farm life brings with it many health benefits, like good nutrition and outdoor exercise, but the lifestyle of rural areas brings its own concerns. Each year 100,000 children are the victims of injuries related to farm equipment.[121] In addition, isolation, boredom, and alienation have been suggested as antecedents of drug and alcohol use in rural youth.[122]

Infectious agents tend to cluster in specific geographic areas and then to spread to other areas via a variety of carriers. A good example is Lyme disease, which causes an acute infection often accompanied by chronic arthritis.[123] Initially, in the 1970s, the disease was confined to the small Connecticut town that gave it its name. With time, the tick, *Ixodes* dammin, the white-footed mouse, and the white-tailed deer that harbor *Borrelia burgdorferi* have shared the infectious agent with their neighbors, and they with theirs. Following the route of disease spread, epidemiologists can almost trace the path of one of the white-footed mouse families. Geography also played a defining role in the spread of AIDS. The HIV epidemic in the United States started on the coasts and did not make its appearance in Midwest cities like Chicago for several years.[124] The SARS experience of 2002–3 demonstrates the effectiveness of quarantining to contain an outbreak.[125] Because families are so globally mobile, it is critical for physicians to find out where children and families are from in order to screen properly for conditions such as tuberculosis and malaria, which though exceedingly rare in the United States remain endemic in many parts of the world.[126] Geography is also a factor in terms of resistant organisms. Because the bacteria in Georgia no longer respond to antibiotics as they once did, physicians practicing in Atlanta need to use substantially higher doses of amoxicillin than their colleagues in Rochester, New York, or Santa Clara, California, to treat the same type of ear infection.[127]

Getting the "lay of the land" in physical, geographic terms aids community leaders, program planners, and policymakers in understanding the distribution of child health concerns. There is nothing like a neighborhood walking or mapping exercise to identify local conditions and to target resources. One of the most effective public health tools available is geographic information software (GIS).[128] This tool allows a block-by-block look at the distribution of health parameters. Using tools like GIS

Figure 3.6. Kids Count map

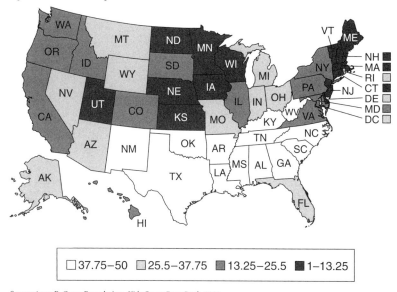

| □ 37.75–50 | □ 25.5–37.75 | ■ 13.25–25.5 | ■ 1–13.25 |

Source: Anne E. Casey Foundation, *Kids Count Data Book, 2004.*
Note: Higher scores indicate poorer health.

and the neighborhood walk allowed groups such as the Harlem Children's Zone to pinpoint areas of the highest prevalence of asthma for targeting neighborhood cleanups.[129] In 1996 a careful geographic look at suicide deaths in the city of Boston identified a series of copycat suicides in a few-block radius in South Boston, stimulating a wide community response.[130]

Figure 3.6, a map of the United States, shows how each state scores on ten child health indicators:

- Percent low-birth-weight babies
- Infant mortality rate (deaths per 1,000 live births)
- Child death rate (deaths per 100,000 children ages 1–14)
- Rate of teen deaths by accident, homicide, and suicide (deaths per 100,000 teens ages 15–19)
- Teen birth rate (births per 1,000 females ages 15–17)
- Percent of teens who are high school dropouts (ages 16–19)
- Percent of teens not attending school and not working (ages 16–19)
- Percent of children living in families where no parent has full-time, year-round employment
- Percent of children in poverty (data reflect poverty in the previous year)
- Percent of families with children headed by a single parent

It appears that children in the southern United States fare worse than children in other regions. The nature of the physical environment contributes to this distribution of health outcomes, but so do many other factors. These include the wealth of the state, the resources available, and the child-centeredness of the state's public policy. Other factors include cultural norms, the socioeconomic circumstances of the families, and the racial and ethnic characteristics of the children.

Health care practice varies by state as well. In some states, there are relatively generous levels of both public and private health insurance, and health services are readily available. In others, medical resources are limited, and it is a Herculean task for families to find and access the financial support required to use them. There are also variations due to less systematically varying factors. In some states, though there is perfectly adequate health insurance coverage and physicians can make a good living, exorbitant malpractice insurance rates drive them to live and practice in another state. Finally, practice patterns vary by state. Using Jack W. Wennberg's methodology, James Perrin and Charles Homer demonstrate that the state you live in determines the chance that you will have an appendectomy or be admitted to the hospital for asthma or other common pediatric problems.[131] Care is driven by custom, and custom apparently recognizes state borders.

Family Income and Health

At the most fundamental level, poverty sets children up for ill health. Families with marginal incomes often must struggle to fulfill their children's most basic needs. While it is rare in the United States to encounter frank starvation among children, there are many families who regularly go without food. In 1996, 15 percent of the parents of children in poverty reported that "sometimes or often" there was "not enough to eat" in their household. Over three-quarters of very low-income renters live in housing with problems, and nearly one-third report that these problems are severe. Poor children live in apartments with inadequately vented room heaters, faulty plumbing, water leakage, open cracks and holes, peeling plaster and paint, and rats.[132]

Douglas Nelson, the president of the Annie E. Casey Foundation, begins the 2003 *Kids Count* report with an eloquent essay on how expensive it is for families to be poor. Everything they do actually costs more than similar activities for people of means. Going to work costs more; child care costs more. The time and energy that go into just subsisting leaves little left over to attend to the needs of children. Nelson says, "Low-income families are commonly one crisis away from economic catastrophe. Even in the best of times, they can't leverage their earnings into real, lasting prosperity for themselves and their kids. Lack of assets means entrenched, intergenerational poverty for millions of Americans, no matter how hard they work."[133]

Poor infants may not get off to a good start. Poor pregnant women often cannot afford to eat well, may not have access to timely prenatal care, and may be at increased risk of prenatal infections (sexually transmitted diseases or urinary tract infections).[134] While substance abuse and domestic violence spare no socioeconomic group, poor women are at higher risk than other women for both of these.[135] As a result of all these factors, the rate of low birth weight among the infants of poor women is 1.7 times as high as that for the infants of nonpoor women.[136]

According to parents' reports, 62 percent of poor children have excellent or very good health, versus 90 percent of children from nonpoor families.[137] Activity limitation for children aged 5–17 with chronic conditions is reported for 10 percent of poor children, compared with 7 percent of nonpoor children.[138] In 2003 completed immunizations (4:3:1:3) stood at 76 percent for children in poverty and 83 percent for those above poverty.[139] Barbara Starfield and Paul Newacheck documented the size and direction of the disparities in health for poor/nonpoor children. Conditions such as teen birth, lead poisoning, and rheumatic fever are three times higher among poor children than among nonpoor children; child deaths are three to four times higher.[140]

Even though many of the disparities in health outcomes can be accounted for by the high risks of poverty, there are also differences in the kind of health care that poor children receive. Compared to nonpoor children, poor children are five times as likely to be uninsured, are four times as likely not to have a usual source of care, have five times as many unmet health needs, and have nearly four times as many unmet dental needs.[141] They rely on safety net services such as emergency rooms and clinics, or they forgo care altogether because of an inability to pay. Major efforts have gone into trying to improve the insurance coverage for poor and near-poor children, but despite this hard work, as of 2002, 8.5 million U.S. children (11%) were without health insurance; the vast majority of these children were poor or nonpoor.[142] The health insurance picture for children reflects just how vulnerable poor children are. As states face fiscal belt-tightening, child health benefits are often the first to go. When states face economic uncertainty, they impose restrictions on health insurance through requiring health insurance premiums and copayments from the families of children in poverty, creating an insurmountable barrier for many parents.

Sara Rosenbaum argues that even if the financial access problem were solved, poor families would still face the problems of "cost, poor services in poor communities, cultural and communication barriers, fear of the health system, and general overall problems in the relationships between patients and providers."[143] Just getting to the doctor is an enormous burden for many families in poverty. A 2003 survey at Children's Hospital in Boston showed that families had to take two or three buses on average to get to the clinic.[144] Then there is the very real problem of areas without any health care facilities. For instance, in isolated, poor rural communities, the pediatrician-to-child ratio may be as low as 1 to 5,555, despite a national ratio of 1 to 2,057.[145]

Affluence may also affect children's health. When parents bring home a combined annual salary of $400,000, the money still may not buffer their daughters and sons from ill health. Several child and adolescent health problems are actually more prevalent among wealthier families. Otitis media, for example, is diagnosed more frequently in children of high socioeconomic status.[146] Acute lymphocyte leukemia is also more likely to be diagnosed in these children. One postulated explanation is that later exposure to infections may be a risk factor.[147] Automobile crashes are the leading cause of death among 16- to 19-year-olds. Nonpoor adolescents are more likely to die as a driver or passenger in a car accident than are poor teenagers.[148] Their greater access to high-risk and extreme sports such as rock climbing, skiing, horseback riding, and boating also puts affluent children more at risk for fatal or life-altering catastrophes.[149] Nor do serious mental health disorders spare the children of the well-to-do. In fact, for some young people, it is their privileged position that puts them at risk of mental health concerns. High-achieving families often are unaware of the stress that their success places on their children, who internalize what they consider to be parental expectations. The escalating rates of mental symptoms on college campuses are attributed in part to such expectations: to be competitive, to get ahead, to win.[150]

The greater prevalence of some conditions among wealthier children and youth may be more a reflection of how often these families seek care than of the actual occurrence of the disorder. The classic example is eating disorders, anorexia and bulimia. When the average person thinks of these problems, the picture that immediately comes to mind is an anxious, overly thin, high-achieving girl living in the suburbs and stressing over Ivy League college admissions. Population-based studies, however, show that eating disorders occur throughout the socioeconomic spectrum and that children in poorer families simply do not get as much attention paid to their problems.[151]

Race/Ethnicity and Health

For years there has been a controversy about whether or not to use racial categories for assessing demographic and health risk. In part, statisticians and epidemiologists have been stymied by serious technical and ethical concerns. It has not been clear what *black* means. If someone has dark skin but traces his ancestry to the Caribbean and not to Africa is she African American? Should the term *African American* be used for a new citizen from Egypt or a white-skinned immigrant from South Africa or Zimbabwe? Are families who speak Portuguese Hispanic? What about people from Spain? Why are they in a different category from people from France or Italy? What are the "racial" similarities between people of Chinese and Vietnamese descent? In Asia demographers and ethnographers make many distinctions, but our census accommodates only the category *Asian/Pacific Islander.*

In the 1970s and 1980s the prevailing wisdom was that putting people in racial and ethnic pigeonholes was potentially harmful. Scholars and policymakers worried that rigid categorization could compound bias, stigma, and profiling. By the early 2000s the wind changed. Gradually, there has been a general recognition that it is not the census that delimits the life chances of various groups; it is the societal structure itself. Accepting the limitations of the methodology and the fact that the tools are not perfect, scientists and policymakers have started describing social and health data not only by income level but also by race and ethnicity to expose disparities for closer scrutiny. Even with the limitations of the methods, the health findings by race and ethnicity are so stark and so disturbing that there is now a national outcry and the beginnings of some action. Table 3.3 presents the breakdown of various health conditions by race and ethnicity, comparing the relative risk of a black or Hispanic individual having a particular condition to the chance of a white person of the same age having the same condition. The use of relative risks and odds ratios allows a quick look at the most obvious outcomes. For each disparity areas, an in-depth analysis—compounding variables and comorbidities—is in order.

Disparities

The infant mortality rate is made up of two components: neonatal (birth to 1 month) and postneonatal (1 month to 1 year). Two-thirds of infant deaths occur in the neonatal period and are primarily the result of perinatal problems (prematurity or low birth weight, congenital anomalies, obstetric complications, intrauterine or birth infections). Black children are at higher risk of neonatal mortality because of a significantly higher proportion of children with low birth weight. Black children also die at higher rates from postneonatal conditions such as SIDS.[152] The black-white disparity in infant mortality has been tracked since the 1940 census, showing a significant improvement in infant mortality rates for both blacks and whites. But the consistent gap suggests that there are still factors that physicians and policymakers are missing.[153]

Somewhat surprisingly, most children of Hispanic backgrounds are not at increased risk of infant mortality. The so-called healthy immigrant effect may hold secrets about essential factors for nurturing healthy pregnancies even in the face of poverty.[154] One explanation for the protective immigrant effect is that the traditional basic nutrition of immigrant families is better suited to fetal development than the American diet of highly processed, fatty, and fried foods. Unfortunately, many studies show that the more acculturated young women become, the more the immigrant protection wears off.[155] In an effort to become more "American," some young people reject the best of their own culture and adopt the worst of the U.S. culture, including cigarettes, alcohol, and drugs. In these situations, the children of the second generation actually have poorer health than those in the first generation. Another problem with looking at Hispanics as a category is that this large and heterogeneous group includes people from the Caribbean, Mexico, Central America, and people of Spanish heritage who have Hispanic surnames but who have lived in the United States for generations. Fine-grained analysis of morbidity and mortality patterns demonstrates disparities among these groups.[156]

As seen in table 3.3, there is considerable racial and ethnic variation in teen pregnancy rates. Compared to white teenagers, Hispanic teens are twice as likely to have a baby and black teens are one and a half time as likely. This point-in-time snapshot fails to show the steady decrease in births to black teens over the preceding decade, with over a third reduction (37 percent). Over that time period the Hispanic rate fell also, but only by 13 percent.[157]

Table 3.3. Racial Disparities in Child Health

Condition and measure	White	Black (risk)	Hispanic (risk)
1 Infant deaths per 1,000 live births (source 1)	5.7	13.6 (2.38)	5.6 (0.98)
2 Very low birth weight (<3 lbs, 4 oz or 1,500 grams) percent (source 2)	1.1	3.1 (2.82)	1.1 (1.00)
3 Teen births per 1,000 adolescents ages 15–19 (source 3)	41.7	73.1 (1.75)	92.4 (2.21)
4 Activity limitation due to chronic illness, ages 0–17, percent (source 4)	6.0	7.3 (1.22)	5.8 (0.96)
5 Assessed health status of not excellent or very good, ages 0–17, percent (source 5)	14.0	25.6 (1.83)	22.3 (1.59)
6 Incomplete immunizations 4:3:1:3, percent (1996 data, source 6)	21.0	26.0 (1.23)	29.0 (1.38)
7 Obesity in boys, percent (source 7)	11.5	12.0 (1.02)	
7 Obesity in girls, percent (source 7)	9.8	16.9 (1.72)	
8 Risk of diabetes, percent (source 8)	29.0	45.0 (1.55)	49.0 (1.69)
9 Asthma mortality, ages 5–14, per million (source 9)	2.5	10.0 (4.00)	
10 Cigarette smoking, 12th graders, percent (source 10)	27.8	7.2 (0.25)	14.0 (0.50)
11 Illicit drug use, 12th graders, percent (source 11)	26.4	20.0 (0.76)	23.9 (0.91)

Sources:

1. Annie E. Casey Foundation, *Kids Count 2003* (Washington, D.C.: Center for the Study of Social Policy, 2003); National Center for Health Statistics, *Health, United States, 2004* (Hyattsville, Md., 2000); *National Vital Statistics Report* 50, no. 12 (2002), tables 3 and B.

2. *National Vital Statistics Report* 50, no. 5 (2002): 77.

3. *Child Health USA 2002* (U.S. Department of Health and Human Services, 2002), p. 35. Rates for Native Americans are 65.7 and for Asian/Pacific Islanders, 20.5.

4. *America's Children: Key Indicators of Well-Being, 1998* (Government Printing Office, 1998), p. 79.

5. National Health Interview Survey, *Vital and Health Statistics, 1999*, table 6.

6. *America's Children: Key Indicators of Well-Being, 1998*, p. 82.

7. Centers for Disease Control, *CDC Fact Book 2000/2001: Profile of the Nation's Health*, p. 28.

8. McConnaughey J, Lifestyle Puts 1 in 3 Kids at Diabetes Risk, speech at the American Diabetes Association annual meeting, New Orleans, June 14, 2003, available at www.drwoolard.com/peinnews/warning_4_children.htm (accessed September 21, 2005).

9. Asthma Mortality and Hospitalizations among Children and Young Adults, United States, 1980-1993, *Morbidity and Mortality Weekly Report*, May 3, 1996, pp. 350-53.

10. *America's Children: Key Indicators of Well-Being, 1998*, p. 87.

11. *America's Children: Key Indicators of Well-Being, 1998*, p. 89.

Note: Relative rate is measured against white referent group.

Teen pregnancy is a complex measure that picks up both those customs that make communities strong as well as those that put little children at hazard. The vast majority of adolescent births are to young women in their late teens who are starting their families. They are taking on adult responsibilities within their communities. Among many cultural and ethnic groups, marriage at age 18 or 19 is the norm, a cause for celebration, not consternation. Families welcome the new baby, and there is multigenerational pride and support. For other groups, young women take on family responsibilities before age 20 at great peril. In some particularly trying situations, having a baby is a one-way ticket out of the neighborhood. Natural supports disappear, and the new mother and her baby are abandoned to the public system of homeless shelters, public assistance, and overburdened social service agencies.[158]

Breast-feeding rates vary by race.[159] In 2000 two-thirds of U.S. mothers nursed their babies, but for most mothers the period was relatively short. In-hospital breast-feeding rates were 72 percent for whites, 71 percent for Hispanics, and 51 percent for blacks. By the time the baby was 6 months old, only 34 percent of whites, 28 percent of Hispanics, and 21 percent of blacks were still breast-feeding. The 1990s saw general improvements in breast-feeding rates across the country, with a concomitant lessening of the disparity between blacks and whites. While the progress is slow, it is most welcome, especially in face of the obesity epidemic and its possible association of overweight with infant feeding practices.[160]

Racial disparities in obesity are becoming increasingly apparent as the national attention is focused on this very serious problem. The children and youth most effected by the obesity epidemic are adolescent black girls, who are one and a half times more likely to be overweight than whites of the same age. Obesity brings with it the increased risk of Type 2 diabetes. Black and Hispanic youngsters are at substantially increased risk for becoming diabetic, with each group having a one and a half times higher likelihood of developing diabetes during their lifetime than white children.[161] These disparities continue throughout the life cycle and help account for the significant racial differences in adult morbidity of heart disease, hypertension, and stroke. Women who are obese are at risk of serious perinatal conditions such as eclampsia, pregnancy associated diabetes, birthing complications, premature delivery, and congenital anomalies.[162]

Some of the most dramatic manifestations of racial disparities are among conditions that affect adolescents and young adults. Although black youth are only a sixth of the population of U.S. teenagers, they constitute over half of young American people with HIV/AIDS.[163] Since HIV is spread through heterosexual contact, the effect is triply bad in racial disparity terms, affecting not only young black men but also young black women, and their babies. While the chance of acquiring HIV has leveled off or decreased for most populations, this is not true for young black women.[164] Babies of color have a strikingly higher likelihood of contracting HIV/AIDS than do white babies (84 percent of the 382 children reported with AIDS in 1998 were black or Hispanic).[165]

The rate for violent death is many times greater among black males than among white males, with a sixfold difference in deaths due to firearms.[166] Black male life expectancy is the lowest among racial groupings in the United States, standing at 68.6 years, compared to 77.2 years for all other groups in 2003.[167]

Racial disparities are documented for many chronic childhood illnesses. Genetically linked illnesses such as sickle cell anemia, cystic fibrosis, and Tay Sachs have a higher predilection for one racial or ethnic group. Acute illness also can vary by race. For instance, Kawasaki disease is twelve to fifteen times more common in children of Japanese lineage than it is among Caucasian children.[168] As the unraveling of the human genome continues, more information will help pinpoint how other diseases vary among racial and ethnic groups. For chronic illnesses with roughly the same incidence, there are troubling differences in the way the conditions manifest in children of various racial and cultural groups. Childhood asthma, for instance, occurs with about equal frequency among children of all races, but asthma mortality rates for black children are four times higher than for white children.[169] The prevalence of childhood leukemia is actually lower among blacks than whites, but black children with the disease have a greater chance of dying of it than do white children.[170] There is a similar pattern with Down syndrome, in which the median age of death for whites is 50 years and for blacks is 25 years.[171]

Explanations of the Disparities

What explains such disparities in incidence, in prevalence, and in the impact of various conditions and disorders? How does the clinician, the scientist, the policymaker follow the path from the initial occurrence of the disorder to the eventual outcome? What place does racism play? Are there blatant instances of unfair, unequal treatment? Is the diagnosis of asthma made later in black children's lives? Do doctors prescribe different medical regimens to different groups of children? Are explanations of, say, the importance of taking the medicines as prescribed as thorough for one group as for another?

Ferreting out the answers to these questions requires a careful look at the interplay of biology, social structures, and individual interpersonal interactions. Some of the possible explanations are straightforward, some more subtle, some quite disturbing. There is no question that many black and Hispanic children grow up with the odds stacked against them: poverty, insecure employment, poor housing, unreliable transportation, and inadequate support networks. Because of de facto segregation in many cities, black families face limited options for housing. Even working families earning a fairly good wage can end up living in poor, dilapidated structures. In cases of extreme poverty, the only choice of housing may be in a neighborhood with a hazardous-waste dump. So-called environmental racism intertwines with the other causes of ill health.

The absence of comprehensive medical facilities in the neighborhoods where black families live compromises their health. Black families turn to hospital emergency rooms and urgent care centers for health services twice as often as white families do.[172] Moreover, black children are much more likely to be uninsured or underinsured than are white children.[173] Uninsured children make fewer health care visits than insured children (figure 3.7). A different pattern of care for blacks than for whites has been documented in studies of care given in university-based emergency departments.[174] Worried about follow-up in the absence of a strong primary care network, emergency room physicians more likely opt for the hospitalization of these patients than for preventive medicines. In an individual instance, this approach might make sense, but on a population basis this differential treatment perpetuates a cycle of inadequate attention to the root cause of the disorder.

Another explanation for health care disparities along racial lines is poor communication. New data are emerging on the miscommunications that occur between health care providers of different racial, ethnic, or cultural backgrounds than their patients. Well-meaning doctors may misinterpret families' questions and needs because they simply do not understand the context of some of their patients' lives. Never having experienced racial slights themselves, some white physicians cannot believe that subtle and overt racial prejudice bedevils the daily interactions of many of the families they care for.

Parents of one racial group may distrust or discount medical advice from health care professionals of a different racial or ethnic background. The powerful book *The Spirit Catches You and You Fall Down* tells of the painful experiences of a Southeast Asian family living in Merced, California.[175] In the family's view, every time their child had a seizure, it was a sign of blessing. They could not understand why the health care workers were adamant that their child was sick and in need of medical treatment. The health care workers found themselves in a net of difficulty trying to do what they thought best for the child. In the end, the clash of cultural beliefs created serious disharmony within the family and the community. This East meets West cautionary tale does not offer all the answers, but it does portray the dimensions of conflict that lie just under the surface in many intercultural interactions.

New theories of cultural variation in the interpretation of scien-

Figure 3.7. Lack of Health Care 1997, by Race and Health Insurance Status

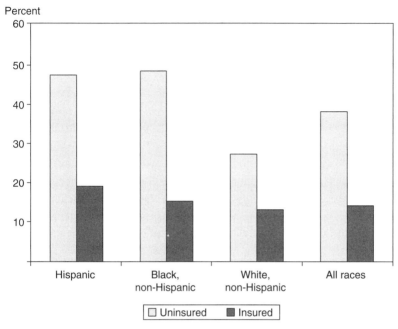

Percent

Source: Centers for Disease Control, National Health Interview Survey 1007.
Note: Figure shows percent of children, ages 10–19, who had not gone to the doctor in the last year.

tific information offer some interesting explanations for communication mismatches. One theory holds that different cultural groups have different notions of time: that the average person of British or Chinese background has a past orientation, that African Americans are present oriented, and that white Americans look to the future. When one thinks about how each of these groups would look at the relevance of preventive services, it would seem that white Americans would put a higher premium on prevention than the other two groups.[176]

A major concern are the frequent racial/ethnic disparities between health care workers and their patients. When a family of color or a non-English-speaking family rolls their baby's stroller into a primary care clinic or arrives at an emergency ward late at night frightened by their child's high fever, chances are that the nurse and doctor who care for them will not be of their racial or cultural group. Nationally, 25 percent of the population is Latino, African American, or Native American, but only 6 percent of practicing physicians come from these groups.[177] Attempts to change this situation focus on the relatively slow process of increasing the number of young people who enter scientific and medical careers. The cycle that stymies progress lies in the fact that nonwhite children tend to be poor and to attend poor schools, where they receive inadequate preparation for entrance into the high schools and colleges that could prepare them for careers in medicine. Until this problem is remedied, there will unfortunately continue to be disparities in the physician workforce mix.

So What Do All These Facts and Figures Mean?

One way of looking at child and youth health conditions at the millennium is to sort them into two clusters, common and complex. Cluster 1 includes health problems that affect many children and often reflect outside social and environmental influences (lifestyle issues, socioeconomic pressures, nutrient availability, acute infectious outbreaks, allergens, pollutants, and toxins). Cluster 2 is composed of many different rare conditions, some of which represent the outcomes of the scientific success of the late nineteenth and twentieth centuries. Other cluster 2 conditions are the consequence of child health care failure to address cluster 1 conditions properly (for example, poor prepregnancy health care, resulting in premature delivery and long-term disability of the child).

A graphic image of these two clusters plotting frequency against cost might look like a sailboat at dock. The broad flat deck represents the fact that cluster 1 conditions are highly prevalent and generally mild to moderate in severity. The costs of these conditions to families and society accrue because so many individual children are affected. The tall, sleek mast represents the cluster 2 conditions. Not many children have these illnesses and disabilities, but when children and youth are afflicted, the problems are serious and the cost to the children and their families can be immense. The average annual health care costs for children in cluster 2 are as much as twenty times that for children in cluster 1.

Children and youth with both types of health condition live in every community, attend every school, call for doctor's appointments at every primary care office, and appear at every hospital's emergency department. The history of modern pediatrics is the history of adaptation to the different (and sometimes contradictory) demands that dealing with these two types of condition places on individual providers, on groups of providers (clinics, hospitals, and so on), and on the entire system of care.

To learn about and truly understand cluster 1 conditions, the child health clinician must be informed about a broad range of issues that span medicine, sociology, current events, and secular trends. Cluster 2 conditions require a highly technical and specialized focus on complex physiologic and biological phenomena. Throughout the modern era of child health, there has been a kind of yin or yang response to the problems encompassed by these two clusters. This is reflected in debates recorded from the annual meetings of various pediatric professional societies. Typically, the incoming president will present a large-scale view of child health and call on his or her colleagues to embrace the totality of child health concerns. Applause. Pause. The first question from the audience suggests hesitancy about the ability of child health professionals to engage in the larger sociopolitical sphere, where the answers to cluster 1 problems may lie. The second responder will express the opinion: "We should focus only on cluster 2 conditions, where we have special expertise. We know how to build hospitals. We don't really know how to build communities."

Increasingly, over the twentieth century and particularly within the past two to three decades, child health as a discipline has begun to confront the tension inherent in the cluster 1 and cluster 2 duality and to articulate the importance of an increased focus on prevention. The child health discipline has begun to combine highly specialized knowledge down to the molecular level with an inflected understanding of how systems interact, how communities are put together, and how families function, bringing the yin and yang together in an integrated picture. A fully inflected response to the child health concerns depicted in this chapter depends on how that picture takes its ultimate shape.

The facts and figures presented here tell a number of stories about the current lives of America's children and youth. Never before have children had such hopes for long and healthy lives. Never before has the food supply been so plentiful or the physical resources and technical equipment so available. Never before has time and space been so compacted and so readily and easily manipulated by human control. And yet despite all of this control of the world around them, children continue to live in a world that is out of control in frightening and threatening ways. It is most discouraging that as a nation, we cannot get a good handle on the disparities in health care and health outcomes and wrestle them to the ground. Without political resolve, a concerted plan, and leadership in the health and political arenas, the situation may not change for a very long time. That is the bad news that these stories tell. But there are also inspiring and positive messages. Most of the good news emerges from

Figure 3.8. Use of Alcohol, Cigarettes, and Illicit Drugs. Among 12th Graders, 1991–2004

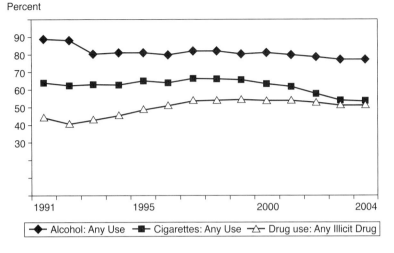

Source: Monitoring the Future, (Institue for Social Research, University of Michigan, 2004). See www.monitoring the future. org (accessed April 2, 2006).

Figure 3.9. Homicide Rate among Males Ages 15–19, 1990–2002

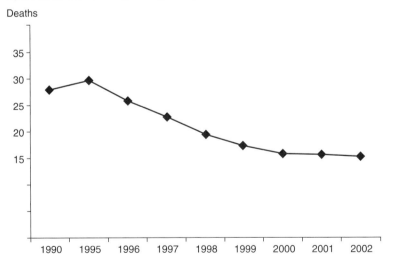

Source: ChildTrends Data Bank, available at www.childtrendsdatabank.org/tables/70_Table_1.htm (accessed October 11, 2005).

the trend data on adolescents: subsiding rates of drug and alcohol use and smoking (figure 3.8); lower homicide rates and gun-related injuries (figure 3.9); fewer teen pregnancies (figure 3.10); and greater use of condoms (figure 3.11).

Figure 3.10. Pregnancy Rate among Females Ages 15–19, 1990–2002

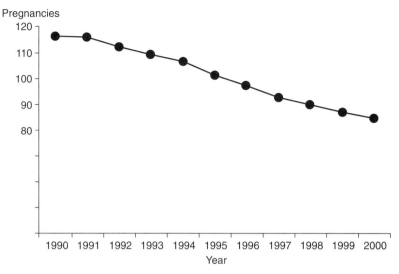

Source: Venture SJ, Abma JC, Mosher WD, Henshaw S, *Estimated Pregnancy Rates for the United States, 1990–2000: An Update,* available at www.cdc.gov/nchs/data/nvsr/nvsr52/nvsr52_23.pdf (accessed October 11, 2005).

Note: Pregnancies are per 1,000.

Figure 3.11. Condom Use, 1991–2003

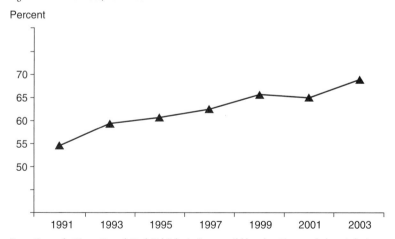

Source: Centers for Disease Control, *Youth Risk Behavior Survey,* available at http://apps.nccd.cdc.gov/yrbss/ QuestYearTable.asp?path=byHT&ByVar=CI&cat=4&quest+Q63&year=Trend&loc=X (accessed October 11, 2005).

Note: Condom use measured by use during last sexual intercourse.

In the chapters that follow, let us explore how advocacy at the clinical, group, legislative, and professional levels depends heavily on the knowledge base of information about what is happening to children and what is (and is not) being done about it. As Lauren Elizabeth and Pete John grow into adolescence and young adulthood, doubtless the facts and figures will be changing. The direction of that change will depend on the use that doctors, other child-helping professionals, community-based organizations, policymakers, and families make of both the bad news and the good.

Clinical Advocacy $\qquad$ 4

ADVOCATING CLINICALLY FOR INDIVIDUAL CHILDREN and their families comes naturally to child health providers. The office, the ward, the nursery, are comfort zones. Nonetheless, it is at the clinical level that many physicians and nurses feel dissatisfied, and even disgruntled, about their inability to make a difference. They worry that they cannot alleviate suffering stemming from family, economic, community-based, and societal influences. The cardiac surgeon thinks to himself, "I know that mom is depressed, but what can I do about it?" The nurse in the neonatal intensive care unit asks, "How can our team be sure that this newborn will be safe at home, when we suspect that his father is a drug addict?" The on-call doctor scans the numerous emergency room visit and notes, "This kid keeps coming in with injuries, but I am powerless to get the slum landlord to fix up that apartment." The pulmonary fellow consulting on the chronic care service muses, "Isn't that something? This family has all the money in the world, but if we don't find a better way to help the parents with the day-to-day care of this youngster on the respirator, their world is going to fall apart."

Across the country, child health providers are creating models to improve and expand clinical care to involve not only the child's condition but also the family's situation and the community's resources.[1] Successful responses involve pediatricians with public health, social services, and education. When practitioners venture outside the clinic they discover opportunities to work with others on systems that diminish health and developmental threats to children.

In this chapter, let us look first at intervention, tools, and models within traditional health care settings, then at models beyond the clinic walls that enhance service availability through partnerships. Together, these models constitute the "medical home," which brings together all the elements of a comprehensive, coordinated approach to care for individual children and their families.

Traditional Health Care: The Basics

In 1978 in Alma Ata in the USSR physicians from around the world met with representatives of the World Health Organization and UNICEF to define the principles of health care delivery.[2] The meeting culminated in the introduction of the "4As" methodology. Using the Alma Ata system, providers are asked, Is the health care you are offering accessible and affordable, available and appropriate? At the most basic level, child health advocacy is about answering yes to all four.

Accessibility

Patients may have trouble gaining access to health facilities for a wide variety of reasons, including the location of the practice. Practice sites with limited parking and accessibility to public transportation may be hard to reach. In some major urban areas, safety issues may present real accessibility barriers. If there is active gang warfare near a health center, parents may be reticent to come to the clinic for well child care. It is not unreasonable for families to miss their children's shots for fear of being shot.

Even the best-placed setting may be inaccessible. Clinics and offices in buildings built before the Americans with Disabilities Act may have no accommodation for baby strollers, wheelchairs, portable suction machines, oxygen tanks, or IV poles.[3] Fortunately, the act's regulations are improving accessibility for children as much as they are for others; pediatricians can even obtain handicapped license plates for the parents of children with disabilities.

Language barriers are the most common accessibility issue. When families cannot grasp what is being asked of them, cannot answer the clinicians' questions, cannot convey their concerns or understand what medicines and regimens are being prescribed, how accessible is the health care? Bringing in the community to help can make an enormous difference; in Boston, for example, translators from Jewish Family Services accompany Russian immigrant families to well child and sick care appointments. Even though no clinic can accommodate ten or fifteen different languages, it can provide translated information for the predominant language groups. A baby book in both English and Spanish, for example, is distributed by the publicly funded Massachusetts Healthy Start program.[4] Private agencies also produce such materials. For instance, the Alina Health System and U-Care of Minnesota have published books on infant feeding in Laotian, Vietnamese, and Hmong.[5] A telephone-based interpreter service is also available, and even though discussing health issues through a third party sitting at a bank of telephones is cumber-some, it can be of great help in complex situations and lifesaving in an emergency. (See www.languageline.com.)

For language accessibility, health care providers may need to adapt more than just the words they speak. Simple cross-cultural misinterpre-tation can compromise care.[6] Saying "You have a beautiful baby" to a mother from some Caribbean cultures is tantamount to inviting the evil eye on the child. In some Native American communities, saying "Thank you" not only ends a series of spoken interchanges, it actually signals the termination of the relationship. It is translated, "We have now finished whatever business or interaction we were meant to have." Physicians and nurses in the Indian Health Service learn this lesson quickly.

Many Latino and Asian parents subscribe to the hot-cold theory of ill-ness, that is, hot conditions respond to cold remedies and cold to hot.[7] To a new immigrant from Guadalajara, the pediatric resident who offers a prescription of a "cold" intervention for a "cold" condition is simply out of touch with reality. It may not be wise to trust her. So it is incumbent on nurses and doctors to learn the theories of illness of the patients un-der their care. This may involve quite a bit of work, because even some-thing as straightforward as the hot-cold categorization of illness varies by region. A condition that is considered hot in San Juan, Puerto Rico, may well be cold in New Delhi, India. There is nothing wrong, however, with a provider showing interest in learning about these beliefs, checking in directly with families. The family's answer to the question "Can you teach me something more about how the hot-cold theory is practiced in your area?" can enrich the therapeutic interchange.

Affordability

The delivery of health care is expensive; costs include staff salaries, office expenses, clinic and hospital maintenance, medical and surgical proce-dures, and on and on. In the absence of universal health insurance, clini-cians are forced to keep close tabs on how many uninsured and underin-sured children and youth are in their care. In some states, such as Florida, the reimbursement rates for children on Medicaid are so meager that physicians cannot afford to have their practices include a large percent-age of such patients. Many families feel beaten down by a system that requires them to reapply for coverage every year (or in some particularly egregious situations, every month). New immigrants often worry that applying for health care benefits will call attention to their legal status and cause more trouble for their family than the health care is worth.

Clinicians who understand these issues ask about health insurance coverage at every visit. By tying themselves in to social service, legal advocacy, and the Department of Medical Assistance, these providers can find solutions that benefit both the patient and the clinic. At the Martha Eliot Health Center in Boston's Jamaica Plain neighborhood, a registration clerk has special training in Medicaid requirements and is able to help families sign up for coverage at the health center, avoiding a trip to the Medicaid office. For his immigrant clients, the pediatrician Robert Karp has created posters showing a copy of his response from the U.S. Department of Justice to his inquiry about these clients' rights to publicly provided health insurance, circling difficult concepts and translating them into layman's terms and in several languages (figures 4.1 and 4.2).

These impediments to health care scream out for both individual and legislative advocacy. In chapter 6 we review the role of legislative advocacy in shaping the current health insurance structure.

Beyond the basics of health insurance availability is the question of what is actually covered.[8] One pernicious problem is that not all medications are paid for by all plans. Each health care office is forced to keep a sheet with row upon row, column upon column, listing which antibiotic is covered by which insurer. Although this is not directly an issue of affordability, it creates an extra step for clinicians, who are trying their best to be efficient and who are watching the bottom line for their patients. The fact that much durable medical equipment and supplies for daily nursing procedures are not paid for at all is more of an affordability issue. The bills for incontinence diapers, for example, can add up substantially for the family of, say, a child with cerebral palsy.

Incidental costs also hinder health care delivery.[9] The financial burden escalates when children require frequent clinic visits, hospitalizations, and therapy sessions. Considerations of affordability include such expenses as transportation or parking fees, as well as missed work and other elements of family life that have been sacrificed.

Availability

Availability refers in part to time. Are the clinic's hours flexible enough for working families? How long is the waiting list for a routine appointment, a specialty care consultation, a radiological examination, or a laboratory test? Where do families turn when their children are sick? Is the primary care office or specialty clinic open twenty-four hours a day or has a clear arrangement been made with a local emergency facility? How

Figure 4.1. Information Sheet on Available Resources (English)

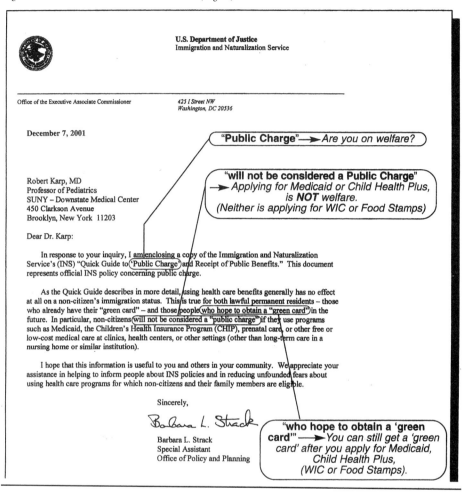

Source: With permission from Robert Karp. Brochures developed with support from American Academy of Pediatrics Community Access to Child Health (AAP-CATCH).

easy or how difficult is it for patients to be seen at this alternative place? Tom Silva of the East Boston Community Health Center has designed an individualized health plan (IHP) for his patients with special health care needs.[10] The written plan contains up-to-date information about the child's health condition, medications, and all procedures in the event that the youngster has to be seen emergently. The Health Center's on-call clinician faxes that information to the emergency service as part of the

Figure 4.2. Information Sheet on Available Resources (Arabic)

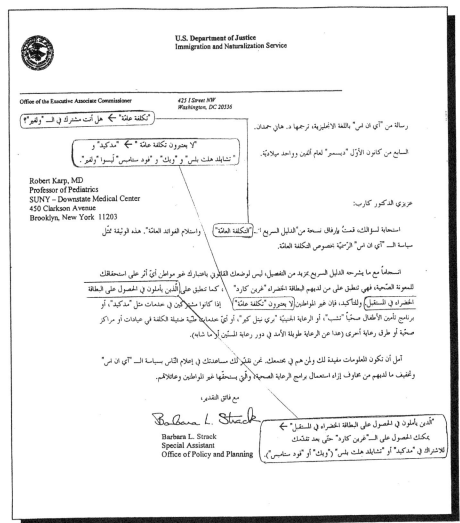

Source: With permission from Robert Karp. Brochures developed with support from American Academy of Pediatrics Community Access to Child Health (AAP-CATCH).

midnight referral. This same plan can be sent along with patients when the child goes to see a specialist for a consultation.

Availability means that patients should not have long waits once they have appeared for their appointment. As part of the Anne E. Dyson Community Pediatrics Training Initiative, the residents and junior staff at Harlem Hospital advocated cutting the waits in the continuity clinic down from several hours to less than an hour. Respect for the patients and concern for a well-run clinic translated into increased availability and a much more efficient operation.[11]

Availability also connotes openness and affability. This may seem a slightly funny spin on the concept, but if parents and children do not feel welcome, they will be less forthcoming with clinically relevant information. When a provider and family have a bilateral, trusting relationship, they can start up a conversation where it left off, the way siblings or old friends do. Not only do families feel better not having to tell their story over and over, but the doctor or nurse practitioner's familiarity with the details of the child's life is a substantial time saver. With children, affability often means the difference between getting a good physical exam and not. Experienced, available, affable clinicians woo little babies with just the right pitch, tone, and inflection. They encourage 18-month-olds to show off: "Point to Jacqui's nose?" "Lets see Manuel's ears?" They tell goofy jokes to ward off a 4-year-old's welling tears.

Appropriateness

Appropriateness in a clinical setting assumes the adequate training and retraining of staff, the use of medical and surgical networks, up-to-date and working equipment, responsive resources, and well-coordinated systems. Physicians and nurses individually attend continuing education courses, pass recertifying examinations, and keep their Pediatric Advanced Life Support certification up to date. So as to maintain competence in ever-changing treatment protocols and regimens, generalists take subspecialty courses, and subspecialists attend on generalist wards. Most practitioners are confident of the appropriateness of the basic health care they deliver, but many are concerned that they are not doing all they can. Part of this comes from a sense that they do not work for the patients but for insurance companies, employers, or the government. In chapter 7 we discuss the way professional advocacy may put health care providers back in the driver's seat.

Practicing Clinical Advocacy Every Day

Even under the most onerous of conditions, forward-looking providers have discovered how to make small adjustments to make their daily practice more accessible, affordable, available, and appropriate. The two biggest problems for most clinicians are (1) a sense that their time is seriously constrained and (2) the concern that they don't have the tools to get the clinical job done. They see the consequences of their rushing and incompleteness in the wary eyes of their patients. To counter such dis-affection and distrust, they make changes in the way they approach the clinic's patient population and in the way they address each individual patient. Here we present innovative solutions that clinician advocates use to address barriers to providing full care.

Knowing the Patient Population

Who are the practice's patients? What neighborhoods and towns do they come from?[12] How many have chronic conditions, and what are they?[13] What are the most frequent complaints and do they vary by season or year? What percentage of patients were born outside the United States?[14] What previous health care have they had? How many of the children have highly successful parents, whose expectations may be causing emotional and physical stress?

It is ironic that insurance company administrators and hospital financial officers routinely conduct demographic analyses for fiscal reasons but that doctors and nurses rarely collect and probe such data for clinical reasons. Providers who can examine patient demographics and epidemiology prospectively are at an advantage in supplying appropriate care, and powerful tools are now available for receiving such data. Steve Downs and his group at the Children's Health Services Research (CHSR) section at Indiana University have applied computer technology to gather such demographics and epidemiology. Their Child Health Improvement through Computer Automation (CHICA) program assesses risk factors, health behaviors, and environmental concerns gleaned directly from parents before the child is seen by the pediatrician.[15] The CHSR section has also combined "geocoded" health data with urban planning data from Indiana University's Polis Center to provide insight into the assets and vulnerabilities of neighborhoods where the children live.[16]

The more that patients can be clustered according to commonalities (newborns, ex-premature babies, children with atopic histories, children with asthma, children with special health care needs, teen parents and their babies, and so on), the easier it is for health care providers to anticipate and prevent negative heath events. A few simple computer programming steps will mine any database for information such as date of birth (to gather the parents of newborns for group well-child sessions), mother's date of birth (to identify teen parents), emergency room and hospitalizations for asthma (to target a group of children with moderate to severe asthma), less than the average number of clinic visits (to find children at risk of poor compliance with health promotion guidelines), and those with more than the average number of clinic visits (to pick up on children who may have underlying disease or disability patterns as well as those children whose parents have greater than average concerns). In most people's minds, the term *managed care* has come to mean cost management, but Robert Ebert's original concept was that of a forward-looking, population-based approach that ensured access to appropriate services for all patients in a particular provider panel.[17] Chapter 5 presents a more in-depth discussion of advocacy for groups of children.

Using Every Minute, Every Wall, Every Chance

Contrary to popular belief, the time pediatricians spend face-to-face with patients has been increasing, not decreasing. Nonetheless, the actual patient-provider interaction is still quite short: less than twenty minutes.[18] Clinicians who plan their patient's entire health care visit, not just the time in the examination room, vastly enhance the care delivered. They make sure that every aspect of the appointment has a purpose and a health care focus. Explicit aspects of health care delivery include how the office is set up, what information is displayed, what reading materials are available, whether or not there is a television in the waiting area and what is on the television; and most important, how the staff in the office interact with the children and with their parents.

Using Every Minute

One of the biggest challenges for child health clinicians is how to use the short time allotted to elicit and listen to the concerns of the families, a big challenge but not insurmountable. Just as surgeons and airline pilots work under the pressure of a ticking clock, many creative child health providers have discovered rigorous methodologies for using each minute to the fullest. They first establish an environment where every exchange produces meaningful information. Eliminating "busyness" allows a great deal of serious business to be transacted.

Asking the right question is often the answer. The well-meaning novice asks the mother, "How are you today?" and for her pains gets, "Oh, fine. The traffic getting here was really awful and I have had a little cold. I am trying to get the kids ready for camp, and there is just so much to do at this time of the year, even though it is supposed to be vacation time. We are just fine thanks." The seasoned clinician, however, asks, "What do you want to accomplish with the visit today?" The mother responds, "Johnny is going to camp next week. I want to make sure that we are doing all the right things so his asthma doesn't come on. I need an extra inhaler to leave with the camp nurse. Do you think I should be sending some prelone as well?" Both conversations take the same amount of time, but there is a world of difference in the quality of the interchange.[19]

"What do you want to accomplish with the visit today?" is the right question because it (1) allows the parent to articulate her concerns immediately, (2) sets the right tone in terms of a shared responsibility between the clinician and the family, and (3) delimits the time that can be used, namely, "the visit today." The message is, "There is a lot we can do together, but not everything under the sun. Let's focus in on the highest priority."

The preparedness of the clinician to address the priority issues by having the appropriate materials at hand also matters. The novice provides the mother a good pat on the back, "You are such an old pro. Just do what you did last year. You know Johnny will do well if he gets regular asthma medicine." The seasoned clinician ensures that there is a clear plan of action and that both she and the family know what that plan is: "This handout gives us the latest asthma recommendations from the National Heart Lung and Blood Institute. Let's run down the checklist together and make sure we are both comfortable about the plan. Here is a written copy for you, and I am putting a second one in Johnny's chart."

Both encounters take the same amount of time, but the second actually saves time because the evidence-based document sheet relieves the clinician from having to write or dictate a note later after rifling through the chart to find out what the heck Johnny actually was taking last year.

Charles Homer and his group at the National Initiative for Child Health Quality (NICHQ) recognize the value of the three maneuvers: (1) asking pertinent questions, (2) offering standardized clinical advice, and (3) customizing the questions and advice to the specific environment. They have prepared training materials and quality improvement forms that save time and improve care through increasing the precision with which clinicians address the concerns that families bring them.[20]

Precise questioning and the use of tools helps with the assessment of children's developmental and educational status as well. Many children's health care providers are beginning to inform themselves better about the children's educational status and ability. The question, "How's school going?" is generally a waste of breath. The typical answers of "Fine," "OK," or "Not so good" give little useful information. The better way to find out if a child is able to read and spell and do math is to give her examples of reading, spelling, and arithmetic. Sean Palfrey in his primary care clinic

Figure 4.3. Example from Development Assessment Book

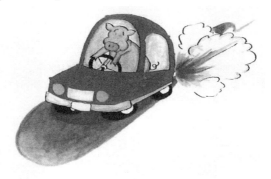

"I saw a red cow jump over the moon.

He hit his big head on a star.

The pig ran away with our little red car.

I hope he will bring it back soon."

Source: With permission from Sean Palfrey.

at the Boston Medical Center put together age- and grade-appropriate short, funny reading passages, thought games, and arithmetic puzzles for his patients. Without adding significant time to a clinic visit, he has found a personal way of letting his patients show off what they know. His congratulations and appreciation have a health- and development-promoting effect. In the case of children who are behind, the two-minute clinician-child interaction can be a wake-up call for further assessment (figure 4.3).

Using Every Wall

Signage conveys a great deal of health and related information inexpensively and often very effectively. Posters that celebrate the special characteristics of the children and youth who attend the clinic can welcome patients who may otherwise feel disenfranchised and scared. Multilingual posters explain crucial health, safety, and social services information to families that are not comfortable reading English. The Injury-Free Coalition for Kids suggests rotating prevention information on a monthly basis and writing the notices at a 4th- to 5th-grade reading level.[21] Many safety programs anticipate a particular hazard of the coming season and feature prevention tactics and materials. In the spring, for instance, they show how to obtain low-cost window guards before the weather turns hot.

Displays and posters can help with sensitive clinical issues. The words "One Day At A Time" on a waiting room bulletin board can send the message to families that the doctors and nurses are familiar with Alcoholics Anonymous, Alanon, and Alateen. Parents and teenagers know that the clinicians and are prepared to talk about alcohol and drugs in a nonjudgmental fashion.[22] Domestic violence experts recommend placing hotline phone numbers on the back of each stall door in the clinic's ladies' room. In the privacy of the stall a frightened woman has a chance to jot down the information. In the adolescent waiting area, a pink triangle tells gay, lesbian, and questioning youth that the clinicians are open to talking about homosexuality and other gender-related issues.[23]

Using Every Chance

Clinical advocacy is about a big objective: the health and well-being of all children. Office staff who share in the vision and feel they are part of the care team add palpable energy and excitement in the workplace. They transmit their sense of mission immediately to the families and children. Nursing staff assistants and clerical aides can play a substantial role in the health care program if they are given the tools to do so. John Knight and his group in the Center for Adolescent Substance Abuse Education and Research show that front-office personnel are not only able but are also willing to administer questionnaires that net important clinical information about alcohol and drug use.[24] This saves time and invests everyone in the clinic in the encounter. Knight has constructed a measure to detect alcohol and drug use in adolescents (the CRAFFT) in such a way that patient confidentiality is maintained and only the primary care provider receives the results. Ensuring patient privacy is the key to expanding the data-gathering role of staff assistants. Structured questionnaires that can be administered in the waiting room by clinic staff are now available for many other topics, including child development, mental health concerns, injury prevention, risk of child abuse and neglect, and youth health behaviors.[25]

The uses of the old faithful prescription pad should not be overlooked. Wherever former U.S. Surgeon General David Satcher goes, he brings his prescription pad. When an admirer approaches him for his autograph, he obliges. With a flair and a fancy pen, he signs the bottom line of a prescription form preprinted with the words "Rx: 30 minutes of exercise each day."[26]

The twenty-first-century pharmacopoeia contains more than tablets and elixirs. Physicians and nurses who are concerned about childhood obesity arrange with the local YMCA and then "order" two afternoons a week of swimming or basketball as part of a weight control program. Developmental pediatricians prescribe karate, skiing, and dirt biking as routine interventions for children with attention deficit hyperactivity disorder (ADHD). As part of the discharge regimen from the newborn nursery, neonatologists list a mandatory infant car seat, and, following guidelines from the National Highway Traffic Safety Administration, child health providers recommend booster seats for older children. A typical prescription for a school-age child is for a really cool, multicolored bicycle helmet to be fitted in the clinic or at the local pharmacy or the neighborhood bike store. Likewise, as a routine part of the clinical encounter, child health care providers often hand out smoke detectors and electrical outlet covers, gun locks and gun boxes, window guards, sunscreen, books and library cards. These prescriptions, just as much as those for an antibiotic or vitamins, are aimed at lowering morbidity and saving lives.[27]

Beyond the Clinic Door

Tom Tonniges describes his first months in practice in Hastings, Nebraska, as a series of neighborhood walks. "I wanted to meet the school principals and the day care teachers of the children I was taking care of." Pediatric toxicologist Michael Shannon says, "The way I find out about what drugs are in the community is I go out and ask the kids. I also keep in close touch with the local police chief." Bron Anders says, "If you truly want to be helpful to the local Native American children, the first stop is with the tribal council."[28] The directors of the University of Rochester, Pediatric Links to the Community—Jeff Kaczorowski and Laura Jean Shipley—advise young physicians starting in practice to visit the Enrico Fermi Middle School Number 17. There they will quickly learn how passionate leadership and community commitment turn despair to hope and discouragement to promise.[29]

It is the actual physical experience that opens the clinician's eyes. It is walking the streets the children walk, seeing the things the children see. When a doctor enters a tenement stairway and feels fear, it is the same fear the little girl feels as she runs up those stairs every day. As a nurse waits while the mother slowly transfers the family's sole light bulb from the lamp in the living room to the ceiling fixture in the bedroom, the minutes tick a new appreciation of poverty. A pediatric intern enters a stuffy, three-room, after-school program for junior high school students and learns why the youngsters are not physically fit. On her disability rotation, a medical student goes to school with a little boy who has spina bifida. At recess she watches him play tag and spin "wheelies." He giggles and laughs with the "normies," as they fight to push him fastest in his chair. When the medical student returns to her campus, she shares with her classmates what an integrated public school really is.

School and Day Care Visits

Periodic school visits alert health care providers to the salient social issues for children and youth. Children, particularly of elementary and junior high age, are deeply affected by both overt and subtle peer pressure. Teachers are attuned to the cliques and clans as well as the identities the children impose on themselves. School-aged children operate within the constraints of elaborate hierarchies. Every 8th-grade girl can recite who in the school is "smartest," "prettiest," "most popular." The students know exactly where they themselves fit in a rank order on these dimensions.[30] Child health professionals who practice in their home community have the advantage of hearing the buzz each day when their own children come home from school: the word of the week (wicked, phat,), the joke of the month, what sports figures are "in," what TV show is "out." They know all about the awesome cartoon character the 1st graders most admire. When these child health care professionals make a school visit, they can compare notes with the teachers about what is valued, what is cool, and how peer expectations are affecting the daily life of the children in the school. Doctors and nurses who practice outside their home communities can profitably use school visits to become more familiar with the current child culture in their community.

Many child health practitioners make an annual trip to the local day care or Head Start center. They want a first-hand look at how the young children in their practice spend their days. The child who is happily chattering away in the dress-up corner at Happy Hillbilly Day Care is the same little 2-year-old boy who cowered, screamed, and clung to his mother's leg during his last clinic appointment. No wonder his parents haven't voiced any concerns. On the other hand, that child crouching over there in the corner is the one whose parents are so worried about autism. He hasn't said a word to anyone. In the examination room, these two children were hard to distinguish. Here amid plastic fire trucks and ring-around-the-rosie, the important characteristics are completely revealed.

City Streets and Foreign Countries

When nurses, doctors, and medical and nursing students explore the community, they discover other things. This is the block where the corner stop sign has been down for three months. The children in this street must pass two drug pushers and three houses of ill repute to get to school. Why are those kids sitting on the back stoop of the restaurant? Are they doing homework, or is this a break from washing dishes at Chef Chiang's? This is a gorgeous neighborhood, but it is 3 p.m., and absolutely nobody is around. What do the kids do in the afternoon? We have driven around this neighborhood for ten minutes and the only stores with any customers are the corner liquor marts. It's such a hot day; look at all those open, unprotected fourth-story windows. I sure hope no children live up there.

The expeditions of child health providers can go even farther afield, especially for those who care for new immigrants. To learn about the culture, the health risks, and health beliefs of the families, some health care providers travel to the country of origin of their most populous group of patients. By asking the simple question, "Tell me where you come from?" Kim Wilson, the pediatric director of the Martha Eliot Health Center in Boston, discovered that the vast majority of her Dominican patients come from Banhi. Some of the children spend six months of the year in Banhi and six months in Boston. Wilson decided to travel to Banhi to learn more about the Dominican culture and experience. She established ties with local nuns, community-based organizations, and health care providers.[31] She now collaborates with the Dominican family doctor of a large number of her Health Center patients and their relatives, creating continuity of care.

By going away, Wilson also learned much about health practices in her own backyard. She learned that merchants regularly transport unregulated antibiotics, steroids, and other drugs from the Dominican Republic to sell in the bodegas just down the street from the Martha Eliot Health Center. Now she has an explanation for the negative throat culture results that have baffled her so many times. Partial treatment, such as her patients were self-administering, covers up important information about bacterial illness. When health care providers make the kind of effort that Wilson made, they notice a new openness from patient families. "If this doctor went to all that trouble to learn about my family, she must value my children and me," and there are grounds for deeper trust and improved communication.

Partners in Clinical Advocacy

All health care providers ideally want their young patients and families to have access to the most comprehensive care. Some offices and clinics coordinate these services within their own walls. Greg Prazar and his private pediatric group in Exeter, New Hampshire, discovered that the addition of a social worker helped them meet the concerns of their families. The improved health outcomes were so impressive that their managed care company agreed to fund the position. At Children's Hospital in Boston school-related concerns were frequent. Joanne Cox worked with Harvard College students to create the Advocating Success for Kids (ASK) program. In conjunction with the Boston public schools, the ASK program provides developmental and behavioral reviews for children teetering on the edge of failure in school. Once a child's plan is delineated, the college volunteers work with the families to carry it out.

Advocating Success for Kids is one of several subunits of Project Health, an innovative program that extends the reach of doctors, nurses, and social workers in the cities of Boston, Providence, New York, and Washington.[32] Other subunits include Asthma Swim, FitNut, STRIVE (a program for children with sickle cell disease), and Help Desks, which help families access information on housing, child care, nutrition, immigration status, and health insurance. Project Health is the brainchild of Rebecca Onie, who was a college student when she began the program. Having read an article in the *Boston Globe* about the multifaceted approaches of the clinics at the Boston Medical Center, she brought her idea to Barry Zuckerman, the chief of pediatrics, who recognized the potential of her idea and who has supported and promoted all of the program's innovations.

In the mid-1980s policymakers and clinicians began experimenting with programs to address health conditions whose roots lay deep in the community and society.[33] Didn't it make sense for a family to come to the same place to obtain help for their children? Following up on this notion, the directors of neighborhood health centers began to locate the offices of the Women, Infants, and Children (WIC) program; the Food Stamp program; early intervention programs; high school completion (GED) classes; and adult literacy projects within their centers. Sometimes, the Department of Welfare and the Department of Public Health combined forces to build their offices and clinics in the same block or even in the same building. Federal agencies promoted the concept with seed grants and other moneys. Offering coordinated services has the potential for cost savings through staff reduction, elimination of duplication, and enhanced communication among child-helping agencies.

The full-service practice and collaboration among appropriate offices allows a nurse practitioner to accompany a mom with a baby who is not thriving down the hall to her colleague in the WIC office. Right then and there, the nutritionist hands the mother cans of fortified twenty-four-calorie-per-ounce formula, and she has plenty of vouchers for more in her top desk drawer. The full-service practice allows an emergency room physician to call in a representative of the Advocacy for Women and Kids in Emergencies (AWAKE) to arrange safe lodging for a child and mother who have been threatened or hurt. Advocates follow up by getting a restraining order on the perpetrator and by helping the women avoid returning to abusive relationships.

A core element of the Anne E. Dyson Community Pediatrics Training Initiative is the identification and cataloguing of community resources.[34] Each training program has a full-time coordinator, who spends a substantial time in the community, networking with the staff of community-based organizations and other agencies. The coordinator shares the lessons with the faculty and the resident physicians, often taking them on guided visits to the local community agencies. The coordinator also works directly with community agencies to make sure that their services are readily available to the residents' continuity or specialty care patients. For example, in Rochester, New York, resident physicians go to the Kids' Café, a subsidiary of the food bank sponsored by Food Link.[35] Equipped with knowledge about this resource, they are prepared the next time they encounter a baby with failure to thrive or a family on the edge of food insecurity. Armed with a good intervention, they are far more likely to encourage families to voice their concerns about food availability.

The resident physician Elisabeth Schainker had a deep commitment to working on the problem of violence. Before entering medicine she had been a middle school teacher and had seen what problems violence could cause in a neighborhood and knew the importance of screening for exposure to violence.[36] During adolescent checkups, she always asked each patient a series of generic questions and would most often receive the socially acceptable answers. "Everything is fine. I only hang out with the quiet guys." In the clinic one day a young Somali boy's sister alerted the doctor to her worries about her brother. Schainker did everything she could through the clinic to work on the problem, but the boy failed to show up again and again. Then one day a headline in the *Boston Globe* caught her eye: the boy had been shot, the victim of rivalry between

African American and African teenagers. Schainker became convinced that the answer for her was in the local community school where she volunteered. There, in the hallways, in the cafeteria, in the gym, she saw and heard the teases and taunts. The precursors of violence brewed just below the surface, infecting the health of all the school children. In the school, there was no coverup. No one needed to please the doctor here.

As the students got to know her in the school, Schainker found that she could work more effectively both in the community and in the clinic. She knew what was going on in the streets, and her patients knew she knew. When she took a history in the clinic, she could use surgically precise probes: "What group are you hanging out with?" "Are the groups fighting now?" "Is anyone out to get you?" With a better appreciation for the roots of animosity, she and Mary Jane O'Brien, the school nurse, partnered on an in-school intervention combined with in-clinic reinforcement. The team engaged in a single mission, to decrease violence.

Community Resources

Unfortunately, huge missed opportunities render health care for individual children less than it could be because there are so few times that community-based organizations, families, and child health providers can compare notes and address common objectives. Each works in isolation, with imperfect knowledge about the capabilities of the others.

Child health providers' conceptions about the community frequently do not include all the formal and informal service networks nor all the designated and nondesignated community leaders. Meaningful collaborations for individual advocacy are a stretch for both the community and the clinical partners; it takes time and the interweaving of clinical and community resources, the giving and taking of control, the establishment of trust. Just as child health clinicians are often leery about moving beyond their usual sphere of activity, community-based agencies often hesitate to approach their medical and nursing colleagues to help with one of the children they are concerned about. They worry that the clinicians are too busy or are not interested in such an interaction. It often takes a number of attempts on the part of both the clinical team and the community group to form a relationship that works for all parties and that meets the individual health needs of the children.

An important "ah-ha" moment for health care providers is when they realize that a critical component of individual advocacy is the dissemination of community resource information through the clinical venue. In almost every town, city, and county there are resources that work and

Table 4.1. Community Resources

Women, Infants, and Children (WIC)	Head Start
Food stamps / food pantries	Schools
Breastfeeding Support (LaLeche League)	Injury prevention programs
YMCA/YWCA	Child protection services
Fitness clubs, after school sports	Behavioral health
Early intervention	Recreation/vocation

those that fail. Some agencies are underutilized; some are full to overflowing; some manage always to have room for one more child or family in need. Families that are familiar with the community generally know which programs to turn to, but the new family in town, the first-time parent, the family under enormous stress may lack those informal networks.

Also, while word of mouth and neighborhood get-togethers work relatively well, no community can rely on Aunt Susie and Cousin Juanita to be up-to-date on all the information. Specialized programs have arcane eligibility rules, procedures for each type of service, and frequently changing criteria. Sadly, many young families are isolated or alienated from their neighbors and relatives. Parents expect their doctor's office and the health clinic to be a place where they can reliably get community resource information. Table 4.1 lists the programs and supports that are likely to be present in most communities. Let's review a few examples of resources that can make important contributions to children's health.

Nutrition, Fitness, Early Intervention

The topics of nutrition and fitness have been moving up rapidly on the list of child health priorities, especially in response to the obesity epidemic. Concerns abound in high schools about serious eating disorders. Child health clinics rarely have on-site nutritionists or breast-feeding consultants. Within the community, the federally funded Women, Infants, and Children program offers food and nutritional consultation as a safeguard against low birth weight and failure to thrive. Nutritionists in the WIC offices counsel young parents about wise food choices and often take teen-age parents grocery shopping.

The health benefits of physical activity are now well documented in both the adult and the child literature.[37] Some health centers have formal arrangements with the local YMCA. At Harlem Hospital, the doctors and local police have established Little League baseball teams.[38] Having the phone numbers of these groups can be as big an intervention as any antibiotic prescription for a possible otitis media.

With less than a quarter of American mothers breast-feeding for six months or more,[39] community lactation supports are a boon to families and doctors alike. Increasingly, nurses and others are establishing private breast-feeding consultative practices. While some proprietary insurance companies will pay for such consultations, it is far more difficult to find community-based lactation support for the mothers of babies who have public insurance.

Since the mid-1980s, as a result of federal legislation, every town and city has a system of early intervention for children with disabilities. Physicians, families, day care providers, and social workers can refer children with disabilities or those at significant risk of developing a disability.[40] Early intervention specialists offer services to diminish the impact of children's handicapping conditions. For instance, through the early-intervention mechanism, children who are deaf or hard of hearing may obtain hearing aids. The children and their families may also learn sign language. Similarly, mobility specialists are available to teach blind infants. Speech/language therapists offer stimulation activities for children who are delayed in talking. Physical therapists work with families on exercises to minimize spasticity in children with cerebral palsy. In most states, the central authority for early intervention rests with the public health department or with education. The referral process is not overwhelmingly complex, but it does require specific knowledge of who to call, when to call, and what forms to fill out. Unfortunately, early intervention programs often reach capacity quickly, and many children end up on waiting lists.

A helpful resource for families of infants and young children with disabilities are family support groups, often called parent-to-parent. No one knows better the shock that accompanies the disclosure of a disability, the "No, no, this cannot be happening to us," than a mother or father who has walked down a similar road. These parents also know that not all is sadness and that there are ways to make the path considerably easier. Parent groups are familiar with all the local resources. They are a tremendous quality check on services, knowing which are well delivered and where the holes remain.

Head Start, Schools, and Special Education
Since the early 1970s, Head Start centers have been key community institutions.[41] Children are eligible to attend Head Start at 3 years of age if their family meets the low income criterion. Head Start reserves 10 percent of its slots for children with disabilities and generally has staff

trained to deal with most common concerns. The comprehensive program offers children and families a wide array of educational, developmental, health, and dental services. The Head Start philosophy is that the precious minds of very young children flourish and grow best when adults have the time and resources to respond appropriately to the children's "readiness moments" with educationally exciting materials and activities; it's approach implies that healthy and nourished children learn better than children who are suffering from a draining ear, an aching tooth, or too little to eat. Head Start centers encourage full family participation. Parent programs focus on skills that mothers and fathers can use to nurture their sons' and daughters' development at home and on into their school careers.

The community agencies that health care providers know the most and the least about are public schools. Understanding the local education system takes patience and perseverance. Health providers may be hesitant to plunge into the education morass, but families frequently ask for help because they are confused. "Shaniqua just came home with this note about an individualized education plan." "Tan failed his standardized test, and Mrs. Miller says he cannot go into 4th grade. We do not understand; he was doing so well." Child health providers who have invested in collaborating with schools can answer some of these questions and steer the families to the principal, dean, or special education official who can help the family.

One way that child health care providers learn the intricacies of the school world is through attending team meetings that map out the individualized educational plan for a patient in their practice.[42] In most cases, the press of the daily office schedule makes it hard for clinicians to accept the school's invitation to a meeting. While it is certainly not possible for health care practitioners to attend these meetings on a regular basis, it is well worth the time spent away from the office once or twice a year for clinicians to see the condition of the schools, to feel the attitudes of the teachers, to hear about their burdens, and to learn about the resources available through the school system. Pediatric trainees benefit enormously from exposure to the real world of the school. The experience helps them differentiate between reasonable and unreasonable requests they can make of the school on behalf of their patients.

When child health providers go out to schools and experience for an hour or so the environment that children spend most of their time in, they see the children they care for from a different perspective. Joey is not sitting all alone with his legs dangling down on the examination table. He is one student among twenty or twenty-five. He is listening intently; he is not listening at all; the little boy next to him just winged a spitball; he just returned fire. There is a little girl in the third row back who looks disheveled. Wonder if she had breakfast this morning. How does the teacher keep all these balls in the air? It makes sense now why she keeps asking me to send information about Joey's seizure disorder. Those times he is spaced out do look a little strange. I'll bet she is scared to death that he will have a grand mal convulsion in the middle of math class, and what will she do then?

Safety, Child Protection, and Teen Services

Recognizing that injuries take a significant toll on children and youth, many American communities have instituted injury prevention initiatives, which vary from city to city.[43] Agencies and groups make available education and safety products with varying levels of eligibility and co-payment. In Osage City, Kansas, the Department of Transportation sponsors driver safety events for high school students. In Cambridge, Massachusetts, the local police station installs and inspects car seats free of charge. In Chicago, Sinai Hospital donates an infant car seat to every mother who has attended at least two prenatal visits and delivers at their obstetric facility. In New Jersey, the Burlington Coat Factory has teamed up with the local group Safe and Sound to conduct in-house safety inspections as a grand prize of a customer contest. In New York City, the public health authority supplies window guards to all families in public housing. A thoroughly American crazy quilt of response, but a response nonetheless. If child health providers are in the loop, they can point their families to available services. They can also work to fill in the gaps.

Often the local chapter of Mothers Against Drunk Driving (MADD) or Students Against Drunk Driving (SADD) will help to arrange driving "contracts" for families. The teenager in the family signs a pledge that he will not drive a car if he has been drinking alcohol and will not ride in a car with a driver who has been drinking alcohol. Parents agree to pick up the student from any party, no questions asked.

Each state has a system to protect children from neglect, abuse, and domestic violence. These offices—often beleaguered and underfunded—are nonetheless the gateway into monitoring, care, and protection procedures and foster placement. Other protective services exist under the auspices of public and private agencies, faith-based groups, hospitals, and women's service organizations. Some multiservice programs offer comprehensive packages aimed at a complex of problems, including parental substance abuse, mental health disorders, and multigenerational violence. Many communities have day care slots set aside for children who have been abused or neglected. Within these settings, trained teachers and counselors observe the children carefully, with the aim of creating an intervention therapy and of being alert to new episodes of abuse or neglect.

Teen behavioral health services are few and far between, but some are very effective. Alcoholics Anonymous groups generally sponsor Alateen in the same location where they meet, usually a church hall. Recovering alcoholics and drug users, even though they guard their privacy and anonymity, are active in outreach and mentorship for young people. The work they do can be lifesaving. Unfortunately, other drug and rehabilitation services for young patients are extremely hard to find. In fact, in some communities, it is virtually impossible to find drug and alcohol treatment for teenagers. By contrast, most communities have readily accessible contraceptive services offered publicly through the health department or privately through groups affiliated with Planned Parenthood. Prevention services for sexually transmitted diseases and HIV usually are offered by the health department because of state and federal mandates. Some of these highly effective reproductive health and STD prevention services for teenagers are being eroded by funding cuts at the federal and state levels. Later chapters discuss the systems-level and professional advocacy needed to protect services that work for children and adolescents.

Recreation and Vocation Services

Healthy bodies and minds need places to go, hoops to shoot, songs to sing, and dances to dance as much as they need medicines, shots, and vitamins. One might even measure the richness of a community by its parks, zoos, sports teams, organized arts, and music classes. Peter Benson of Search Institute and John McKnight at Northwestern University have demonstrated that such resources can prevent substance abuse, violence, and early and unprotected sexual activity.[44] The consequences of the lack of recreational activities are demonstrated by children's poor physical and mental health: inactivity tightens tendons and ligaments and turns muscles into flab; boredom sows the seeds of mental and behavioral health disorders and feeds a sense of defeat and depression.

Recreational resources for child health include swim programs to build physical strength, pulmonary residual capacity, stamina, and self-esteem; karate schools for teaching self-control, particularly for conditions like attention deficit hyperactivity disorder; theater programs for building self-confidence and social poise; inclusionary sports programs for junior and senior high school students to help them build their skills; and specialized sports competitions (such as Special Olympics) for children with special health care needs. After-school programs also offer valuable opportunities for children to exercise and to play sports.

Uncertainty about the future plagues the adolescent years. Although schools do have the societal responsibility for steering their students along career paths, other community agencies also have proved helpful in this regard, especially for young people who have unconventional interests.

Vocational planning can be particularly challenging for adolescents with disabilities. Resources for the transition of youth with disabilities do exist in many communities, but they are often offered only at the state level. With cohort survivorship and the longer life expectancy of young people with mental retardation and physical and developmental disabilities (see chapter 3), these issues present themselves with increasing frequency to primary care and specialty physicians. Internists and family physicians encounter questions about vocation from 25-year-olds who present them the Social Security Income Catch-22. "Dr. Generalinternist, I would love to get a job, but if I do I lose my Social Security income and my health insurance benefits and will not be able to come to see you again for the control of my seizures." The balance stick to walk this tightrope does exist in most communities. Finding it takes some concerted searching.[45]

How Partnerships Work

Partnerships among health professionals, parents, community agencies, community-based organizations, volunteers, and youth groups provide direct, personal clinical care for children. Working in concert, each partner makes a specific contribution, efficiently focusing precious time and energy. Health care providers know the discrete medical profile of each child. An active partnership with social and educational services allows them a range of services and opportunities to enhance and reinforce the care plan for individual children. Together, the partners share a vision. They move toward the goal of a seamless system of services for their common constituency. Partnerships that allow for the coordination of services do not emerge simply because it is the thing to do. Two or more parties come together because they are concerned about an issue—something that is hurting children and youth. Several examples:

In San Diego in the late 1980s a state highway cut the Mid-City area off from the rest of the city.[46] Living conditions in Mid-City deteriorated to intolerable. Drug pushers arrived from all over Southern California and terrorized the families in this isolated area. Crime flared. Children's health and development were literally under attack. Recognizing that it was time for action, the neighborhood association, the police, and the Pediatrics Department at the University of California at San Diego formed the Mid-City Community Partnership. It took about a decade for the coalition to reclaim the neighborhood, but by the early 2000s they had built a school and a police station. A spanking-new public library became the pride of the neighborhood and the hub of community life. The partners also opened a clinic in the revitalized area.

In the mid-1970s, the cardiologist Donald Filer took stock of children's heart cases in New England and decided to increase the effectiveness of the Children's Hospital Cardiology Department by taking the clinical show on the road. Working with community partners throughout New England, he founded the Pediatric Cardiology Network. Through the network, Filer saw to it that whether a child had a small atrial septal defect or transposition of the great vessels, he received individual care with a specially tailored cardiac health plan. Once the plan was written, community physicians, public health nurses, and local social workers implemented the plan.

In the mid-1980s, in upstate New York, David Olds was struck that clinicians were not able to detect the early signs of child abuse when they saw babies for well-child visits in their offices. The time was too short, the questions were too closed-ended, and there was little opportunity for clinicians to understand the daily stresses and strains of each new parent. He began a nurse home-visiting experiment for young mothers; here was a way that a clinical team could really practice individual advocacy. Several models of home visiting have proved successful in preventing child abuse and promoting healthy parenting.[47] Home visitors can document the actual living conditions of the babies' families, assess the mother's knowledge of child development, make sure that the home is safety proofed so that toddlers can toddle and 2-year-olds can explore their world. The visitors help parents to anticipate their children's changing growth and behavior, to deal with tantrums, to take time to cool down when the children "push their buttons."

Some health problems, like teen pregnancy, cry out for individual advocacy through partnerships. Adolescent providers who braid together their efforts achieve much more than when they operate out of their separate silos. Girl by girl, individual case by individual case, the multidisciplinary partnership can figure out what will work best and implement the specific plan. Is this a youngster who will respond to counseling? Is she a candidate for birth control pills, for Depo-Provera, for barrier methods? What about an abstinence pledge? Should we involve her partner? If so, how do we get him in? What is going on with her family? Are they pushing her out? Is she being abused? What is happening with her education? Work by partnership programs like the Center for Adolescent Pregnancy Prevention in western Pennsylvania have contributed to a 13 percent decline in the national teen birth rate as well as to a truly stunning 39 percent drop in the teen abortion rate.[48] Results like these draw new allies, such as faith-based organizations eager to help teenagers but opposing abortion.

One of the biggest concerns that child health clinicians voice about venturing into the community is that doing this will bring them more work. Yes, perhaps. But with work comes help—often lots of it—in the form of community agency personnel; community-based organization workers; volunteers from churches, elder organizations, and colleges; and the police and the courts. The learning curve for incorporating this help into daily clinical care can appear steep at first, but those who have climbed the hill find themselves with a new vantage and enormous advantages for their work with children and families.

When Children's Hospital in Boston began its window guards distribution, the planning committee worried about who would install the guards in the families' homes. Emergency room nurses and intensive care unit physicians know more about children falling out of windows than anyone, but it is surgery and splints they manage, not housing codes and carpentry. A partnership with the Boston Public Housing Tenants Association solved the dilemma. Here were workers who knew their business, and here was a critically important source of jobs for community residents. In concert with the Boston Public Health Commission and the Boston Medical Center, the Boston Children Can't Fly campaign logged successes comparable to those in other cities that have mounted window fall prevention projects.[49] Now when a clinician asks if a family has window guards and gets no for an answer, there is a specific response of individual advocacy to protect that child and his brothers and sisters.

The co-location of community agency personnel into child health clinics can be a boon to everyone. In New York City, Children's Hospital of New York (CHONY) has established a partnership with Alianza Dominicana, a community-based social service agency located in the heart of the Dominican community of Washington Heights. Milagros Batista, the co-founder of Alianza Dominicana, is a faculty member in the CHONY resident continuity clinics. Her presence in the clinic has sharpened the observational acuity of the resident physicians and honed their interviewing skills. Knowing that there are resources available for their families, the doctors now readily ask parents about domestic violence. If they detect a problem for a particular family, they make a referral and Milagros Batista and the program staff are immediately ready to meet the family.

Parent-professional partnerships expand the capacity to help individual patients. Groups like Family Voices, Family TIES, and Parent-to-Parent help the parent who faces the news of disability in a newborn or a child who has suffered a serious accident. Together with physicians, social workers, and nurses, these parents provide a range of advice on resources. The parents share among themselves and with the professionals the availability of a new support, which can then be offered to the next family that comes into the office for a routine physical. In Sacramento, California, Head Start Alumni Parents formed a partnership with the Department of Pediatrics at the University of California at Davis. They set their sights on ensuring the health and safety of all the young children in Sacramento.

So if clinicians act on the need to get out of the office on occasion, and if community and family partners are interested in working with clinicians, how do these partners pull it all together? The answer is that all partners must truly believe that they can do a better job for children and youth by working together than alone. They must find the lacunae, the missing pieces, those activities or roles that the other partners can fulfill. Using a sports' team analogy, suppose the health center clinicians cover the pitcher's mound, the plate, and the infield, but they keep losing games because there is no one in the outfield. Community-based organization members can get out there and protect individual children and youth against drug use, teen pregnancy, early smoking, and peer violence by catching some fly balls.

Who Gains?

There are many types of partnership, from the most informal to those that involve building community centers for the physical co-location of services. Partnerships work best when there are explicit terms for the relationships between the partners with a well-delineated understanding of what each partner brings to the enterprise.[50] This can be written in the form of a contract or a less formal memorandum of understanding. For example, subcontracts can indicate that the residents from the medical center will perform the state-mandated physical exams for the young men in the juvenile detention center and that they will also participate in group rounds so that the information they have gleaned is put into a larger context.

Collaborative arrangements succeed best when all parties benefit from the arrangement:.

1. Health providers benefit from more effective efforts and twenty-four-hour access to community services for children with chronic health and social conditions.
2. Community agencies and volunteer can attend more directly to their focus areas, such as education. There is easier access to training and information for staff, especially around children and families who are having problems. In addition, children are healthier and more poised for education, recreation, and other activities.
3. Families have clearer information on who does what and on where to go for services. In addition, the range of services is greater. In addition, fewer school and work days are lost.
4. Government and business experience a more efficacious use of money and more satisfied and productive employees.

The Project Health volunteer model is an example of how a clinical partnership can benefit all the participants. At the Boston Medical Center Pediatrics Clinic, Harvard College volunteers coordinate a resource data bank for families: the Help Desk. They assist parents in obtaining child health-relevant services such as housing, immigration information, schooling, literacy programs, and de-leading programs. The college students are rewarded when a family has a breakthrough with the housing authority, the school, or the local truant officer. Nonetheless, the battles they fight with irrational regulations and irascible bureaucrats can be daunting, with few personal payoffs.

To reinforce the good work of the volunteers and to plant the seeds for ongoing clinical advocacy and larger-scale systems advocacy, Project Health includes two components focused on the college students themselves: mentoring and reflection sessions. Faculty mentors meet regularly with the students to anticipate the swerves in the road ahead and to help solve problems when they arise. The professional mentors are always available by beeper. Several times during the year, they arrange coffee or a meal to check in with the students and to steer them toward networks and resources. The professionals often get as much out of the meetings as the students do: perhaps at the community interface, the volunteer has learned of five slots for children with autism at the YMCA's Saturday recreational program, information welcome to the professional with autistic patients.

The volunteers also participate in reflection sessions with their professional mentors and guest speakers. Each week, in the late evening, the volunteers can be found sitting on couches and wing chairs in an Adams House common room, eating pizza and discussing in-depth the social, economic, and political surround that dictates the conditions and experiences they encountered over the past few days in Roxbury and Jamaica Plain. These reflection sessions reinforce learning by putting the individual clinical encounters into a larger context. The final picture fits into the larger worldview that the college students are creating for themselves as they read the classics of sociology, anthropology, history, literature, economics, and government.

Measuring the Effects of a Partnership

For partnerships to last, there must be measures of their impact. Does it continue to make sense for us to work together? Did we establish the right goals? Are we gaining from the work together or are we spending more time and energy on the intricacies of the collaboration and not enough time on the end results? The only way that these questions can be answered is by a rigorous evaluation of the impact of the work.

From the inception of any partnership, data can document the progress of the partners' work. When Harlem Children's Zone and Harlem Hospital began their collaboration under the auspices of the Robin Hood Foundation, they established the prevalence of childhood asthma in Harlem as a key concern. No one was quite sure how many children in the area met criteria for asthma, but schoolteachers, Head Start directors, karate masters, and pediatric residents were certain they were seeing a huge amount of disability from wheezing. It was time to find out, to count. With such a clear need, it was relatively straightforward to come up with a community-based plan of attack.

The Harlem Children's Zone (HCZ) is a geographically delimited area with no limits on the aspirations of its community members. They want success for the families and children who live there. Leader Geoffrey Canada stresses four key points: (1) there are best practices for services for children and youth, (2) all children have a right to these services, (3) communities can deliver these services, (4) this happens when community members own and operate the services. Harlem Hospital is one of the precious resources of the community. To carry out the first step of the HCZ asthma project, Geoffrey Canada and Stephen Nicholas, the director of pediatrics at Harlem Hospital, formed an alliance. The pediatric staff and residents from the hospital then conducted an asthma needs assessment in Harlem schools. To everyone's surprise and consternation, they discovered that asthma was far more prevalent than anyone had predicted. Nearly a third of the children in Harlem Children's Zone met the Asthma Initiative criteria.

By interweaving the partnership from the beginning and by establishing an original database, the Harlem Children's Zone Asthma Initiative started on a firm foundation of clinical advocacy principles. The entire community is now engaged in the identification of risk factors for asthma in homes and schools. Services in primary care are integrated with community health workers, home visiting, and visiting nurse interventions. Community members are employed in the improvement of housing stock and living conditions. Trainees are learning about what triggers what in ways that no textbook could ever describe. The group is also aware of the discussion of environmental-genetic factors that may influence the disease. This high-level clinical advocacy is improving individual children's lives.[51] Six-year-olds are breathing better. Young athletes are throwing more basketballs. Little children are sleeping through the night.

Clinical Advocacy Principles: The Medical Home

The principles of clinical advocacy for children and families have been eloquently articulated in pediatrics under the rubric of the *medical home*.[52] The medical home concept is that the provision of health care for children must be an integrative endeavor, pulling together aspects of biology, environment, culture, socioeconomic realities, insurance, and national standards for primary and specialty care. The seven key components of the medical home are

1. Accessibility
2. Family centeredness
3. Continuous care
4. Comprehensive services
5. Coordination
6. Compassionate delivery
7. Culturally effective understanding

The ten parameters of the medical home as published in the American Academy of Pediatrics 2000 policy statement are

1. Provision of family-centered care through developing a trusting partnership with families, respecting their diversity, and recognizing that they are the constant in a child's life.
2. Sharing clear and unbiased information with the family about the child's medical care and management and about the specialty and community services and organizations they can access.
3. Provision of primary care, including but not restricted to acute and chronic care and such preventive services as breast-feeding promotion and management, immunizations, growth and developmental assessments, appropriate screenings, health care supervision, and patient and parent counseling about health, nutrition, safety, parenting, and psychosocial issues.
4. Assurance that ambulatory and inpatient care for acute illnesses will be continuously available (twenty-four hours a day, seven days a week, fifty-two weeks a year).
5. Provision of care over an extended period of time to ensure continuity. Transitions, including those to other pediatric providers or into the adult health care system, should be planned and organized with the child and family.
6. Identification of the need for consultation and appropriate referral to pediatric medical subspecialists and surgical specialists. (In instances in which the child enters the medical system through a specialty clinic, identification of the need for primary pediatric consultation and referral is appropriate.) Primary, pediatric medical subspecialty and surgical specialty care providers should collaborate to establish management plans in partnership with the child and family and to articulate everyone's role.
7. Interaction with early intervention programs, schools, early childhood education and child care programs, and other public and private community agencies to be certain that the special needs of the child and family are addressed.
8. Provision of care coordination services in which the family, the physician, and other service providers work to implement a specific care plan as an organized team.
9. Maintenance of an accessible, comprehensive, central record that contains all pertinent information about the child, while preserving confidentiality.

10. Provision of developmentally appropriate and culturally competent health assessments and counseling to ensure successful transition to adult-oriented health care, work, and independence in a deliberate, coordinated way.[53]

The medical home encompasses the full range of clinical service provision for individual children. It is the ideal that child health providers aspire to and that child health advocates continue to fight for. Not all children have access to a medical home, and many practitioners find that they have to justify the work that they do over and over to insurers. It is somewhat ironic that payers, many of whom clamor for "managed care," seem to have trouble grasping the notion that the coordination of care that can be accomplished through the medical home has huge cost saving implications. Chapter 7 is a discussion of the professional advocacy needed to translate to insurers and business people the value that they will purchase by supporting high-quality clinical care as delivered through the medical home.

Group Advocacy 5

ADVANCES IN CHILD HEALTH often depend on someone recognizing a pattern. John Snow discovers that all his patients with debilitating diarrhea obtain their water from the Broad St. pump;[1] Martha Eliot observes that children from the cold, dark north are far more likely to suffer from rickets than children from the sunny south;[2] Steven Gortmaker and William Dietz find that boys and girls who watch many hours of television are heavier than their peers who spend time playing outside.[3] Patterns, commonalities, associations, group characteristics—they may be so clear that any alert high school senior can appreciate them or they may be so subtle that only health service researchers using statistical analyses can discern them. However the pictures emerge, clinicians respond by tailoring interventions to alleviate common problems. This is group advocacy.

By aggregating children and studying their similar experience, advocates find the point where change can happen. If the middle school principal discovers that a high proportion of her students are complaining of headaches, then the group who need attention are all the children in that school. If the problem is that all the 8th graders have jumped two percentiles in their BMI (body mass index) weight category, the group is those children as well as the students in the two grades below. The younger children belong in the group because weight gain is the result of long-term exposure and well-established eating habits. Group response also has built-in efficiencies and economies of scale. Why should a pediatrician's office assistant spend time translating the same document into Creole each time a Haitian family turns up? Doing the work once, printing it up, and making the information available to all patients from the same ethnic group saves everyone time and effort.

Children and youth can be grouped by a variety of characteristics, including the nature of their biological impairment, their age, socioeconomic status, and cultural heritage or the language that they or their parents speak. Groups can be based on a particular outcome, such as failure to thrive or conductive hearing loss. Grouping may also be intervention based. Groups may be large or small, multiproblem or single focus. Child health advocates often define a group in response to a service concern, but forming a group also greatly facilitates research opportunities.

In all fields of medicine, subspecialists routinely use grouping techniques. By bringing patients with similar characteristics together, clinical investigators improve their observations, generate hypotheses, and test new interventions. One might well ask, how advocacy for a class or group of children is different from traditional subspecialty care. The answer is that there are many similarities but two substantial differences. Group advocacy expands the domains of investigation and calls on expertise from community members and families.

What do we mean by expanding the domains? In group advocacy, child health professionals look for patterns beyond those defined by organ systems. A 2003 Commonwealth Fund study shows that adults with cardiac disease benefited enormously from new high-technology interventions.[4] That was the subspecialty look. The authors then imposed the category *insurance status* on the data analysis and found that high technology was saving lives but not of those without insurance. Heart attack victims who were uninsured were 7 percent less likely to have access to invasive cardiac care than insured patients. The authors estimated that this lack of high technology treatment led to a loss of $6 million to $28 million in medical and death-related costs, a societal cost over and above the burden the patients had to bear. Here is the expansion beyond subspecialty care. A new element of group or subgroup advocacy is required to deal with the insurance dilemma, which is a very real and measurable contributor to morbidity and mortality.

The other element that makes group advocacy different from standard subspecialty care is the explicit construction of partnerships among clinicians, community-based organizations, and families. In subspecialty care the doctor is generally the expert on most topics, but in group advocacy the expertise is shared. Clinicians who succeed in group advocacy recognize that they have only a limited number of puzzle pieces in their own hands. To complete the picture, they enter into partnerships with the community members, family experts, and sometimes with children and youth as well.

Problems of Grouping

Chapter 3 presents contemporary child health trends. The patterns that the demographers and epidemiologists see on the national level play out on the local level as well. Poor children in inner-city Detroit have more health problems than affluent children who live in Grosse Pointe. Racial disparities are present in every community. The Hmong children in Minneapolis have more health problems than children in the general population, and the Hopis in the four-corners states are far more likely to be hospitalized than the Anglos who live there. Language barriers affect patient-professional communication in Los Angeles as much as they do in Honolulu. The patterns are all there, but they are not all the same. There is a local flavor and a particular spin. One community is child friendly, another community is indifferent to children and families, and still another is actively hostile to young people. Because of all of these local factors, the way program planners go about assigning identity to a group matters.

Amartya Sen, the Nobel laureate economist, warns about identity assignment. He says of himself, "I can be at the same time an Asian, an Indian citizen, a U.S. resident, a British academic, a Bengali with Bangladeshi ancestry, a graduate of two colleges in two different countries, an atheist with a Hindu background, a non-Brahmin, an economist, a researcher and teacher in philosophy, a Sanskritist, a married man, a feminist, a defender of gay rights, a nonbeliever in afterlife and also beforelife, and a nonbeliever also in frequent visits by extraterrestrial aliens in austere spaceships, but a believer in the view that if such aliens do exist, they ought to make their spaceships a lot jollier and more colorful."[5] Any individual, Sen says, has multiple simultaneous identities, none of which defines him but all of which taken together describe his life experience. Although categorization allows us to gather people into useful associations, it carries with it the risk of setting Hutu against Tootsi, North Korean against South Korean, Kurd against Turk. There can be interminable conflict when the identity of one group is defined by a common hatred of "the other."

For clinicians, there are tensions in placing children in groups. The trick is to use identifiers for grouping but to not to allow them to constrain. Clinicians want to be able to use similar characteristics to target appropriate services; at the same time, they want to avoid stereotypes and biases. Complicated at best. To see just how complicated, let's think about a child and play out Professor Sen's argument about multiple identities.

The child is a schoolboy of Chinese heritage living in a wealthy Midwest neighborhood. He has a chronic illness. His parents and grandparents are professionals; in fact, all six are in dentistry. The child speaks only English; he does not know a word of Mandarin or Cantonese. Based on these facts, the child would fit into many identities: he is school-aged, male, a child with special health care needs, an Asian American. He is nonpoor and nonbilingual. He may be pre-professional. Each of these descriptions might lead us to classify the child into a particular group. Some of the characteristics might help us classify him correctly and help us design a good program for him; others presume a great deal about him, may or may not be true, and may lead us to make some very bad choices.

To get a full picture of what grouping might be beneficial for this boy, we need to know a great deal more. How severe is his chronic illness? Do his parents have adequate health insurance; have they reached their insurance cap? Does the boy also have a cognitive deficit, physical limitations, or emotional problems? Is he gifted? What grade is he in? Is it the right grade for his age? Does he want to learn more about his cultural background? Is he crazy about the Ohio State football team?[6] Is his family eager for him to be in the mainstream or do they want more specialized services for him? The answer to each question will determine whether he fits one or another category. As Amartya Sen points out, identities can be useful but only when their full impact is carefully considered.

Program developers often use grouping techniques for child health projects but not without substantial stress and strain. The planners know how important it is to identify the children and youth correctly, how essential it is to secure community and family support.[7] They also fear selecting one worthy group at the expense of another. They spend hours, weeks, or even years trying to decide what issue to go after, which group to serve, and how to be fair in divvying out whatever dollars, time, and talents are available.

Sometimes this process is so cumbersome, with Gaston waiting for Alphonse and Alphonse waiting for Gaston, that the planners actually waste precious time, energy, and talent. When such paralysis occurs the answer is for the planners to start somewhere, anywhere. Getting started on even the most meager something has the potential to improve conditions in general. Often when the program planners launch a new system for one group, it can be adapted for another group. Forward movement of any kind for anybody inspires others to get involved in group advocacy for children and youth.

This chapter discusses a number of successful group programs that have used age, socioeconomic status, culture, and clinical conditions as their organizing categories. No matter which classification is chosen, there are two principles and three steps that apply to all group advocacy. Let's look at these elements and then view how they play out in some exemplary group programs.

Guidelines for Grouping
Two Principles

Professional, Community, Family Partnerships

Chapter 4 includes a discussion of the importance of partnerships for individual advocacy. Partnerships are equally important for group advocacy. Partners work together to break traditional molds, to open up new possibilities, and to reinforce each other's initiatives. To form a partnership for group advocacy all of the members need to define clearly what the enterprise is and what part each will play. Forming partnerships depends on listening, translating. and time. Often a person who has traditionally been a leader has to relinquish the director's role. Frequently, funding compromises are required. Despite these complexities, there are success stories: all over the country organizations are forming partnerships, creating synergies, and flexing their collective muscle for the health of groups of children and youth. Community-based organizations, legal advocacy teams, the county public health department, the PTA, and the local Family Voices affiliate are combining efforts with child health practitioners in academic and community-based practice. Together, they tap latent energy and unleash power for change.

Sustainability

One of the biggest challenges for group advocacy is keeping the intervention going. When demonstrable concerns come to the forefront, imaginative program planners may respond with an intervention. The drama of the moment attracts attention and funding. The persuasive personality of the advocate gets an exciting group program off the ground. What is much more difficult is sustaining the effort over the long haul. To maintain the group advocacy program, the planners will do well to address several questions right at the beginning: Is there a specific end date for the intervention? Or do we want this program to go on indefinitely? Are there markers to indicate that the intervention is having its desired effect? What funding streams are available? Are there other groups who could benefit and what would it do to take this effort to scale?

Three Steps

Identifying and Naming the Group

The first step in groups programming is defining an equitable and reliable identification process. How does the school health team find all the students with asthma? How does the local chapter of the American Academy of Pediatrics go about identifying recent immigrant children who are behind on their immunizations? What is the best way to locate all the children with special health care needs in the pediatric practice?

During the past ten to fifteen years, a number of clinical investigators have designed rigorous screening tools that neither underidentify nor overidentify a specific group of children and youth. Standardized and practical schemes are now available to identify children with special health care needs,[8] children with behavioral concerns,[9] children with missing immunizations,[10] children with developmental concerns,[11] adolescents who are experimenting with alcohol and drugs,[12] and for children in families experiencing domestic violence.[13] These tools exist and are standardized and validated, but putting them to use is a huge hurdle for advocates. Chapter 7 discusses this issue as one of the biggest current problems for professional advocacy.

Child health advocates find that naming the identified group can be helpful. The name should convey why the group has been formed without imposing unnecessary or incorrect labels on the children and youth. Conscientious program planners vet the name with families, clinicians, and policymakers to prevent misinterpretation. While terms like *at risk* and *underserved* may be true descriptors, they have a negative ring. Families do not like to hear their children being identified as *asthmatics* or *diabetics.* Person-first language, such as *children with asthma* and *children with diabetes,* acknowledges that the disease is only one characteristic in the child's makeup.[14] Using the group's name to communicate a sense of hope about the children and youth can be a constructive part of the intervention process. For instance, at the Children's Hospital Primary Care Center, the obesity group program is called One Step Ahead. The Massachusetts Foster Care program is Special Kids, Special Care.

Defining the Intervention

It is wise for program planners to ask themselves some hard questions about group intervention. Are we enhancing routine services? Is the program supplanting another program? Are we introducing new services? If so, what are they? Can we succinctly describe what we are doing? What do we plan to achieve and what is the time line for seeing a difference? What will the participants get? Who will conduct the intervention? How much input will there be from the participants? Who else can help with this?

The most successful group programs concentrate energy on one type of child or problem, but they derive that energy from multiple sources. To battle childhood obesity, the staff members in the clinic, the teachers in the school, the YMCA director, the church pastor, and the families all deliver the same message. They serve the same balanced nutrition. They all show up at the fitness fair. Activities are aligned and mutually reinforcing. Coordinating their separate actions is like using a magnifying glass to pull sunrays into a point. Anyone who has ever burned his name into a piece of wood using this technique knows how potent focused energy can be.

Monitoring and Evaluating Results

Documentation is a tedious chore, but it is essential to the long-term viability of any group program. Zealous program planners want to right wrongs as quickly as possible. In their hurry, they are at hazard of bypassing critical steps in the process. Preintervention assessments paint the picture of unmet needs: this many toddlers living in the 17th St. housing project are undernourished; the 8th graders of Central City have nowhere to go after school and the rate of teen violence is three times higher than in Jollyville; the use of steroids and strength-enhancing substances among high school athletes has skyrocketed in Middleton County. Preassessment figures like these are the "down" to go "up" from. They document the cold, hard facts.

The other set of helpful numbers are the benchmarks or goals. By three years from now, 95–100 percent of the children in the 17th St. housing project will have achieved a normal height and weight (individual outcomes); every six months there will be the addition of twenty more after-school slots in Central City (proxy, process measure), and three years from now the number of arrests for violent crime by teenagers will be half what it is today (program outcome); as a result of the project, coaches will be held liable for any infraction of the interscholastic drug ban and may lose their jobs if the ban is not enforced on their team (associated program outcome).

Systems of Grouping

Program planners who follow the two principles and the three steps spelled out above avoid serious pitfalls in group advocacy. Below, are examples of group advocacy programs that are making a difference with long-term, high-impact interventions. They address a variety of conditions and problems, but all do so with a systematic approach and careful attention to history, current context, and community liabilities and assets.

There are many different ways to think about organizing groups and, as Amartya Sen points out, putting any individual into a classification immediately delimits and excludes basic characteristics of that person's being. But when the sun comes up, the day needs to get started, patients are lining up at the registration desk; the practical reality is that it can be very useful to group by common characteristics such as age, experience, social situation, and clinical condition. Below are some examples of group programming and advocacy.

Grouping by Age

Advocacy for groups may quite naturally be based on age. Children and youth at the extremes of the age spectrum have significantly different health concerns. Advocacy for young children might focus on outcomes such as language development, linear growth, appropriate weight gain, and kindergarten readiness, while the staff of a teen enterprise might aim to address coping with peer pressure, comfort with body image, and healthy decisions regarding drugs, alcohol, and sexuality. Programs for very young children incorporate family and community in decisions. Programs for adolescents direct all decisions to the young person but encourages them to check in with their family and community.

Early Childhood

Early childhood is a prime time for health and developmental intervention. As young families welcome their new baby, they need encouragement, information, and role modeling. They are eager to get together with other new moms and dads. Parents are their children's best teachers and advocates. In general, parental instinct guides young mothers and fathers fairly well. But not all child rearing is intuitive, and even the most knowledgeable parents encounter situations that stump them, be it establishing and maintaining breast-feeding, consoling colicky 3-month-olds, settling toddlers to sleep, or managing the inevitable temper tantrums in 2-year-olds.

Good evidence establishes the short- and long-term payoff of multidisciplinary early childhood activities.[15] In addition to routine health care maintenance, early childhood program staff deliver nutritional counseling, breast-feeding support, immunization assurance, developmental and educational input, home visiting for safety reviews, literacy enrichment, and parent behavioral education. Successful early childhood enhancement activities take advantage of the strengths and resources in families and communities. No two early childhood programs are completely alike, but all of them emphasize teaching parents about child developmental stages.

One example of a popular early childhood intervention is the Touchpoints model developed by Berry Brazelton.[16] As a result of years of private practice and getting in tune with babies and their parents, Brazelton believes there is an enormous payoff when adults "listen to the child." Using his observational skills and deep understanding of child development, he has taught several hundred thousand parents the impressive repertoire of the young child's behavior. At the first pediatric checkup, he plays a little game. He deftly places the baby between himself and the child's mother; then he and the mother hold a whispering competition in the baby's two ears. When the mother "wins" as the baby turns his head preferentially in her direction, Brazelton points out that the baby is making distinctions between the two voices. The infant is drawing the first broad outlines of the sensorineural map that he will add to for the rest of his life. At subsequent well-child visits, Brazelton uses similar demonstrations of the child's emerging behaviors to help parents anticipate the growth and development that lie ahead. His Touchpoints system is incorporated into early childhood and clinical programs throughout the United States.

This all sounds nice, but what does it matter if a parent listens to her child? What difference does it make if there is a mobile above the baby's bassinette? How can it possibly be important that a baby learn to soothe himself or that the toilet training process goes off without causing too much family turmoil? These things do matter, profoundly. For many years, child development theory has held that what happens in infancy and early childhood sets the emotional and cognitive stage for later developmental outcomes. Building on the Freudian model, Erik Erikson published his now classic "Eight Stages of Man" in 1956.[17] His developmental theory provides the conceptual framework for most subsequent child development work. Erikson contends that the task of infancy is to resolve the conflict between trust and mistrust and that all subsequent human interaction derives to some extent from how this most basic interaction plays out.

Absence of a positive early experience can be disastrous. Children suffering from severe neglect (such as children in orphanages) do not establish basic trust. Lacking early physical and cognitive stimulation, they do not grow well. They can even be so starved for emotional engagement that they die. New evidence from Felton Earls's work on the Chicago Longitudinal Study gets at the mechanism of how abuse and neglect effect development.[18] Punitive treatment of young children teaches them to see themselves as "bad." Never experiencing attention for what they do right, they lay down patterns of behavior that too often lead to negative long-term consequences, the worst of which is criminality.

The actual structure of the young baby's brain forms in response to external stimulation.[19] Brain interconnections are constructed during fetal life and on into the first few years of life. Early in gestation, neural cells differentiate and find their anatomic homes in predictable spaces in the brain. The developing cortex seeks and receives information from the outside world. The 7-month-old fetus, in training for life outside the womb, thrusts his little fist or foot. These movements also represent actions directed by the developing brain. Action, reaction, stimulation, information: that's what happens if I kick, that's what happens if I jab.

When the baby is born, the full interaction of neural tissue and outside world comes to fruition. Outside the protection of the uterus, the baby is immediately exposed to massive stimulation. Flashing lights, darkness-brightness, the strong odor of delivery room disinfectants, voices, beeps, clicks, the delicious taste of the mother's milk, the feel of tender stroking on the newborn skin. Each of these sensations telegraphs direct signals to the baby's relatively unorganized cortex. Not much of the barrage makes sense to those naïve cells. Over the millions and billions of subsequent nanoseconds, the baby's brain begins to sort through the chaos of the short electrical messages coming from the music box, Uncle Scott's tickle, and Aunt Noriko's perfume.

Mothers always win Berry Brazelton's whispering contest because even the smallest baby can distinguish signal from noise by recognizing recurrent patterns. The consistent and familiar frequency of the mother's voice elicits an, Aha, I know that JodieJodieJodieJodie from somewhere. Signals transmitted to the cortex in the same way over and over predominate over the background confusion. The familiar signals add up to build something bigger and more permanent. To incorporate these recurring messages, the brain begins to manufacture the chemical and electrical scaffolding of dendrites and neurotransmitters and synapses. Out of disorder, slowly, steadily, predictably, order emerges.

In 1981 David Hubel and Torsten Wiessel won the Nobel Prize for their elegant research demonstrating that the order in the cortex, its very physical structure, *requires* the bombardment of outside stimulation.[20] Without sights, sounds, and smells the alert and ready neurons wither; they have no connections to make. The brain does not organize; it cannot grow. Hubel and Wiessel's work shows that if a newborn kitten's eyes are deprived of light, their occipital cortex will not develop. The neurophysiologists won the world's most prestigious prize in science because they proved that what happens outside the baby's body—in the nursery, in the kitchen, on the street—literally, physically, determines how the child's neurons and brain are assembled. When Dad takes Junior in the Snugli to the neighborhood grocery store the experience helps construct the template for all further development and cognitive understanding. Every experience matters.

Early childhood programs are built on an understanding of the critical nature of such early experience. Throughout the United States these programs are constituted in a variety of ways. Some are based in health departments, some in primary care centers. Some are the outreach arm of a nursing program or a local school. The programs derive their funding from various sources, including philanthropy and local, state and federal funds. The names of the programs are upbeat: Healthy Families America, Healthy Child Care America, Early Head Start, Healthy Steps, HIPPY, Parents as Teachers. They have in common the goal of making sure that young families have what they need to celebrate the unfolding of their young child's abilities.

Premature Birth

Born too early, before their parents or the community are ready, premature infants do constant battle just to stay alive until their due dates. High-frequency ventilation, emergency surgery, exquisite management of fluids and nutrients, treatment with antibiotics and anticonvulsants rescue them in many life-threatening situations until, alive, little, and kicking, they are ready to graduate from the neonatal intensive care unit (NICU). And then what happens? We actually know the answer to that question because of group advocacy. That advocacy has taken two forms: the meticulous tracking of data bases and the institution of NICU follow-up care.

Maureen Hack, Marie McCormick, and others have compiled data on the outcomes of neonatal intensive care.[21] Through grouping children by birth weight categories (less than 1,000 grams, 1,500 grams, or 2,000 grams) and by time of delivery (less than 27 weeks, 30 weeks, 34 weeks, 37 weeks, and so on), epidemiologists have provided the field of neonatology with invaluable information about NICU care. These data assist advocates for group programming and inform arguments for health care and research dollars.

Doctors and psychologists in NICU follow-up clinics monitor the babies' health, growth, and development. NICU graduates who had respiratory disease as a result of their premature birth are at risk for long-term lung complications. They need careful pulmonary monitoring. Limited external contact and the prophylactic use of monoclonal antibody prevents life-threatening infection with respiratory syncytial virus infection in many of these children. Children with cardiac and gastrointestinal concerns also benefit from NICU graduate follow-up in coordination with the subspecialty care they receive from their cardiologists and gastroenterologists. In general, premature infants are more prone to the ear infections and hearing loss secondary to such infections than are babies born at term. NICU follow-up programs alert the babies' physicians and day care centers about this so that they will note signs of poor hearing or delayed language acquisition.

Many babies with very low birth weight will "fail to thrive"; all of them will be stunted as young adults.[22] As many as 20 percent of children who were less than 1,000 grams at birth will have significant developmental delay and ongoing central nervous system disorder such as cerebral palsy and seizure disorder.[23] Long-term follow-up into school age demonstrates a recurrent, clear pattern of learning problems and behavioral concerns among NICU graduates.[24] Premature infants have spatial difficulties and math-related learning problems. In some series, as many as 16 percent are diagnosed as having ADHD.[25] Now that researchers and clinicians recognize these patterns, early childhood specialists and special educators are designing preschool and school-based approaches that take their specialized learning styles into account.

Teen Parents

When a 15-year-old patient sits in the pediatric waiting room holding her newborn on her lap, the normal celebration that attends childbearing is muted. Caregivers, parents, friends all know that the new mother has foreclosed options for personal growth and that this new baby is at high risk. Everything may seem fine, but the odds are not in his favor. Group advocacy for teen parents can change those odds.

In the 1980s adolescent medicine physicians argued that teen mothers were not getting the special attention they needed when they were pitched, undifferentiated, into ob-gyn prenatal and postpartum clinics. The alternative of having them cared for by their pediatricians was no better. As pregnant women and as mothers, the girls required specialized treatment, which pediatricians were ill equipped to offer. The "teen-tot" model solved the dilemma. A specially designed clinical program could address the health and social care needs of both the young mother and her baby.[26]

Typically, in group programs for teen parents, the mother comes to the same team of doctors and nurses for her postpartum checkups as for the baby's well-child appointment. In addition to gynecologic assessment, the team social workers arrange for high school completion classes (the GED) and vocational training. They advocate for the mothers not to lose out on the chances that other girls their age have. A key component of the model is parenting classes. The new role of mother is hard for any woman but especially hard for teenagers. Curricula such as the one designed by HighScope in Ypsilanti, Michigan, are tailored especially for teenage parents.[27] The young mother's focus on her own development is very intense. She is preoccupied and scared. The program staff must handle the teenager's concerns about her relationship with her boyfriend, her teachers, and her parents before they introduce the lessons about the baby's emerging development.

Advocacy for teen parents and their babies is accomplished by arranging community-based parenting classes at times and places that make them easily accessible. The work is compelling but exceedingly hard. Imagine ten 16-year-olds with babies in tow from ages 2 weeks to 2 years. One of the mothers lives with her boyfriend, one with her husband. Three of the young women are still at home with their own parents. Three move again and again between the streets and homeless shelters. The other two are fairly settled with grandmothers and great aunts. They speak of the "baby's father." In some cases the young parents' relationship has been casual at best. In others it has been turbulent, even violent. The parenting educator talks about routine and stability and the importance of consistency to nurture the baby's sense of trust. And she will wonder if there will ever be any such stability in the world of either the child or the mother.

Recognizing that teen fathers often abandon girls when they become pregnant, some young parents' programs are reaching out to these fathers, who are disenfranchised with regard to health care and other social services. Programs focusing on them offer classes on relationships, parenting, job opportunities, and other age-relevant topics.

Gay and Lesbian Youth

Most gay and lesbian youth are as healthy as any other teenager. They have normal questions about their height, their size, and their zits. They have the same aspirations for success in school as the straight students sitting next to them in the boring 11th-grade biology class. They want to find fulfilling relationships and lifelong stability with a partner who shares their values and joys. They are aware that there are ways to stay healthy, and they are more than willing to receive health education, to use condoms, to avoid smoking, to respect state laws regarding underage drinking. Too often the media, and even the medical literature, portray the dangers of the gay lifestyle. Such scary publicity unfairly marginalizes these young people.

The newspapers, magazines, and health journals are not entirely wrong, though. There is a subset of gay and lesbian youth who do have very serious health and mental health problems. Among this group, rates of drug abuse, alcoholism, unsafe sexual practices, depression, and suicide are high.[28] These teenagers may be running away both figuratively and literally from real and imagined demons in their lives. Some gay and lesbian youth have long histories of rejection and even abuse. Some come from family situations that are rife with conflict, violence, drugs, and alcohol. Other young people struggle continually with understanding their sexual orientation and are severely confused about what the changes and feelings in their bodies and minds mean. Finally, no matter how healthy and well-adjusted gay and lesbian youth are, almost all have periodic worries about where they fit and how others perceive them. Because of these special health and mental health concerns for gay and lesbian youth, there is a need for specialized health services delivered by doctors and nurses who understand the complex interplay of biology, emotion, cognition, and social elements.

The sad fact is that gay and lesbian youth are tremendously medically underserved. They can be socially segregated and disenfranchised in many communities. In urban areas, adult gay community agencies may proffer a small nod to the health care needs of teenagers who are going through the throes of gender identity confusion, but teenagers are often uncomfortable or even wary of such programs. In rural areas, even such minimal services are generally not available.

Fortunately, there are hopeful signs on the horizon. Little by little, around the United States, child health advocates are launching experimental projects to provide health care services for gay and lesbian adolescents. The Sidney Borum Health Center doors are open to gay and lesbian high school and college students in the Boston area. At Children's Memorial in Chicago, the Adolescent Medicine Division has extensive community-based ties with organizations run by gay and lesbian youth. Physicians at the Kapiolani Medical Center in Honolulu are working to understand how culture and minority gender status intertwine as either risk or protective factors.[29]

One of the most difficult dilemmas for clinicians who open up their doors or go out seeking to provide health care services to gay and lesbian or other disenfranchised youth is getting paid to do this work. It can be an enormous task to convince health insurance companies to pay for services for young people who are adamant about keeping their health and social information away from their parents.

Grouping by Social Factors

Foster Children, Adopted Children

Children in foster care are at risk of a large number of health, developmental, emotional, and cognitive problems.[30] While not all children in foster care have suffered previous abuse or neglect, many have. Moreover, the very process of being in substitute care or up for adoption is fraught with difficult passages. Two steps forward toward potential placement and one step back to try reunification is the dance pattern that many small children know all too well. The steps and the music are both familiar and menacing.

Most children in foster care move helter-skelter from one health clinic to the next. As the doctor thumbs through the child's chart, she knows she is in for a difficult encounter. She will take the history from the new foster mother, who will do her best but will have only partial information. The doctor must search through the scattered notations of two or three other physicians, who have had the same experience. Nobody is quite sure if the child had too many or too few shots. To be certain that the child is fully immunized, the doctor will probably institute the catch-up series, without any assurance that someone hasn't done that six months ago. When the nurse arrives with the needles, the child's grimace may tell all—but then the child has been through so much anyway.

Anybody with half an eye can see the waste and frustration in such a nonsystem of care, but inertia is the world's strongest force and "we've always done it this way" the commonest theme song. Heather Forkey and several residents in the community-based clinic affiliated with the Children's Hospital of Philadelphia (CHOP) finally got fed up with the same old, same old. The situation was disheartening for them, for the foster parents, and for the children.

Forkey worked with the clinic and with the Philadelphia social service agencies to arrange a primary care group program for children in foster care. As a result, CHOP faculty and residents now serve their patients in foster care in a much more coordinated fashion. They keep careful and detailed records and educate the foster parents about the children's health histories and current health conditions. They look for signs of developmental delay or emotional aggression. They document any history suggestive of behavioral outburst, sleep disturbances, and incontinence. The doctors systematically review the children's immunization and medications histories and update any vaccinations that are missing. By building a special foster care primary care approach, the hit-or-miss aspect of health care for the children and youth is gone. Working together, the social service agency and the health care providers designed a straightforward process that (1) identifies the children, (2) enriches the health intake session, and (3) documents that session at both the health site and the foster care agency.

Forkey reports that the scale of the CHOP program is small compared to the foster care needs in Philadelphia. An advocacy coalition she and others began as residents in 1996 still meets regularly to improve overall conditions for children in foster care. While their work on health care is far from finished, the standard for clinical care has clearly been established.

Uninsured, Displaced, and Homeless Children

In 2002 more than 8 million American children were uninsured. Although this is appreciably better than the 11 million children and youth who lacked health insurance in the late 1990s, it is still an unacceptable number. It is particularly unacceptable in light of the State Child Health Insurance Program (SCHIP; see discussion in chapter 6), which should have remedied the health insurance problem among children. The experience with SCHIP has proved the adage that no matter what happens in the halls of Congress, all real solutions happen at the local level. Once the SCHIP program was passed, it was imperative that community-based group programs reach out to families and children in a concrete, step-by-step fashion. Here was another critical type of group advocacy for child health providers.

In 1997 Joseph Carrillo, the medical director of the Martha Eliot Health Center in Jamaica Plain in Boston, formed a coalition with parents and with representatives the Bromley Health Housing Development, the Head Start agency, the local Boston public school, and several other community-based organizations. The coalition mapped out a strategy to enroll at least a thousand children in Medicaid over the next nine to twelve months. They printed brochures and fliers; they silk-screened the logo, *1000 More Healthy Kids* on T-shirts and baseball caps; they showed up everywhere: PTA meetings, church suppers, basketball games. Before their deadline, they had enrolled more than 1,300 children. Perhaps as gratifying, they had also signed up hundreds of parents. Their group advocacy worked because they were sure of the need, had a clear message, and persisted until they reached their goal. They also succeeded because they approached the same problem from every angle they could think of and made the most of the community's strengths and resources.

Delivering health care to unserved and underserved has been brilliantly addressed by the Mailman Center for Child Development at the University of Miami Miller School of Medicine. Several mornings a week, Arturo Brito reports to the loading dock where the Pediatric Mobile Clinic is parked. He jumps inside the cab alongside the driver and literally rides his clinic to work. The Mobile Clinic regularly visits areas of Miami-Dade County where nearly half the children and families are classified as undocumented aliens. These are families from all over the Caribbean and Central and South America who have made the journey to Miami with the hope of making a new life, free from political oppression, poverty, hunger, and despair. They have found less than they dreamed of. But for underinsured, uninsured, and undocumented children, this clinic offers comprehensive and extended primary care, including basic screenings, immunizations, diagnostic workups, and management of common and complex illnesses. Without this clinic, many children in South Florida would otherwise remain invisible to the conventional health care system. By focusing his energies on and documenting the status of children living in these circumstances, advocates like Arturo Brito are able to go the next step toward larger solutions.

Children who are homeless are the most disenfranchised of all. Nothing in their lives is stable or regular. They shuttle from one temporary setting to another. One week they are sleeping at the domestic violence shelter; the next week it is a welfare motel; before you know it they are tripled up in their cousin's apartment. They attend one school for two or three months, and then the vagaries of the complex situation they are in send them packing to another town and a whole new set of books, teachers, and classmates. Their health care is completely disrupted, with no continuity between providers.

In Sacramento, California, homelessness contributes significantly to children's disease and maladaptation. Many of the homeless families and youth are newly arrived immigrants from Southeast Asia or Mexico who have found their way to the fertile farming area of Northern California. Unfortunately, population growth has outpaced the housing and social service capacity. In 2000 between 400 and 1,000 children and youth ages 12–20 were homeless, with more than 200 being turned away from shelters each month.[31] Clifford Yee, a physician in training at the University of California at Davis, decided to advocate for this a group of homeless children and youth. He collaborated with the state public health authorities and Health Care for the Homeless to establish a pediatric well-child clinic in an old firehouse. The HOPE Clinic became an integral part of the training program for all residents at the medical school. In their third year of residency, the doctors provide well-child examinations, immunizations, and vision and hearing screening two days a week to a children who otherwise might not interact with the health care system for years— and then most likely for a preventable condition.

Grouping by National, Ethnic, or Cultural Attributes

In Indianapolis Sarah Stelzner began to notice that many of her Spanish-speaking patients were children of Mexican farmworkers who move up and down the Mississippi River Valley. Probing more into the situation, she learned of the Texas Migrant Council, a multistate, binational association. By thinking of the children as members of a group, she was able to establish a medical home for them at the Wishard Memorial Hospital. Through the medical home, the children have electronic medical records accessible to families and health providers along the migrant route. Stelzner was also able to access educational programming for her patients through the Texas Migrant Head Start Program. It wouldn't matter now if in July Juan's family were working in the rice paddies of Mississippi or in May if they were picking corn in Iowa. Wherever the family was along the route, their little boy would be able to continue his preschool learning in a safe and accommodating Head Start classroom.

Nicole Prudent grew up in Haiti and still has family roots there. She knows the ins and outs of the politics that have caused nightmarish disruptions for families on an almost annual basis. She knows when there is likely to be an influx of families arriving from Port-au-Prince desperately seeking a new life, often without legal documentation, without jobs or transferable skills, and often without having finished their education.

Prudent arranges medical and social programs to help parents cope with the new pressures they face raising their children in a new culture where the opportunities and customs clash with the old. She developed a program to help families who have children with mental retardation overcome stigma and find appropriate services. She spearheaded a system of support for Haitian youth who have lost their parents to HIV disease. She reaches out to women with HIV disease and uses group dynamics to increase adherence to medication. She also creates mentoring opportunities for youth interested in a health careers; many of them are her patients.

In San Francisco, the Tung Wah Dispensary (later named the Chinese Hospital) was established in the early twentieth century by missionaries because Chinese patients could not receive care in the traditional health facilities in the city.[32] When the bubonic plague was introduced from Asia into the Bay Area in the early 1900s, a complex of political, business, and public health factors led city authorities to decree a quarantine on the Chinese workers. Overt racism exacerbated an already difficult and dangerous situation by further limiting the access of Chinese families to San Francisco's health care institutions. In the early twenty-first century the citizens of San Francisco's Chinatown would, of course, not be excluded from health care clinics or hospitals because of their ethnic background. But lack of insurance could keep them away. Many families in Chinatown run small businesses such as restaurants, laundries, and small grocery or specialty stores. A small business often means no health insurance coverage, and lack of insurance puts a big damper on access to health care. In the early 1980s, by pulling together a large group of Chinese families, the Chinese Hospital was able to work with Blue Shield of California to form the Chinese Community Health Plan. Here was group advocacy creating an innovative health maintenance organization (HMO) for patients who wanted to receive their health care within a health system built around their culture.

Grouping by Clinical Conditions

Children with HIV/AIDS

By 2002, 9,300 U.S. children under age 13 had been diagnosed with HIV, nearly 6,600 youth (13–19) were reported with HIV/AIDS, and 80,000 children and adolescents were AIDS orphans.[33] HIV is not one problem. It is the confluence of medical troubles, family devastation, and community disruption. Group programming is a practical response that can take into account the health of the parents; the health of the child; contingencies in the case of the death of the parents; premorbid conditions such as drug abuse among family members; living conditions; access to food; the willingness or the ability of the caretakers to administer complex drug regimens; the cognitive, developmental, and emotional status of the children; and stigma and community intolerance.

The challenges of HIV infection are so all encompassing that the solutions have to come from many sectors. In Wisconsin, public health, specialty and primary care providers got together in 1991 to form a statewide network with responsibility for the care of all children with HIV.[34] Data suggested that there would be 200 pediatric patients by 2000 but that they would be located all over the state. Solo, rural practitioners might have one or two youngsters with HIV in their practice, but the distance to Milwaukee would prohibit frequent visits to a medical or social care center. Mindful of the high costs of caring for children with chronic conditions, the planning committee wanted their network to fit into to the existing HMO infrastructure. At the same time, they wanted the HMOs to work through a centrally coordinated network to optimize the specialty and social service consultation available to the children

To ensure high-quality care, the Wisconsin HIV Primary Care Support Network built a team and clearly specified the roles of each player. The central team took on the functions of gathering data, updating clinical protocols, and ensuring that each child was receiving the most effective treatments and appropriate monitoring. The local providers ensured local care and culturally appropriate community support. When there were extraordinary circumstances (hospitalization, death of a parent), all team members would collaborate to augment the medical and social care. Keeping an effective program like the Wisconsin Network together is a tall order, involving high staff input and considerable energy. Funding for the coordination of the network is always at hazard, and program directors continually need to justify the program to keep external funding coming in. Chapter 7 discusses how professional advocacy is required to make the case over and over again.

Pediatric HIV group work also focuses on those young people who are at risk of acquiring AIDS, especially homeless youth, runaways, and throwaways. School and street outreach approaches have been highly successful in containing the HIV epidemic among teenagers. In 1985 statisticians were drawing frightening graphs with logarithmic growth of HIV cases, predicting that there would be massive spread among adolescents and young adults. A popular AIDS awareness poster traced the infection from John to Sam to Bill to Susan to Greg to Aisha, and on and on. In the face of crisis, there was a prompt marriage of public and private health interests and resources and an all-hands-on-deck mentality that led to a general willingness to follow the leadership of Surgeon General C. Everett Koop. While Koop's leadership facilitated a response, it was the creativity of those who put together group programs at the local level responsive to local conditions that made the difference.

In downtown Boston, Maurice Melchiono, a nurse practitioner with the newly formed Children's Hospital AIDS Program, and the leadership of BAGLY (the Boston Alliance of Gay and Lesbian Youth) arranged the first-ever installation of condom machines in the gay bars. In Jamaica Plain, with its large Latino immigrant population, Cathy Samples began Project Protection, a community-based HIV prevention-education program. The owners of bodegas, barber shops, beauty parlors, check-cashing establishments, and clothing stores joined the campaign, putting a red *Use One/Usalos* condom sticker on their shop windows and made condoms available to their customers. In adolescent clinics, prep schools, and college health centers, nurses placed large goldfish bowls filled with condoms in the waiting rooms and lavatories. In large ways and small, each of these activities added to an enormous, national group program to stem the tide of HIV.

While the success of these programs is apparent in the improving health statistics in the United States, the problem of HIV/AIDS is far from solved and the salience of programs of outreach and education is as high as it was at the height of the epidemic. In the absence of continual reminders, celebrity spokespeople, and a steady stream of media spots and news stories, there is the possibility of an increase in the virus's spread. In the absence of public outcry, the job of the public health and pediatric communities is to make HIV/AIDS prevention a routine part of health care maintenance. Thus the special group emphasis finds its way back into the general clinical service provision. Children who have contracted HIV/AIDS require intensive group advocacy. Clinical advocacy is also needed to make sure that other children and adolescents never enter that specialized group.

Children with Special Health Care Needs

Children with special health care needs represent 13 percent of the nation's child population.[35] These children have ongoing demands for health care that are more than those required by an average child. While two-thirds of these children have only moderate and intermittent needs, the other third are quite incapacitated and depend on daily medicines or procedures. Because of their medical conditions, these children face uphill climbs in most aspects of their lives. The path is made smoother by accommodations in the community and at school.

Group advocacy for special-needs children at the community level can ensure that a teenager with end-stage renal disease can receive peritoneal dialysis in the school health office and that another child can receive gastrostomy feedings at the local Head Start. Group programming involves a complex array of activities that muster the help of family members, physicians, nurses, and community agencies. Having the community ready and prepared saves children and families from lost school and work hours and keeps the children's daily schedule as regular as possible.

Child health providers who care for large numbers of such children quickly find that if they want to serve their patients well they must speak up. To get the equipment and supplies for the children on a timely basis, they perfect case arguments. They learn how to say, You must! when the insurance companies say, We can't. They say yes more forcefully when they hear no from nursing companies and community agencies that say they are not equipped to include the children on their rosters. To deal with the needs of the families, advocates experiment with expanded hours, with health care information data sheets, with call-in hours.

Six Boston-area physician practices recognized the commonalities in the advocacy approaches they were taking and banded together to develop a loose association called the Pediatric Alliance for Coordinated Care (PACC).[36] Together with physicians at the Children's Hospital they designed a group program that expanded their capability to care for the children needing special health care in their practices. The PACC physicians formalized a number of components of care, including (1) an identification system to flag children with complex health care needs, (2) case coordination by a specially trained nurse practitioner, (3) use of an individualized health plan (IHP) for each of the children, and (4) regular input from a family consultant.

The nurse practitioner advocates on an individual basis for each of the children in the group but also leverages services and resources from the community for the group as a whole. The nurse practitioner is the point person who performs a triage function for a large number of children. Nursing agencies, public health personnel, and insurance company case managers respect her assessment of the general situation and are likely to follow her suggestions.

The individualized health plan is a powerful advocacy tool. Written by the health care provider along with the child's parents, the IHP contains information on the child's condition, his most recent health procedures (or hospital admissions), his medication, and any emergency procedures and therapy (occupational, speech, and physical) he has undergone. Each IHP contains a section on goals for the future, the road map for advocacy. As the health care provider works with numerous patients, he hears one after another parent report their dreams. When the third or fourth mother voices the wish that her child could attend a particular after-school program, just the way other kids in town do, the pattern is clear and the advocacy moment has come.

Family consultants associated with clinical practices for children with special health care needs advocate for individual children as they usher new families into the program, give them the telephone number of a willing listener, and share parenting tips. As part of the PACC project, Linda Freeman, the family consultant, produced a disability etiquette sheet that helps practitioners check themselves on how savvy they are about what makes for a disability-aware setting and what doesn't. This tip sheet has helped practitioners identify simple situations that make families of children with disabilities feel uncomfortable.

In group advocacy, each experience builds on the last, to create a system of expertise. The clinicians, families, and community representatives who work on each problem learn to count on each other, to know when to call, to know when to expect a call back. The team aspect of group advocacy allows a full range of health and community services for children and families.

6   Legislative Advocacy

THERE ARE AT LEAST THREE REASONS to confront child health problems through the policy route: social justice, administrative burden, and creative pragmatism. Driven by concerns for justice, some child health advocates deem that societal forces are hurting rather than helping children. They find it unfair that any child lacks health insurance or that any family is forced to choose among fundamentals such as food, shelter, day care, and health care. Appalled that children are denied resources, they look to the promises of the Constitution to address basic human concerns. Administrators and health care managers select the legislative path when the poor functioning of their systems convinces them that the general health care system is out of kilter. When their clinics and hospitals are subsidizing health care services that others should be paying for, these managers quite naturally look to the legislature for fiscal relief. Innovative program planners move to the 20,000-foot view and ask basic questions about how societal priority is driven. These activists suggest legislative and systems solutions that churn up the old order. They dare to design new policies. They propose change through stepwise action.

Table 6.1 lists federal legislation passed between 1916 and 1997 that supports the activities of child health clinicians. These laws set standards and regulate public and private systems. They provide money and personnel to health care agencies to immunize children, build clinic buildings, screen for hearing problems, and test for lead poisoning. The laws launched discretionary programs for babies with thalassemia, for example. They allowed for pilot testing of health surveys in school and alternative therapies at home. Through the policy route, advocates have made sustainable change for children and youth on the local, state, and national levels.

The chapter outlines the legislative process and defines principles of legislative and systems-level advocacy. A review of four major pieces of child health legislation (Title V, Medicaid, SCHIP, and IDEA) illustrates these principles. Literally thousands of child health advocates worked to establish these major laws. Knowledge of the provisions of these four

144

Table 6.1. Major Child Health and Health-Related Federal Legislation, 1916–97

Year	Legislation	Impact or Outcome
1916	Child Labor Act, P.L. 64-249	Prohibits interstate commerce of items produced by the labor of children under 16 years
1935	Title V of the Social Security Act, P.L. 74-271	Maternal and child health services, services for children with disabilities, child welfare
1946	Hospital Survey and Construction Act, P.L. 79-725	$75 million for the construction of hospitals after World War II
1955	Poliomyelitis Vaccination Assistance Act, P.L. 84-377	Virtual eradication of polio in the United States
1961	Community Health Services and Facilities Construction Act, P.L. 87-395	By 2005 there were 1,000 federally qualified health centers serving 15 million people in the United States
1962	Vaccination Assistance Act, P.L. 87-868	Control of diphtheria, tetanus, measles, mumps, rubella
1962	Establishment of National Institute of Child Health and Human Development, P.L. 87-838	Research on childhood illness with subsequent interventions to counteract disease
1965	Amendments to the Social Security Act Title XIX, Medicaid, P.L. 89-97	Established a program of health insurance for the poor
1966	Head Start as part of Economic Opportunity Act, P.L. 88-452	Over 1 million preschool children served in comprehensive education and health programs annually in 19,000 centers and 829 home-based programs
1970	Lead-Based Paint Poisoning Prevention Act, P.L. 91-695	Provided funds to treat victims of lead poisoning and established procedures for lead paint removal
1975	Education for All Handicapped Children Act, P.L. 94-142	Ensured a free appropriate public education for all handicapped children
1989	Early Intervention, P.L. 99-457	Authorized an early intervention program for handicapped infants
1990	Ryan White CARE Act, P.L. 101-38	Grants to improve care for individual and families with HIV disease
1990	Individual with Disabilities Education Act, P.L. 101-476	Reauthorization of the Education for Handicapped Children Act
1997	State Child Health Insurance Program (Title XXI, of SSA), P.L. 105-33	Extends insurance benefits to children above the financial eligibility line for Medicaid

laws gives child health advocates a foundation for securing the health of children. Understanding the process by which the laws are passed gives some pragmatic hints for future action.

The Legislative Process

Figure 6.1 maps the progress of a bill from the day it is introduced until it is signed into law. The bill makes its way by separate tracks through the House and the Senate, from committee to subcommittee and back again to the full committee, before the full House or Senate ever discusses it. Because a bill can be substantially modified at each stage, the House and Senate versions may differ greatly when they are passed. A conference committee reconciles the differences and presents a final version to the House and Senate for their approval. The bill is then sent on to the president for him to sign or veto. Each of the ups and downs, twists and turns offers opportunities for child health advocacy.

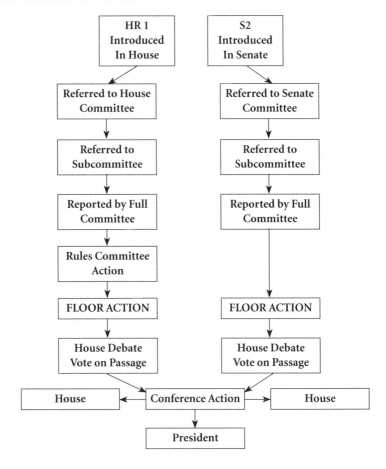

Figure 6.1. How a Bill Becomes Law

What the diagram does not convey is the very long time the passage of legislation takes. The slow pace is particularly disconcerting to clinicians. A pediatric intern may be motivated to take political action after a month or two of trying to procure early childhood services for a 2-year-old with cerebral palsy. But by the time the intern's idea has been transformed into a legislative package, her little patient could be on the way to elementary school, facing a host of new clinical and societal problems.

The temporal disconnect accounts in great measure for the larger and more fundamental disconnect between the different types of advocacy discussed in this book. Clinicians on the front lines want action this minute, for this child. Pressed for time to meet the continual stream of patient concerns, busy clinicians cannot sustain the battle at the statehouse.

The Health Care Committee in the legislature may have the time, but often the members do not have as great a sense of urgency. Not seeing the children day to day, they often do not see the areas of greatest need. The solution to the time problem is getting clinicians together with policy-makers to form partnerships to engage the legislative system for the long haul.

When the legislative system works at top form, all citizens receive a good hearing. In the best of all possible political worlds, there is a wide range of exposure of new ideas and options; there is room for the full participation of parents, teenagers, teachers, pediatricians, and other involved parties. Unfortunately, the legislative process rarely attains the ideal. Substantial flaws render the system less than it could be.

An uneven balance of power favors those with wealth, access, and in-sider information. Those "in the know" get to have their ideas and influence felt. If no one looks out for children, the powerful can easily manip-ulate the system. Perhaps unwittingly, the strong heap more harm on the downtrodden—by zoning laws that forbid the construction of special clinics, by rules that restrict state subsidization of urban school districts, by regulations that protect special interests over individual rights. The legislature passes laws that penalize schools for not educating children but do not provide adequate funding for them to do their job. They grant exemptions for unfettered growth to certain corporations without mea-suring the environmental impact on neighborhoods. Who really cares if a few kids get respiratory ailments? Children are too often the weak, the unheard, the forgotten. They depend on outspoken advocates to keep sounding out their issues.

Principles of Legislative Advocacy

There is a common assumption that the weight of a just cause is power-fully persuasive. Unfortunately, simply being right is not sufficient in the competitive world of legislation. With all of the other priorities in front of the legislators, they do not pay attention to weak arguments or quiet persuasion. The power to make a difference through legislation depends on having a strong team, a clear message, practical ideas, and a plan for protecting the flank against attack.

Building a Strong and Effective Team

The first principle of legislative advocacy is that it is a team affair. No one can effect systems change alone. Only a team of leaders, partners, experts, and part-time and full-time players can devote the time, have the skills, and carry out the actions that create sustainable change. Legislators act when they hear from their constituents—parents, grandparents, providers, neighbors, the butcher, the baker, the local librarian. It is not enough for a child psychiatrist to have a good idea about a new rural mental health center. To raise public dollars, Dr. Winslow needs to find people in the coastal town of East Ossingham who can convince their elected representative to vote for this line item for services in West Arundalvania County, even though it is 150 miles away. He needs a team.

Creating coalitions for children is very difficult because children do not vote. They cannot unseat an unresponsive state representative nor elect a child-friendly candidate. Infants and toddlers cannot argue for themselves as the laws that affect their futures are crafted, debated, and enacted. Children need groups of adults to speak up for them and keep speaking up. Once a coalition is formed, someone must support and nurture it. Sustaining the political will of such a group is a gargantuan task and requires skill, experience, and a tough stomach for the twists and turns of the long ride to get a bill through.

Unlikely partners strengthen coalitions as long as they share a common agenda. Having helped create the Massachusetts Legislative Children's Caucus and working for years in the state legislature, Margaret Blood knew, for instance, that child advocates alone would never persuade the legislature to vote for a universal early childhood education bill. She pulled together a coalition of business executives, policymakers, pediatricians, educators, and families. She equipped them with cogent, interlocking arguments. The widened constituency—with their concerted campaign of phone calls, letters, editorials, e-mails and personal visits to their state legislators—could make the elected officials sit up and take notice. This broad-based coalition helped develop and advocate for a state legislative proposal—An Act Establishing Early Education for All—significant portions of which were passed into law in 2004 with the creation of the first-in-the-nation Board and Department of Early Education and Care.[1]

Advocacy coalitions depend on the involvement of many, many people. Some of the people, the Margaret Bloods of the world, must devote more than full-time effort, but they depend on an hour here, a five minutes there from parents, neighbors, doctors, lawyers, ministers, nurses, and on and on. Legislative advocacy for clinicians involves a willingness to help out in small ways and large.

In addition to advocacy leaders and their large band of partners, there is often an advantage in including an advocacy expert who can monitor legislative activity and stay on top of the general legislative agenda. Built into each piece of legislation and regulation is a regular cycle of review. These reviews are opportunities for improvement, but they also present the possibility of losing ground. As a result, those concerned about child health advocacy can never rest content that a good piece of legislation has been enacted. Before too many years, that law will be on the docket for its periodic reauthorization and appropriation. The bill's detractors will be working their hardest to water it down. During the battles for continued budgetary support of initiatives, opponents will do everything they can to cut funding. At the time of this writing, many child-oriented health, education, and development programs are under attack and, in the absence of significant intervention, stand to lose both authority and funding.

Recognizing the complex demands of monitoring legislative activity, most large child health professional organizations have established offices of government affairs and advocacy. In general, the staff members in these offices have extensive experience in health care policy and the legislative process. Increasingly, hospitals and other health care organizations are setting up such offices because they recognize the impact that specific legislation has on their ability to operate effectively. Although the highly technical aspects of advocacy belong in the hands of these expert advocates, the experts also rely on the teamwork of parents, medical professionals, and community-based organizations for clout.

Presenting a Clear Message

Elected officials cannot possibly know everything that is happening in the communities they represent. Newspapers tell them only part of what is going on. An advocate is another pair of eyes and ears. Child health clinicians, parents, and community-based organizations report the real scoop. Bearing witness is the most fundamental form of advocacy. There is nothing like the authority of a pediatrician describing the brain injury of a child who has fallen six stories from an unguarded apartment window, or of a mother telling what it is like to water down formula for her 3-month-old because she cannot afford to buy more at the end of each month. A high school junior reporting that he cannot take biology because the lab door is too narrow for his wheelchair vividly illustrates the importance of reducing physical barriers in public places. When each state senator and representative finds a tiny diaper pinned to a paper on his or her desk, the realization dawns that this one-inch-by-one-inch piece of cloth covers nearly half the body of a premature infant. Aha!

the Ourtown Children's Hospital really does have different technical and resource needs from those of the Veterans Administration. Bearing witness involves translating clinical information into a clear message that everyone can understand cognitively, respond to emotionally, and act on practically.

Table 6.2 outlines the American Academy of Pediatrics' suggestions for activities that send the message: I care about this legislation. My patients care about it. My husband cares about it. It would be well if you, Ms. Elected Official, took a serious look at it. At the end of the day, when legislation is pending, staffers actually do count the for and against calls, e-mails, and faxes. If too many days go by without any endorsement for the fluoridation bill, the senator gets the feeling that she should put her energy elsewhere. If she doesn't hear from the child health dentists, why should she stick her neck out? The John Birch Society has certainly made their opinion known.

Child health advocates sometimes flounder in their attempts to garner public support because they garble the message they are trying to deliver by reverting to technical jargon. Most educated people do understand the fundamentals of health, physiology, anatomy, pharmacology, immunology, and increasingly, genetics. The advocacy challenge is to find the common ground where child health professionals, families, legislators, and the general public are talking about the same fundamental issue and plan. This is far from a clear-cut task.

Simple words are not so simple when they are used differently in general parlance and in the technical language of different disciplines. For example, a straightforward word like *development* means vastly disparate things to an economist, a fund-raiser, a child psychologist, and an embryologist. Put these four people in a room together and try to make sense of the initial conversation. Until there is greater clarity, the push for national programs that enhance "early brain development" are likely to encounter continued uncertainty and weak commitment by program sponsors.

Once advocates find the words that ring true to the ears of multiple listeners, they can make great progress. The early success of the anti-tobacco campaigns came when advocates constructed clear messaging about the physical effects of smoking tobacco. Health professionals and affected persons now present an allied front, iterating and reiterating the same facts. Like the consistent and focused drip of water, that message is eventually boring its way into the rock of the public conscience.

By its very nature, witnessing connotes emotional impact. Advocates

Table 6.2. Key Steps in Doing Effective Advocacy

Make a Visit to the Hill
Be prepared!
Coordinate your presentation
Present the most important points first
Present the facts concisely
Share your expertise
Be constructive, be honest, and be familiar with the opposition
Leave fact sheets on your issues
Follow up your visit!

Advocacy Skills
Presentation—brief and clear
Be firm and persuasive not confrontational or abrasive
Personalize your message, share anecdotes
Know the opposition's arguments

Leaving a Phone Message
Identify yourself and indicate you are a constituent
State the bill(s) you are calling about and your position on the bill(s)
Leave a substantive, short message; don't get too technical
Provide a contact information so they can call or write you

Advocacy Strategies
Writing letters
Voter education
Filing a lawsuit
Testifying before a state or federal legislative body
Focus groups
Write an editorial or letters to the editor
Press conference
Invite celebrities to join the efforts

Source: American Academy of Pediatrics, courtesy of Karen Hendricks.

speak out intending to move their listeners. Playing on emotions involves many unknowns, and the public response can be completely unexpected. In the mid-1950s a radio announcer was doing a story about the Red Sox program for visiting hospitalized children with cancer. At the end of a bedside interview, he said, "Anyone wishing to help kids like little Jimmy here, send in a check." The next day, a huge pile of mailbags filled with generous donations greeted the medical chief resident at his office. That was the day the Jimmy Fund to support research in childhood cancer was born.

But emotions are quirky. Nerves get hit, and some outcomes are not so good. For instance, there is the experience of pediatricians who were concerned about children exposed to crack cocaine. The doctors were as troubled about the complex inequities that placed poor women at the mercy of drug warlords as they were about the potential effects of cocaine on the newborns. But the story they told was only half heard. The mothers (victims in the minds of the child health advocates) became villains in the lay press; even worse, their children were labeled as severely damaged. All sense of humanity and hope went out of the picture, making it increasingly hard to get the very drug treatment that could help both mothers and babies. Because the emotional impact can be so important, advocates should pilot their messages with small focus groups of listeners before launching wide advocacy campaigns.

Often coalitions of health care providers, families, and community leaders venture into the halls of the statehouse or of Congress. The building is imposing. The legislator's office is impressive, its walls lined with photographs of the representative meeting with famous people. After a few minutes, they are ushered into a small office with more pictures and a round conference table. More waiting, and then the legislative aide walks in. Bright, energetic, and young, the aide is all ears, at least initially. He is not Senator Z; the wall photographs are most likely all the child health delegation will glimpse of Senator Z; it is this young person who will be drafting the ideas for Senator Z's consideration.

These sessions are most effective when the visiting advocates have done their homework. The aide is looking for practical suggestions for legislative change. If the visitors present an idea that is too big and amorphous, the aide listens politely, checking the clock so that he can sit through the full ten minutes that politeness dictates, but his mind is on the next problem. If on the other hand the delegation brings a targeted proposal that has clear benefit not only for children and youth in general but also for the constituents of the legislator's district, the clock doesn't matter and the aide steers the group discussion toward the next steps to move the idea forward. The next section details some of the practical details the aide will be listening for.

Developing and Translating Practical Ideas

Transforming dreams into policy terms is a multifaceted task that profits from the energetic input of all team members. From the earliest brainstorming to the concept formation to the drafting of the legislative language, there are crucial times when the ideas of clinicians and families strengthen both the process and the product. Policy formulation must be informed by answers to the question, What do we actually want?

Dr. Simpson may know that he really hates the new Medicaid guide-lines for prescription drugs. Mrs. Takihama can describe precisely why it is unsafe for her daughter to ride her bicycle home from school. Clinicians and families can almost always say what is wrong, but that is not enough for legislative child health advocacy. The crucial contribution is the construction of a new plan, a new system, and a new way of doing things. Dr. Simpson needs to come up with a better scheme for prescriptions. Mrs. Takihama needs to describe in detail a new bike path through Lincoln Township.

One of the skills that successful child health advocates develop is to package their request as a clearly delineated program or policy. In the Anne E. Dyson Community Pediatrics Training Initiative, one of the many ongoing activities among the faculty and residents has been the detailing of the elements of successful projects and programs. Articulating these elements using the appropriate terms refines program planning. The "goals and objectives" of the project become the *preamble* of the bill. The "descriptors of the patient population" become the program *eligibility criteria.* The personnel needed to carry out the project become the designated *agents* of the federal or state authority who will execute the government's mandate. The "budget" for necessary supplies and services becomes the *authorization,* which must be placed under the aegis of one or another state or federal agency.

Savvy advocates know that the choice of the governmental agency that will have authority for their proposed program is critical to the program's success and long-term viability. The bill may pass, but the program will languish without a champion. Choosing the right agency protects the program and can have the added benefit of increasing the number of influential people who want programs for children to succeed. For example, the placement of the Women, Infants, and Children's nutrition program (WIC) in the Department of Agriculture immediately added the farm lobby to the voices speaking up for children. Nothing like powerful allies to keep milk and cereal flowing to the homes of poor women and children.

The idea for a particular project or program may come from a child health advocacy team, but the packaging and shepherding of the bill rests with the staff members of the senators and representatives who sponsor the bill. Effective child health advocates work with the legislative staff to predict any obstacles to the passage of the bill. Together, they conjure up the potential roadblocks to the successful conduct of the eventual program. Will this new program effect constituencies we haven't thought about? Can we conceive of any negative consequences for children and families, for child-serving agencies, for others? Will this new state-run clinic for children with special health care needs be competing with the clinics at the academic health center or the local Shriners' hospital? Will the proposed window guards meet fire codes for easy removal? Will the emancipated minor legislation impinge on family rights and responsibilities? Will state payment for immunizations decrease the funds available for newborn screening? Will the addition of folic acid to foods, with the aim of helping women of child-bearing age, negatively affect the health of elderly people? The answers to these questions strengthen the proposed law and immunize its regulations from encroachment.

Most legislative programs are categorical in nature. The bills are the response to one type of problem (e.g., substance abuse, mental illness, thalassemia), or the answer for one group of children and youth (e.g., newborns of teenage moms, Hispanic girls). Many observers of state and national child health policy argue that there are inherent inequities and problems built into categorical service delivery. Care is doled out in fragments. Families must turn to one program for well-child health care, to another for adjusting their child's leg braces, to another for physical therapy, another for the child's specialized diet, and still another for genetic counseling. Tight criteria for eligibility for categorical programs can also create complicated service delivery patterns. Children whose families meet certain income criteria may be eligible for services that are not available to their neighbors because they are in a slightly higher income bracket. These latter families may not be eligible for any services because their incomes are too high for public subsidy, even though they are far too low to allow them to purchase the services privately. The pragmatist, however, recognizes that targeting facilitates the legislative process. The easier it will be for lawmakers to claim a specific local impact of their work, the more likely it is that the legislation will pass.

There is clearly a role for policy development of a comprehensive nature as well. Fundamental social justice changes are unlikely to emerge from the incremental ward-by-ward, county-by-county, state-by-state programmatic approaches. Fair enough. But without the demonstration that small steps work, the naysayers and risk avoiders have stronger ammunition and more persuasive arguments than do the reformers. Large policy change happens when small streams of movement finally align at the right moment, with the moon in the right phase and the right person sitting as the chair of the right committee. The stories of Title V, Medicaid, SCHIP, and IDEA later in this chapter illustrate this point.

Protecting the Flank

Legislative advocacy is as much about protecting children and youth from the passage of laws that hurt them as it is about passing new laws. Some attacks on children's health are subtle, the by-products of unrelated matters. Others are the result of unfortunate competition with worthy proposals that pit the child population against some equally deserving group (frequently, the elderly). Still others are direct and overt attacks designed to undermine well-established child health practices. The legislature, with its floor available for public debate, is appropriately the scene for skirmishes of all kinds. Child advocates who do not engage at this level leave health policy open to infringement by special interests, the misinformed, and even the truly crazy.

In the legislative process, entrepreneurial interests easily drown the voices of children's advocates. Better prepared, better funded, and better connected, the lobbyists for infant formula companies, tobacco companies, paint manufacturers, the film and television industries know how to get what they want. Over and over, these companies are rewarded with tax breaks and regulatory exemptions despite the adverse effects their unfettered business has on the health of children and youth.

Undoubtedly, the fiercest special interest group with antichild health positions is the National Rifle Association. Repeatedly, child advocates have sought legislation to limit the sales of handguns and to enforce stricter monitoring of access to guns. Repeatedly, the special interest lobby has been able to outargue, outwangle, and outspend the child health advocates. Through deft self-promotion, the gun industry has prevented the passage of standards on the domestic production of Saturday night specials (a cheap, easily concealed handgun). It has restricted the federal Alcohol, Tobacco, and Firearms agency (the ATF) from monitoring gun production, and it has made sure that the Consumer Product Safety Commission would not be allowed to comment on the hazards of firearms and ammunition. In sixteen states, the industry had gone so far as to obtain legal mandates granting gun manufacturers immunity from lawsuits.

David to the gun industry Goliath, groups like the Million Mom March and HELP, led by pediatrician Kathy Cristoffel, have kept alert, documenting the extent and seriousness of the problem and seizing every opportunity to chip away at the NRA's hold on the legislative process. Since the early 1990s gun control advocates have made slow, steady progress, to the point that by 1999 thirty-one states had statutes or executive orders that built on and strengthened the federal legislation regulating licensed gun dealers. The impact of the regulations is seen in the decrease in gun sales and in the slowly falling rates of child gun fatalities.[2]

Simply setting the factual record straight about medicine and child health is not a small matter. Misinformation is available in large supply. Passionately engaged but poorly informed special interest groups badger their elected representatives on a regular basis on topics of enormous importance to child health. Their loud voices show that they care and will vote. Such groups often mount campaigns to oust elected officials who do not vote their way. These groups are formidable forces. They understand that, at the state level, three to four phone calls can win the day. As a result, it is critical that there be countervailing forces of information, so that legislators and their staffs are not hearing only from people whose information is derived from the latest pseudoscience being promulgated on the 11 a.m. TV talk shows.

In recent years, many of the topics that have been engaged in this way have involved post hoc ergo propter hoc arguments (it came after A, therefore it was caused by A), alleging that one or another childhood vaccine is the causative agent of a serious childhood disorder. In the late 1980s Phil Donahue used his powerful position on television to publicize the theory that DPT vaccine (for diphtheria, pertussis, and tetanus) induced seizures and neurological damage in children who received it. Since no biologic relationship is simple and the form of whole cell vaccine at the time did have the potential of aggravating a latent, existing neurological condition, there was a kernel of truth in the claim. Its unfortunate consequence was that families all over the United States kept their children from receiving vaccines of all kinds, unknowingly placing their children at far greater risk of serious life- and brain-threatening disorders than the DPT vaccine ever posed.

Similarly, although no credible link has ever been established between autism and the administration of MMR vaccine (for measles, mumps, and rubella), several groups claim such a causal relationship. The fact is that children begin to show the full-blown symptoms of autism around 18 months, several months after the routine administration of the MMR vaccine.[3] There is thus a temporal relationship, but there is no other credible link. One might just as well blame the introduction of whole milk or the child's first step or a new toy as the inciting agent. Epidemiologic concepts are complex and dry and require understanding and acceptance of variation around means and some level of uncertainty about all interrelationships. In statistical terms, there is always a vague, distant, potential, possible, maybe chance that something is related to something else, but that relationship can become so remote and so unlikely as to approach zero. It can be hard for the general public to bend their mind around such concepts. It is much easier to believe what they see or hear in emotionally depicted fashion: Johnny received the MMR vaccine; Johnny developed autism; the MMR vaccine is bad and no one should receive it.

The sadness for the family of the child with autism is profound. What is forgotten in all of this, however, is the many children who died from measles in the prevaccine era, the 800 annual new cases of congenital rubella in the 1960s, and the countless days of illness and suffering of children with catarrh and pneumonia, encephalitis and orchitis and other symptoms of these once devastating and now almost unheard of illnesses. Keeping these and other facts front and center is as critical as any role in child health. If parents become blasé about the importance of preventive efforts and keep their children away from care, there is the serious possibility of the reemergence of these childhood illnesses and the breakdown of the protective herd immunity.

The unfortunate reality in the world of child health advocacy is that some groups take uncompromising positions. These groups can be radicalized to the point of being dangerous, resorting to personal threats and attacks. The Church of Scientology has been increasingly active in the promotion of a legislative agenda against the medical treatment of childhood mental and behavioral disorder. Their position is that there is no such thing as mental health disease and that children should not be subjected to psychiatric care.[4] Mental health problems in children are on the rise, and there are far too few services already. An active lobby such as the Church of Scientology places one more obstacle in the path of those who wish to assist children and youth with serious health conditions.

Divergence of opinion on child health issues can be the stimulus for provocative debate and productive argument. By putting concepts through the paces of public discussion, new components or new adaptations can greatly improve upon the original thought. Compromise and reconstruction can make the end product more politically viable and can sometimes (but not always) make the program better.

Health Advocates and Policy Development

Child health advocacy has been critical in creating the current child health delivery system. Imperfect as they are, the standards and regulations of four major pieces of federal legislation have played an essential part in improving American child health services, access to care, and outcomes. Here we review the history of the passage of

- Title V of the Social Security Act
- Medicaid
- State Child Health Insurance Program
- Individuals with Disabilities Education Act

Title V of the Social Security Act, 1935

In 1929, when the stock market crashed and the Great Depression caused massive unemployment across the country, communities were literally torn apart. People lost their jobs and homes. Hundreds of thousands of parents were incapable of feeding and clothing their families. Mothers and fathers could not afford medicine for sick children. To bring the nation back together, the president, the Congress, and the citizenry determined to reorder priorities and to rearrange structures. Franklin Roosevelt's New Deal included specific legislation to protect the vulnerable and to plan for a safer future for all Americans. The centerpiece of his legislative agenda was the Social Security Act.

Title V of the Social Security Act of 1935 was one of the most important pieces of legislation ever passed for children's health. Advocates took full advantage of this defining moment in American history to introduce language about children's health into the New Deal legislative agenda. They made sure that the federal government would be committed to more than a casual role in the oversight of children's health and development.

For their time, the provisions of Title V were far-reaching, but they were a clear outgrowth of the 1930s mentality. They reflect the ambivalence of a country pulling itself out of the depths but concerned about maintaining the primacy of individual rights. Some politicians like Huey P. Long spoke of sharing the wealth, but others were unwilling to vote for anything that smacked of socialism. Congress reacted with a compromise: they would provide limited federal support to the country's most vulnerable individuals through a state-level program.

Title V's grants to states for Maternal and Child Health services funded child health services in two separate, well-demarcated areas: Maternal and Child Health and the Crippled Children's Service. Welfare services were also originally funded through this provision. Let us look at the health care provisions and their evolution to the present.

Sowing the Seeds

The seeds for federal child health legislation had been planted long before the Depression.[5] In the early 1900s, Progressives, muckrakers, and other movers and shakers identified infant mortality and child labor as rallying points for social reform. They could not convince the nation as a whole of the need for a governmental focus on children, but they did get the attention of Theodore Roosevelt, the father of six boisterous sons and daughters. As one of his last acts in the presidency, TR hosted the first White House Conference on Children, setting in motion the establishment of a federal Children's Bureau.

In 1912 Congress enacted legislation to create the Children's Bureau in the Department of Labor to address a wide array of problems, including child health, child labor, dependency, and delinquency.[6] To do all this, however, Congress provided a very limited budget and feeble authority. Even with these constraints, the early Children's Bureau accomplished amazing things. The first director, Julia Lathrop, made the strategic decision to spend the bureau's few dollars on gathering information about infant mortality. Imagine a time when the only recording of birth was in the family Bible. Until Lathrop and the staff of the Children's Bureau began a ten-state pilot birth registration project in 1915, there was no systematic federal data collection documenting the circumstances of birth for America's children.[7] Once Lathrop could demonstrate the hard facts—14 of every 100 Americans infants were dying before their first birthday—she could ask Congress for more support.

In 1918 the first woman member of Congress, Jeannette Rankin,[8] introduced the Sheppard Towner Act to increase the Children's Bureau's funding and establish a federal-state matching program for maternal and child health services. Despite the early successes and growing prestige of the Children's Bureau, the 1921 passage of the Sheppard Towner Act came at an enormous price. Almost from day one, the Children's Bureau was attacked on all sides. The directors were forced into a continuous trench warfare that made forward progress and creative achievement difficult, if not impossible.

Many Americans did not like the idea that the federal government was telling them how to raise their children. Vince Hutchins captured those feelings in the words of social commentator and cowboy comedian Will Rogers: "I am mighty glad so many people in America are taking up the children work. Being a ranchman and a farmer, and also a child owner, I have often wished that when one of my children got sick, I could wire or call some Government expert and have him look after them, like I can do if one of my cows or pigs get some disease. If your fertilizer is not agreeing with your land, the Government will send a specialist, but if the food is not agreeing with the baby, why, we have to find out what's the matter ourselves, and lots of times parents mean well but they don't know much. It's not a bad idea whoever thought of doing something for the children. If it works and you improve them, I will send you mine."[9]

Most of the criticism of the Children's Bureau was not so lighthearted. The statements were often couched in anti-Bolshevik language. Opponents of the bureau included influential groups such the Daughters of the American Revolution and the Catholic Church. They argued that setting federal standards for decent child health, education, and welfare for every child was an encroachment on the privacy of families.

Against the backdrop of inadequate support and outright antipathy, the directors of the Children's Bureau (child health advocates Julia Lathrop, Grace Abbott, and Martha May Eliot) realized that they must garner the authority and funding that stronger legislation would afford them. Without such backing, they would never accomplish any substantial change for children. In the 1920s Martha Eliot began the careful behind-the-scenes advocacy needed to position the concerns of children and mothers more centrally. When the time came, she was ready with specific language relating to mothers and infants to fit into the Social Security legislation. She knew that "chance favors the prepared mind."[10]

Maternal and Child Health Services

A prime function of Title V of the Social Security Act was the provision of direct health care services to mothers and children. An odd conglomeration of health clinics, charity outreach services, and child health dispensaries, some affiliated with medical schools, some free standing, dominated the health scene in the mid-1930s. There was no consistent funding for these enterprises, nor were there standard operating guidelines.

As a result of Title V, states were enabled "to extend and improve, as far as practicable under the conditions in such State, services for promoting the health of mothers and children, especially in rural areas and in areas suffering from severe economic distress." Previous federal child health endeavors had been minimally funded, but the appropriation for Maternal and Child Health (MCH) services of Title V was a more substantial sum ($2,800,000). For the first time, the MCH directors of the Children's Bureau could embark on innovations with financial support to some child health providers in the field.[11] But even this funding was inadequate. Primary care services continued as a patchwork quilt made up of health department clinics with limited hours and staffing, mobile units making erratic visits to rural sites, and urban storefronts struggling day to day just to pay the rent.

By midcentury some of these clinics found better sponsorship by allying with universities or social service agencies, but it was not until the introduction of neighborhood health centers during the Lyndon Johnson administration that there was a formal, coordinated structure of clinics with mandated responsibility for the care of poor children and mothers (see chapter 2). Locally controlled and operated, these neighborhood health centers were not directly under the jurisdiction of the Maternal and Child Health Bureau, but increasingly over the 1970s and 1980s they became the homes for MCH programming and often the recipients of MCH grant funding.

In 1989 the goals for MCH services were laid out in the Omnibus Budget Reconciliation Act (OBRA '89). Each state should be in a position, it says,

> to provide and to assure mothers and children (in particular those with
> low income or with limited availability of health services) access to qual-
> ity maternal and child health services [and] to reduce infant mortality and
> incidence of preventable diseases and handicapping conditions among chil-
> dren, to reduce the need for inpatient and long-term care services, to in-
> crease the number of children (especially preschool children) appropriately
> immunized against disease and the number of low income children receiv-
> ing health assessments and follow-up diagnostic and treatment services,
> and otherwise to promote the health of mothers and infants by providing
> prenatal, delivery and postpartum care for low income, at risk pregnant
> women and to promote the health of children by providing preventive and
> primary care services for low income children.[12]

Using the opportunity presented by OBRA '89 to rewrite the regulations, Vince Hutchins and Merle McPherson, the directors of the MCH Bureau, made a significant shift in emphasis for the public health authority. Although the vulnerable must be protected first, language in OBRA '89 on health promotion suggests that the federal government should ensure health services for *all* mothers and children. Although the bureau would never have adequate dollars to invest in service delivery improvement, the OBRA '89 language strengthened its hand.

State MCH directors carry out the mandates of Title V in a variety of ways.[13] Since the Reagan era, their budgets have come as block grants to the states. In general, the bureau's departments distribute these dollars through a competitive process, with agencies submitting grant proposals and bids for contracts. Many neighborhood health centers have expanded their clinical capabilities by adding a nurse or a social worker or outreach staff to perform so-called wrap-around services, such as nutritional counseling, injury prevention, home visiting, housing and food security interventions, and drug abuse treatment and prevention. During the height of the HIV epidemic, for instance, Title V dollars were often used for HIV education and counseling. When state and professional organizations introduced new immunization plans or prevention campaigns like the effort to prevent sudden infant death syndrome, Title V funds have added a boost to staff auxiliary activity.

The close alliance of Title V with neighborhood health centers makes MCH funds a vital component of health center support in the 2000s. Typically, health insurance (such as Blue Cross or Medicaid) pays the centers for individual encounters only on a fee-for-service basis. Those funds do not support the centers in carrying out all the tasks required of them, let alone outreach. The centers use MCH money to build the infrastructure necessary to conduct comprehensive individual and public health activities.

One way to think about infrastructure support is to consider what it would be like if all policemen were funded on a fee-for-service basis. Imagine the situation if the only time the cop on the beat got paid was when he nabbed a burglar in the act of robbing a convenience store. The policeman's total presence as he patrols, chats on the sidewalk, and looks out for unusual patterns affords the crime deterrent that the public wants. The specific arrest is only a small part of the picture. And yet in the health care arena both private and public insurers generally limit their payment to "encounters," "procedures," and face-to-face "relative value units." Such individual visits actually could not occur at all without the support of nursing and ancillary staff. Title V ensures that medical providers can walk the "child health beat" fully prepared and backed up.

Periodically, the dollars for MCH programs and neighborhood health centers come under attack at the executive and congressional level. During periods of fiscal retrenchment, they are viewed as expendable. When this happens, if child health advocates are not poised for an all-out effort, children lose vital services. During the Reagan-Bush era there were large and damaging cuts to the neighborhood health center infrastructure. Funds for the health centers were restored with a fair amount of flourish under the George W. Bush administration. Child health advocates at the state and federal level protected the essential services by relying on the fundamentals written into legislation. Title V's mandates for monitoring and oversight of child health provisions put advocates in a much stronger position than if they were starting from scratch. Martha Eliot's legacy is a legislative contract for maternal and child health. Advocates can count on the terms of that contract as society's commitment is put to the test time and time again.

Crippled Children's Service

The Crippled Children's Service (CCS) provisions of Title V were designed to support states in locating "crippled children" and improving the medical care available to them. The large polio epidemics of the first half of the twentieth century reached a peak of 21,000 new cases in 1952.[14] In the prevaccine era, children and young adults with paralytic polio faced enormous challenges, and states had few resources with which to respond. Initially most states used their CCS money for children suffering from polio: the federal regulations governing the program left it up to each state to define the eligibility criteria for funding. This flexibility turned out to be both a boon and a liability. It allowed states to adapt to the changes in child disability prevalence over time, but it caused substantial state-by-state variation in the types and severity of conditions covered as well as the state responses to the needs of children with disabilities.

During the mid- and late-twentieth century, significant shifts occurred in the population of children with disabilities (see chapters 2 and 3). Polio came under control as a result of an aggressive national vaccine campaign. The combined efforts of the scientific research community, federal and state public health authorities, and the March of Dimes virtually eliminated the disease by the late 1960s. Iron lungs were no longer a necessary adjunct to care. It looked as if units in special children's and orthopedic hospitals were going to be able to close up shop, but that was not the case at all.

Just as the scourge of polio began to disappear, other chronic conditions started to increase. Graduates of neonatal intensive care units, children with surgically corrected congenital anomalies, and survivors of severe chronic illnesses were living longer. As medical knowledge and surgical acumen saved more children, the need for continuing health and developmental services grew proportionately. In the mid-1980s, the HIV/AIDS epidemic added another group of children with disabilities.

Children with Special Health Care Needs

In 1985, in recognition of the evolving pattern among children with disabilities, Merle McPherson began the effort to change the term *crippled children* to one that accurately reflected the contemporary situation. McPherson and others proposed a new designation for the group: children with special health care needs (CSHCN). Noncategorical wording was incorporated into the Consolidated Omnibus Budget Reconciliation Act of 1989 (OBRA '89). Each state retained the right to create its own eligibility criteria, but OBRA '89 encouraged them to use broad general categories for programs rather than discretely defined ones like the thalassemia program, the HIV program, the phenylketonuria program.

Despite OBRA '89 it took almost fifteen years for the noncategorical approach and the CSHCN terminology to earn common acceptance. It was an uphill battle for McPherson and her colleagues because the concept was elusive to most people. *Crippled child* conjured up the image of a child on crutches; *CSHCN* lacked an obvious association. Over time, though, policymakers, clinicians, and families began to agree that children with conditions as heterogeneous as maple syrup urine disease, traumatic brain injury, cerebral palsy, and autism had similar special health care needs for health promotion, subspecialty care, medications, therapies, and coordination of services. The usefulness of the term *CSHCN* became increasingly evident. The MCH definition since 1998 is, "Children who have or are at risk for chronic physical, developmental, behavioral or emotional conditions and who also require health and related services of a type or amount beyond that required by children generally."[15]

Once the definitional issues were clarified, McPherson went on to launch a national survey that would allow comparability across states and across time in the monitoring of both the prevalence of and services for CSHCN. The survey documented that 13 percent of the U.S. child population met the criteria for CSHCN, with states varying relatively little in their estimates.[16]

Healthy Children 2010

In 2000 Merle McPherson and her staff put into place a forward-looking plan for children and youth with chronic illnesses and disabilities; Healthy Children 2010 fits into the Healthy People 2010 objectives for the nation. These goals guide all of the systems-building activities that

Table 6.3. Healthy Children 2010 Goals for Children and Youth with Special Health Care Needs

All children with special health care needs will receive regular and ongoing comprehensive care within a medical home.

All families of CSHCN will have adequate private or public insurance to pay for the services they need.

All children will be screened early and continuously for special health care needs.

Services for children with special health care needs and their families will be organized in ways that families can use them easily.

Families of CSHCN will participate in decision making at all levels and will be satisfied with the services they receive.

All youth with special health care needs will receive the services to make appropriate transitions to all aspects of adult health care, work, and independence.

Source: www.mchb.hrsa.gov/programs/specialneeds/measuresuccess.htm (accessed September 21, 2005).

the Maternal and Child Health Bureau sponsors to improve the health of CSHCN (table 6.3).

In chapter 4, there is a detailed discussion of the components of the medical home. The goals of Healthy Children 2010—sponsored by the MCH Bureau and endorsed by the American Academy of Pediatrics—set the standard for the type of comprehensive and coordinated medical care that is expected for children with special health care needs. The specifications of the medical home include primary and specialty care and coordination of services across sectors in the community.

The goals also include an emphasis on family-centered care. This concept acknowledges both the needs of families and their considerable strengths for working in partnership with health care providers on creative solutions. Family-centered care means that health care providers and parents work together to promote health with forward-looking services rather than responding only to crises. Tools like the individualized health plan (IHP) allow providers and parents to anticipate health, social, emotional, educational, and vocational needs and to plan for them. Family-centered care also means a more flexible deployment of health care dollars.

Because of the late-twentieth-century advances in education, rehabilitation, and medicine, young people with disabilities are more capable of living productive lives in community settings than they have ever been in the past. Unfortunately, communities are often ill prepared to nurture such young people's strengths and abilities. For the transition goal to succeed, pediatric and adult health providers, business, and industry need to adopt new attitudes and new behaviors. This requires training and preparation as well as substantial systems-level cooperation and the creation of appropriate fiscal relationships and dollar flows.

The MCH dollars committed to programs for CSHCN in the year 2000 were sufficient for direct services to only about a tenth of children with special health care needs.[17] There is still a long way to go. In fact there are still significant challenges for the entire community of people with disabilities. The 1999 Supreme Court case of *Olmstead v L.C.* brought a public spotlight to bear on the failure of state systems to design and fund community-based services for people with disabilities.[18] Justice Ginsberg reported the court's decision that states must provide community-based services in the least restrictive settings for people with disabilities (including mental health disabilities). The Bush administration responded with the New Freedom Initiative, which sets the goal of helping "Americans with disabilities by increasing access to assistive technologies, expanding educational opportunities, increasing the ability of Americans with disabilities to integrate into the workforce, and promoting increased access into daily community life."[19] It remains to be seen if these words will be matched with the dollars that would make the goal a reality. Success depends in large measure on the degree to which Title V federal and state agencies are supported with the authority and financial backing to carry out the mandate they have been given.

Medicaid, 1965

Child health advocates have had a long and involved love/hate relationship with Medicaid, but substantially more love than hate. Passed in 1965 as Title XIX of the Social Security Act, Medicaid funds the health care of nearly a quarter of America's children, to the tune of almost $27 billion a year.[20] But Medicaid is a poor people's program, a compromise at best, a last-dregs program at worst. The strings attached to its bureaucratic requirements often constrain even the most willing child health practitioners from taking Medicaid recipients, creating barriers to health care for poor children. Over the years, child health advocates have needed to tread delicately in moving forward with Medicaid, hoping to optimize its assets while minimizing its limitations.

For those concerned with child health advocacy, it is essential to understand the historical roots of Medicaid, the forces that created both its adequacies and its inadequacies. Financial access to health care has never been a universal right in the United States.[21] Rather, most health insurance has been privately bought and sold. The first health insurance companies began to spring up in the early 1900s. Entrepreneurs operated them like other businesses in a market economy, competing openly, winning and losing their share of the action. Eventually, as small companies merged into larger and larger conglomerates, the private health insurance industry became a multi-hundred-billion-dollar operation. Health insurance became entwined in employer-employee contracts and complex salary negotiations. Because most Americans receive health insurance as a consequence of their job status and not as a consequence of being a U.S. citizen, the majority of health insurance for children comes from employer-based benefits. However, there has been a steady erosion of private coverage over the past decades. In 2002, 64 percent of children under the age of 18 had private insurance coverage, down from 73 percent in the early 1980s.[22]

The U.S. government has always sponsored some publicly funded health care for select groups of citizens. For instance, ever since the Pilgrims battled the Pequots, veterans of armed conflict have received government-funded health care and disability benefits.[23] Step by slow step, the government has added other groups, such as the merchant marine, federal government employees, and U.S. senators and representatives. When World War II broke out, Children's Bureau director Martha Eliot took advantage of these precedents to establish the Emergency Maternity and Infant Care Program (EMIC). Using the language of Title V that charged the Children's Bureau to "extend and improve" health care services for children, Eliot obtained authorization for federal funding for health care for the wives and children of servicemen. With their husbands and fathers on the beaches of Normandy and in the air above the Pacific, mothers and children were stranded in the unfamiliar surroundings of army bases all over the United States. Martha Eliot made her case to Congress so effectively that, by the end of World War II, EMIC had logged more than 1.5 million cases; one in six U.S. births had been covered by government funds.[24]

Soldiers and their families applauded EMIC, but obstetricians and pediatricians did not. Many doctors were outraged by government interference in their professional affairs. They objected to the Children's Bureau setting standards for medical care and fixing medical fees without means testing. Many members of the American Academy of Pediatrics (AAP) were so incensed by what they considered high-handed tactics that the Executive Committee of the AAP voted in 1944 to cut off relations with the Children's Bureau. Fortunately, Henry Helmholz, president of the AAP, maintained a calm head. The relationship between the practicing community and the Children's Bureau had often sparked debate, but Helmholz knew that a formal disengagement of the two groups would be damaging to children. He and Martha Eliot designed a creative solution to the dilemma. Together, the academy and the bureau would sponsor a national study to document the health needs of America's children. Out of the dispute over health financing came the first step toward a complete cataloguing of the health of America's children.

It has never been clear whether Senator Claude Pepper's 1945 proposal to keep EMIC going during peacetime was a backdoor attempt by Eliot to begin the process of universal health insurance coverage for all children. Certainly, the idea sounded like something she would endorse. It was also almost too convenient that the national study included just the information that any program planner would need to inaugurate such a program. If this was Eliot's plan, the time was not right. Pepper's message found far too few supporters in Congress to move the agenda forward. Not for another fifteen years would the nation address the issue of children's health insurance, and even then the program would only cover children in poverty.

Pepper and Eliot were ahead of their time and so was a most important ally in the White House. President Harry Truman was determined to take more dramatic action in support of government-sponsored health insurance for all Americans. During each of his years in office, Truman introduced health insurance bills, but each time there was bitter opposition to the idea, spearheaded by the private insurance industry and the American Medical Association. The United States was simply not going to move to universal health insurance access except possibly through incremental change.

In 1965 the incremental approach finally resulted in a movement for substantial health care legislation. With a strong economy and a Democratic majority in Congress, Lyndon Johnson proposed legislation that would allow the United States to be a Great Society.[25] He believed it was time to use the power and resources of the government to offer basic health services to all Americans regardless of income, color, or creed. He called on the nation to "build a society where progress is the servant of our needs." He worked with the Congress to commit federal government support for health care insurance.

The person who took Johnson's Great Society rhetoric and turned it into a feasible program was Wilbur Cohen, the assistant secretary of Health Education and Welfare. A behind-the-scenes pragmatist, Cohen was an economist-turned-professional-bureaucrat. He was only 21 years old when, as a member of the Committee on Economic Security, he helped draft the Social Security Act of 1935. He had promoted the provisions of the act since that time, so much so that his nickname became

Mr. Social Security. Cohen knew when, where, and how to cajole the Dixiecrat from Alabama and the Republican from Illinois. Together with President Johnson, he knew which legislator owed who what and which vote could be exchanged for what promise. Cohen understood just how far he could push the Great Society agenda. He also knew a great deal about the opposition in the form of the American Medical Association. He and the president would compromise, but they would not give way on the central objective. The federal government was going to provide health care coverage for all of the citizens of the United States, not just those employed by the federal government.

During his presidential campaign, Lyndon Johnson promised that he would create a national insurance program for the elderly. Termed *Medicare,* this insurance would not only address the health care needs of the nation's elders but also alleviate poverty among the 20 percent of the nation's older people who were poor. Health care costs were escalating, and many older citizens were falling into poverty as a direct result of their medical bills. Medicare would be part of the arsenal in the War on Poverty. What came as a surprise to Johnson, to Wilbur Cohen—to everyone—was the action of Wilbur Mills, chairman of the House Ways and Means Committee. Mills was a late convert to the idea of public accountability for health care, but once he got religion he was totally committed. He added provisions to HR-1 not only for the elderly poor but for all of the poor. Mills's actions introduced *Medicaid.* It was time for bold action. The forces were aligned and the energy was there. The strategy team in the White House, the Department of Health Education and Welfare, and the Congress decided to move ahead with full force.

In July 1965 Congress passed two amendments to the Social Security Act. Title XVIII created Medicare, the all-encompassing health insurance program for persons 65 years old and older. Its companion, Title XIX, initiated the Medicaid program, a federal-state matching system of health insurance coverage for the poor. Medicare and Medicaid were passed together, but they were very different. Medicaid was Mills's afterthought, something that had to be done for the poor. There was little or no celebration of Title XIX's passage. In writing the history of Medicare and Medicaid, Rashi Fein points out the profound discrepancies in the conceptualization and the enactment of the two bills.[26] He shows how they continue to be perceived in the government and by the general populace. Medicare is for everyone; it provides *care.* Medicaid is for the indigent; it provides *aid.* Fein dubs Medicaid "the poor relation," the program that belongs to "them," not "us." Poor families need fundamental protections in the increasingly expensive health care market, and they will be protected but in a grudging, often unfriendly manner. The poor will wait on hard wooden benches, stand in long lines, and fill out innumerable forms. Over and over, they will declare their poverty, and then they will receive Medicaid.

Unlike Medicare, which is administered uniformly to all states by the federal government, Medicaid is administered by each state.[27] Under Medicare, the eligibility and benefits are the same whether a 65-year-old lives in Boca Raton, Florida, Rattlesnake Gulch, Montana, or Fairfield, Connecticut. By contrast, if a poor family moves from Oakdale, Texas, to Oakdale, California, it will find completely different Medicaid eligibility, benefits, and reimbursement rates. As the saying goes, when you have seen one Medicaid program, you have seen one Medicaid program. Because the territories and the District of Columbia also have jurisdiction over their Medicaid offices, there are actually fifty-six Medicaid programs.

Medicaid is an insurance program that grants money to individuals (and families) to spend on their health care, either on a fee-for-service basis or, increasingly, as a part of a managed care plan. The funds for the insurance come from a federal-state match determined by the federal medical assistance percentage (FMAP) formula, which compares the state's per capita income with the national per capita income. The federal:state match varies from 1:1 (Maryland, California, New York) to 3:1 (Mississippi, Alabama, Montana, New Mexico). Although the formula is designed to favor poorer states, some states are so disadvantaged that they even have trouble raising their 25 percent share. Larger states question the FMAP match because the formula does not take into account the number of poor people in the state. As a result, some of the more populous states like California and Florida have far less to spend on each individual than states like Wisconsin and Iowa.[28]

Since Medicaid funding depends both on appropriations at the federal level and on determinations at the state level, each state's Medicaid agency is constantly at the mercy of Congress and the state legislature. Commissioners of such state programs are hard-pressed to keep within their allotted budget and still meet the needs of the assigned families. Some states run out of money midway through the fiscal year and are forced to stop paying providers. Advocates for children sometimes align themselves with the Medicaid director to get the word out to the public that every time the state cuts $1 of Medicaid funding they are actually losing an additional $1–3 in matching funds from the federal government.[29]

To receive federal matching funds, states must ensure Medicaid funding to certain federally designated groups. These include low-income families on Temporary Assistance for Needy Families (TANF), Supplemental Security Income (SSI) recipients, infants born to Medicaid-eligible mothers, and recipients of adoption assistance and foster care under Title IV-E of Social Security. States must provide Medicaid coverage to pregnant women and to children under the age of 6 whose families are at 133 percent of the federal poverty line. All children born after September 30, 1983, who live in low-income families must also be covered until they are 19 years of age. At their own discretion, states may also offer Medicaid coverage to pregnant women and children whose families earn more that 133 percent of the federal poverty level and to some children with disabilities. This accounts for the wide state-to-state variability in eligibility.

Medicaid eligibility for children is erratic because states are allowed to modify the criteria. Also, a given family can go on and off the Medicaid rolls as a result of changes in their own economic status. This is such a common occurrence, affecting so many children, that scholars who track Medicaid routinely include "partial year coverage" as an analytic category.[30] One particularly pernicious practice occurs in some beleaguered states: to maintain the minimum number of eligible families, they require monthly or quarterly in-person reenrollment at the welfare or Medicaid office.

States vary also in the benefits delivered under Medicaid. On the books, Medicaid has a rich set of potential provisions that are as good as if not better than what is available from any private insurer. Medicaid's optimal service plan includes primary care and preventive services; consultation with medical and surgical subspecialists; the provision of occupational, physical, and speech therapy; counseling and family counseling; as well as emergency room, hospital, and home nursing services.[31] In the heady days of the health care reform debates, several major health care advocates, most notably Sara Rosenbaum, argued for basing all of children's health care planning on a Medicaid model, largely because of the careful thought that had gone into the design of the optimal package. The problem is that states are not held accountable for their benefits offerings. Margaret McManus and Harriette Fox have tracked the wide variability of the state plans, from the enormously generous to the unbelievably meager.[32]

All Medicaid packages include a poorly understood feature, the Early Periodic Screening Diagnosis and Treatment (EPSDT) provision. EPSDT is a far-reaching effort to expand the screening function in primary care.[33] Child health providers are encouraged (and paid an enhanced fee) to conduct systematic screening for vision and hearing, developmental delay, language impairments, and lifelong physical conditions with their origins in childhood (e.g., hypercholesterolemia, scoliosis, hypertension). When EPSDT functions properly, treatment of the detected problems is ensured. In some states treatment is not always guaranteed, engendering skepticism in the ranks of child health providers about the whole EPSDT procedure.

The biggest problem with Medicaid is that there simply is not enough of it. The funding levels for Medicaid have always been insufficient, missing the mark by billions of dollars each year. Medicaid does not compensate physicians adequately (not even to Medicare levels).[34] Doctors in private practice who take on indigent patients are put in a compromised position. Not only are they taking on cases with a high potential for health, social, and emotional problems, they are also settling for poor pay. When the state Medicaid agency does not pay its bills, the physician has to take a personal pay cut to pay her secretary's and nurse's salaries. Even physicians of good will are going to live through that scenario only once or twice before wanting to call it quits.

Large health maintenance organizations, hospitals, academic health centers with large training endeavors, and neighborhood health clinics may be less reluctant to accept Medicaid rates because they can rely both on cross subsidies from private insurers and from other government programs (such as Medicare, Graduate Medical Education payments, and Title V) and on various grants and contracts. The disincentives to private practitioners to accept Medicaid are so strong that poor children and families are more likely to find care in settings such as training clinics and neighborhood health centers. Much of this care is of excellent quality, and the situation for poor families is far improved over the situation two to three decades ago. Nonetheless, the care is different from that delivered in a private office, and the question remains whether the coexistence of private and public insurance systems means the existence of two levels of service for children.

Medicaid is far from perfect, but it is also far better than nothing. Medicaid has been successful enough that Congress created the State Child Health Insurance Program (discussed below) to extend and expand its reach. At the time of this writing, because of state and federal cutbacks, Medicaid is under attack at all levels. Over the next several years, there is the threat of retrenchment rather than outreach, maintenance rather than innovation. Like Title V, Medicaid does afford basic federal assurances that allow it to serve a safety net function. Advocates for children recognize that the most damaging thing that could happen to Medicaid would be a gutting of the federal assurance function.[35] Only time will tell whether Medicaid expands or contracts as an insurance scheme for children, but even with all its imperfections it is likely to be the major vehicle for health insurance for poor children for the foreseeable future.

State Child Health Insurance Program, 1997

A Japanese Haiku says, "O little snail by nature weak and lowly, Climb up the cone of Fuji, slowly, slowly." Sometimes it feels as if the issue of access to child health insurance is like that little snail, plodding inch by inch toward a clear and inevitable goal. Leaders in child health have made the compelling case for universal health care access for children, but time and again they have been forced to take a compromise position and work toward an incremental solution. The State Child Health Insurance Program, also known as SCHIP, is such a pragmatic answer.[36]

Passage of Medicaid greatly improved health care access for poor children, but it did not ensure health care coverage for all children. In 1995, 10 million children and youth in the United States (the richest nation the world has ever known) had absolutely no health insurance and no prospects of obtaining any. In general, the parents were employed (sometimes both parents were working two jobs) but were making just a little too much money to meet the Medicaid eligibility cutoffs. So they lost out there. In addition, they were working for employers that did not include health care for dependents as one of the benefits of employment. They lost out there as well.

The passage of SCHIP needs to be seen in the political context of its time. The Clinton administration came into office in 1993, promising health care reform. They would overhaul a health care system that was incredibly costly, complex, overly bureaucratic, and unfriendly. The plan was to create "managed competition" that would control costs, simplify administrative hassles, cut down on burdensome paperwork, and put patients back in control. Clinton was committed to insuring as close to 100 percent of the nation as possible. For the first time in a long time, child health advocates saw an opportunity to join a general reform movement. The president and the first lady were going to make the health system more transparent, more rational, and more compassionate. Kids issues would fit right in.

Unfortunately, in the complex political milieu of the United States, where proprietary health insurance has held sway for so long, a program of sweeping health care reform was doomed from its inception. To "simplify" the existing system, the Clinton administration produced an 1,800-page document with flow charts and algorithms. Patients were to follow one set of instructions, doctors another; the dollars would flow according to still other instructions. It was difficult for the administration to attract support for the plan. The health insurance industry countered with their "Harry and Louise" television ads, spreading alarm about health care if the Clinton plan passed. Enthusiasm for all-encompassing reform died.

During the height of the health care reform debates, many child advocates worried that children's issues would get lost. Nonetheless, they put away their "Children First" buttons in the hope that the larger movement would be successful. They decided that it was politically astute to build a coalition with adult-oriented groups. When it became apparent that all-out health care reform was going to fail, child health advocates changed tack again. Here was the opportunity to save the administration a little face and to close the enormous gap for kids. Out came the "Children First" buttons, on came the arguments for universal coverage for children, in walked two skillful child health advocates: Teddy Kennedy and Orrin Hatch. From widely divergent geographic and political backgrounds, one of the Senate's most liberal standard-bearers could agree wholeheartedly with one of the Senate's most conservative ideologists on the importance of child health insurance coverage. They created a new state-based child health insurance program and fought for its passage as Title XXI of the Social Security Act.

SCHIP was incorporated into the Balanced Budget Act of 1997 to enable states "to initiate and expand health insurance coverage for uninsured children. The funds cover the cost of insurance, as well as outreach services to get children enrolled and reasonable costs for administration. Funds must be used to cover previously uninsured children and not to replace existing public or private coverage."[37] Like Medicaid, the SCHIP program is a federal-state partnership with both the benefits and the liabilities of that system. SCHIP ensures that individual states have a good deal of flexibility. They can expand Medicaid, or they can create new insurance delivery vehicles, or they can create a combination program. The states can also select from "several benchmark benefit packages, develop a benefit package that is actuarially equivalent to or better than one of the benchmark plans, or use the Medicaid benefit." Eligibility determination is also left up to the states.

State flexibility builds into SCHIP the same state-to-state variability that bedevils Medicaid. The inequality has actually been exacerbated in SCHIP because the states that have used their funds wisely have been able to recruit additional dollars for outreach and service while those states that have poor systems lag further and further behind. As a result, there are many more uninsured and underserved children in some states than in others. In a classic move, the State of Florida solved its dilemma of having large numbers of children on a waiting list for health insurance by simply doing away with the list.[38] This may have made their numbers look better on the national scorecard, but it did absolutely nothing for children.

It is a little difficult to know how positive or how negative to be about SCHIP. In some ways it has been a glorious achievement; in others it has been a big disappointment. SCHIP has not accomplished its primary objective of closing the health insurance gap for children. In the late 1990s there were 10 million uninsured children; in 2002, despite the availability of SCHIP and associated outreach activities, there were still nearly 8.5 million.[39] What is the problem?

There are a number of explanations. First, it is important to understand that the uninsured pool of children has always been dynamic, with families moving on and off the rolls of the insured from year to year and month to month. Second, there is the issue of accountability. In a way, what SCHIP has done is to expose the weakest link in the American health care system. There is private insurance. There is public insurance. There are all sorts of regulations about who can get insurance, for how long, for what conditions, and for what procedures. There are rules and regulations. But there is no absolute accountability. There is no desk in the country where the child health insurance buck stops. No person, no agency, no elected official is responsible for the health of the nation's children. In the absence of such accountability, employers will not be admonished if they drop family health insurance benefits when an alternative government program is available.

Ironically, instead of correcting the problem of private companies divesting from family health insurance plans, the very fact that SCHIP existed allowed employers to cancel policies. The "crowd-out phenomenon" accounts for a substantial amount of the uninsurance among children and youth. Mr. Seven Figure CEO can use the money he saves to protect his company's assets and pour the profits back into the economy to make it healthy. Just think how many more jobs the fast food chains and mall markets can create if they aren't fettered by the extra cost of insuring Sammy and Bobbi and little Terrance.

SCHIP requires that immigrants be in the United States for five years before they are eligible for health insurance benefits. This limits access to preventive care and the care of chronic conditions. Federal law prohibits hospitals from turning away any child or family in a dire emergency, but reliance on crisis-oriented health care drives up the costs of medical care and imposes burdens on the health care system. A very disheartening aspect of the SCHIP experience has been its inability to track down new immigrants who do qualify and encourage their participation. Many qualified immigrants fear signing up for anything that might be a one-way ticket out of the United States. Since the new immigrant families represent a significant population expansion, particularly in border states, this problem of uninsured children is a constant and growing one.

The SCHIP story is not over. No, SCHIP has not cured the serious dilemma. In fact, it has been little more than a finger in the dike. Nonetheless, SCHIP has brought the nation one step closer to a system of full coverage for children and youth. In a country that moves by small measured steps, that is a big accomplishment.

The Individuals with Disabilities Education Act

The Individuals with Disabilities Education Act (IDEA) was originally titled The Education for All Handicapped Children Act of 1975. This special education legislation emerged in the 1970s as a natural step in the progression of American civil rights legislation. The story of its passage demonstrates the power of parent-professional-policymaker collaboration. Several strands of activity braided together a national response that fundamentally changed the circumstances for children with disabilities in the nation.

In the 1950s and early 1960s parents and advocates for people with physical and developmental disabilities were increasingly dissatisfied with what they saw as substandard, socially isolating, services for children and youth with disabling conditions.[40] In the early 1950s parents of children with mental retardation had begun meeting together in a group then known as the National Association of Parents and Friends of Retarded Citizens. They determined that it was critical to base their advocacy on facts and science. Forming a group called The Arc, they set out "to promote and stimulate needed research into causes, cure and prevention of mental retardation."[41]

The Arc parents were able to enlist research scientists from Harvard, Yale, and Johns Hopkins to conduct descriptive studies of mental retardation. The first report from the Arc, "A Survey of Research in the Field

of Mental Deficiency," was followed by a series of more basic investigations on the causes of mental retardation and developmental disability.
Among the scientific findings were two key ones: (1) many causes of
retardation are preventable, and (2) youngsters with developmental disability still can progress developmentally, especially when provided the
appropriate environmental stimulation.

Armed with these basic facts, the coalition of parents and researchers
was equipped to advocate for congressional support of a major research
effort on childhood disabilities. In 1960 The Arc formed a partnership
with the American Academy of Pediatrics to strengthen the base of support. Whether it was serendipity or just the way things should happen,
the project found a ready and willing listener in the White House: President John Kennedy knew the impact of mental retardation on a child and
her family. His sister Rosemary suffered from mental retardation, and
the Kennedy family had founded the Kennedy Foundation to improve
the community's advocacy for children with disabilities. Robert Cooke,
who was a leader in pediatric research and academics, was the medical adviser of the Kennedy Foundation. Cooke was also the parent of
two children with disabilities. He knew how important a firm evidence
base would be for moving an advocacy agenda forward. In large part
because of his urging, the Kennedy administration proposed a major
expansion of NIH's program in child research, with a specific emphasis
on the causes of mental retardation.

John Kennedy convened the first Presidential Panel on Mental Retardation. Within a short time Congress passed bills to sponsor research on
the causes of mental retardation. An explosion of information followed
with the publication of articles on lead poisoning, phenylketouria, and
toxoplasmosis. In 1965 Goodman published the first information on the
genetic basis of Down syndrome.[42]

After President Kennedy's death, Cooke remained one of the most
trusted advisers to Lyndon Johnson and Sargent Shriver, John Kennedy's
brother-in-law.[43] He was in the situation room as President Johnson and
his team devised their battle plans for the War on Poverty. Poverty and
disability are linked in a myriad of ways, and Robert Cooke made sure
that research into the prevention of disability was front and center of the
national agenda.

As the research community compiled the scientific case, other activity
unfolded on the public policy front. In the early 1970s, in the state-level
suit *Pennsylvania Association for Retarded Citizens (PARC) v. Pennsylvania,* the court ruled that children with disabilities should be included in

public education. Another case, *Mills v. the Board of Education of the District of Columbia*, established the principle that school systems could not use "special education" placements as a form of de facto segregation. As important, the *Mills* judgment said that schools could not claim that financial burdens precluded them from offering necessary services. These state-level legal precedents created just enough pressure to induce the Congress to take a long look at the rights of children with disabilities.[44]

At the time, two high-ranking members of the Senate, Hubert Humphrey and Lowell Weikart, were very familiar with childhood disability. Both had children with Down syndrome, and their personal experience paralleled the tales they heard in parent's testimony. One mother recounted how her 6-year-old son stood at the bus stop every day with his brother and cried as the bus pulled away, leaving him behind. Every member of Congress had constituents whose children were getting the short end of the educational stick—at least 1 million children were not receiving the educational services they were entitled to under the Fourteenth Amendment to the Constitution. As Congress heard from parents, physicians, teachers, nurses, and therapists, they became convinced that there was need for fundamental reform in the way communities designed services for children with disabilities. Viewing the special education legislation as a vehicle to right many of the wrongs of the past, Senator Harrison Williams and Representative John Brademas introduced the bill. In 1975 members of Congress, by an overwhelming majority, passed P.L. 94-142, the Education for All Handicapped Children Act.

The basic tenet of the Education for All Handicapped Children Act is that all children in the United States deserve a full, appropriate public education no matter how severe their physical, cognitive, or emotional disability. The states must provide services and remove barriers so that all children can be educated.[45]

The special education law rests on four cornerstones: identification, evaluation, related services, and due process. The law requires states to *identify* all children and youth with disabilities as soon as possible so that the children do not regress further in the absence of state-of-the-art education. The *evaluation* requirement of the law ensures that the schools, working with appropriate consultants, make a timely, proper, and unbiased assessment of the educational and related services needs of the children. The resulting individualized education plan (IEP) contains the educational goals and the specifications for educational services the child will receive. The school also must provide *related services* such as transportation, therapies, counseling, and school health care so that all children can attend school in the least restrictive environment. Finally, the law affords *due process* rights to the parents of children with disabilities, rights that other parents do not have. Until a child's parents signal their satisfaction with the IEP by signing it, the process of evaluation, review, and planning is not over. If a child's parents are very dissatisfied, they can call for arbitration and even take their concerns as far as the United States Supreme Court.

Subsequent amendments and refinements have maintained the law's core tenets and extended its reach to infants, toddlers, and preschoolers with disabilities. In 1986 Congress passed P.L. 99-457 to make educational services available to children with disabilities from birth on.[46] The preamble to the legislation documents the part that science and advocacy played in moving legislation forward. In 1990 Congress reauthorized the special education law and took that opportunity to amalgamate the regulations for children of school age with those for infants, toddlers, and preschoolers. The Education for All Handicapped Children Act was renamed the Individuals with Disabilities Education Act (IDEA), which now includes provisions for children ages 3 to 21 years (Part B) and for children ages birth to 3 years (Part C).

In November 2004 the reauthorization of IDEA updated the language of the law to acknowledge the increasing diversity of the child population and to alert the special education community to the persistence of racial, ethnic, and socioeconomic disparities among the children covered.[47] Of greatest concern was the finding that there are disproportionately high numbers of minority students in schools where the teachers and students are predominantly white. This led to the call for the recruitment, training, and promotion of special education professionals from minority backgrounds.

IDEA 2004 calls for high-quality assessments and scientifically based curricular input. The law also raises the expectation that all children will succeed in their educational pursuits. This new language brings IDEA into line with the requirements of the No Child Left Behind Act (the Elementary and Secondary Education Act). The emphasis on high-quality education and improved preparation of teachers is considered a good step by most observers, but concerns remain that children with special education needs may not fare well in an atmosphere in which the major mark of accomplishment is a score on standardized achievement tests.[48]

One of the main areas of focus in the revisions of IDEA 2004 is transition for youth with disabilities. IDEA 2004 makes a specific recommendation that transition planning for youth must begin by age 16. The planning functions are spelled out in detail and involve a description of the student's strengths and needs and the development of "appropriate measurable postsecondary goals based upon age, transition assessments related to training, education, employment, and where appropriate, independent living skills."[49]

IDEA 2004 addresses the complex issues of behavior problems and discipline among children with disabilities. Handling discipline for young people with acting-out behaviors can be especially thorny. When the child threatens or hurts another child or a teacher, the answers about the best placement for the child are never easy. IDEA 2004 spells out the procedures for placement in alternative settings and for assessment of the child and the situation in great detail. Because each case is different, the law still leaves room for a variety of interpretations. As a result, some children who are hard to manage may unfortunately end up in more restrictive environments than necessary.

Although the new language of IDEA 2004 is largely clarifying and adds flexibility for families and schools, some of the changes in the law could have problematic consequences. The law calls for a reduction of bureaucratic tangles and paperwork and introduces a pilot program in fifteen states to allow school systems to offer three-year individualized education plans. This risks the elimination of one of the IDEA's strongest provisions, namely the annual monitoring of the educational progress of children with disabilities.

The federal special education legislation has enjoyed broad bipartisan support in the Congress despite periodic attempts (mostly by the executive branch) to weaken its provisions. The most dramatic confrontation came during the Reagan administration when Secretary of Education Terrance Bell was thrown out of the congressional chamber because he came to recommend substantial cuts in the special education program.[50] The honorable secretary and his message were not welcome: Congress is committed to the rights of children with disabilities. But the real question is how committed are they? A fundamental concern with IDEA is that Congress has never appropriated the full federal funding originally envisioned for the program.

When the special education mandate was passed in 1975, the funding formula obligated the federal government to provide 12 percent of the additional costs that local education agencies would incur as they fulfilled the requirements of the law. The states and localities would pick up the rest. To ease the financial burden on states, cities, and towns, the federal portion of the cost of special education was supposed to increase each year until it ultimately reached 40 percent. That never happened. The federal contribution remained close to 12 percent from 1977 through the 1990s, leading critics of IDEA to call it the one of the largest unfunded mandates of all time. During Newt Gingrich's tenure as leader of the Congress, special education legislation came in for a great deal of rhetorical invective.

In the late 1990s and early 2000s several parent groups joined forces with Senator Jim Jeffords of Vermont to call for the full funding of IDEA. Jeffords became so impassioned about the problem and the unwillingness of his Republican colleagues to face the issue of Congress's disappointing performance on their promise that he left the Republican Party to become an Independent, thus denying the Republicans a majority in the Senate. This may have been the first time that a child issue literally redistributed the power in the legislative branch.

The battle around full funding is still waging at the time of this writing. The 2006 appropriation for IDEA is nearly $12 billion, which is approximately 20 percent of the excess costs to educate a child in special education. This is a major improvement over the original funding of 8–10 percent. Over the next few years, the House and Senate will continue to deliberate and act on proposals to reach the full federal funding levels initially spelled out for special education.

Living in a democratic nation is about deciding what you are for and speaking out about it. This chapter outlines the ways in which advocates show that they are for children and youth. Legislative advocacy allows large-scale policy change that affects the lives of children now and for many years to come. Title V, Medicaid, SCHIP, and IDEA have established fundamental safeguards for children's health and development, but there is still a long way to go before all children benefit. Every phone call, every e-mail, every testimony counts.

7   Professional Advocacy

THIS BOOK'S CHAPTERS DISCUSS how professionals, families, and community organizations collaborate to improve the health of children and youth. In the best of all possible worlds, child health professionals act on their convictions with few constraints. But in the real world, forces within and outside the profession often prevent child health professionals from using their talents to the best advantage for society. When poorly aligned incentives, senseless customs, or irrational standards affect the ability of health professionals to act on behalf of children and youth, a reexamination of what it means to be a professional is in order. There are times when advocacy is called for to keep the profession true to its original charge.

To understand the call for professional advocacy, the first question is, What does professionalism entail? That question was the topic of the April 2004 Old Docs Dinner at the Harvard Faculty Club. Amid the bouquets of spring flowers, the linen tablecloths, and the fine china, ten deans and professors of the Harvard Medical School devoted their formal after-dinner discussion to delineating their thoughts about professionalism. Dean Dan Federman had given each of the Old Docs a homework assignment of defining the construct. Like medical educators around the country, he was reaching out to wise colleagues to help him come to grips with how to teach the core competencies now required by the Accreditation Council for Graduate Medical Education (table 7.1). Professionalism, according to the council, is "manifested through a commitment to carrying out professional responsibilities, adherence to ethical principles, and sensitivity to a diverse patient population."

Some of the Old Docs had gotten out their Webster's and Oxford English Dictionaries; others had Googled the Internet for the latest definitions. The discussion was far-ranging and at times deeply moving, as these medical experts, the educators of the next generation, probed the heart of the matter. The upshot of the discussion was that professionalism involves actions that will advance the larger field and benefit the wider society. As clinicians, physicians should be striving to improve

Table 7.1. Accreditation Council for Graduate Medical Education, Competencies

---

Patient care that is compassionate, appropriate, and effective for the treatment of health problems and the promotion of health

Medical knowledge about established and evolving biomedical, clinical, and cognate (e.g., epidemiological and social behavioral) sciences and the application of this knowledge to patient care

Practice-based learning and improvement that involves investigation and evaluation of their own patient care, appraisal and assimiliation of scientific evidence, and improvements in patient care

Interpersonal and communication skills that result in effective information exchange and teaming with patients, their families, and other health professionals

Professionalism, as manifested through a commitment to carrying out professional responsibilities, adherence to ethical principles, and sensitivity to a diverse patient population

Systems-based practice, as manifested by actions that demonstrate an awareness of and responsiveness to the larger context and system of health care and the ability to effectively call on system resources to provide care that is of optimal value

---

Source: Accreditation Council for Graduate Medical Education, Program Requirements for Residency Education in Pediatrics, available at www.acgme.org/outcome/comp/compFull.asp (accessed September 22, 2005).

health. As scientists, medical doctors should be committed to seeking new knowledge of basic biological mechanisms and new cures for disease. The Old Docs all shared the belief that the fruits of science and medicine belong to everyone. As a consequence, a commitment to equity through social justice is a key element of professionalism.

There was general agreement among the Old Docs that a profession has rights and responsibilities as well as limits and boundaries. Members of the health professions experience life in a very special way. Few others enter the most personal spaces and times of people's lives. Few others have the powerful tools of biology, chemistry, physiology, anatomy, and pharmacology at their disposal. Few others are able to affect individual lives so directly. Despite this, the doctors expressed frustration that insurance companies and government regulators interpose stumbling blocks between health care providers and their patients.

The Old Docs were also worried about ethical issues. As keepers of the professional charge, they were concerned about an erosion of professionalism in the generation of new knowledge. The health care arena is changing into the health care industry, with large sums of money in play for those with new ideas and technical innovation.[1] The rules of the game are in flux, and the stakes are high. The deans watch as some of their brightest and best scientists are lured out of the universities into biotechnology and pharmaceutical companies. They agonize about the dangerous liaisons with business when patients are the subjects of research ventures. Discussions of who owns various forms of intellectual property dominate university agendas and appear in investigative journals.

The deans were discomfited also by the inability of the profession to tackle the persistent inequities between poor and rich, black and white, the forgotten and the privileged.[2] They were mindful of the diverse and changing demographic makeup of the United States and of the new data linking disease states to community and cultural factors.[3] They also were all too familiar with the imbalance between the racial and ethnic characteristics of their faculty and the population of patients who seek care in the hospitals served by the medical school.[4] They were encouraged, though, by the increasingly diverse student body in medical schools and by the eagerness among incoming students to learn about cultural forces and their impact on health and illness.

The Old Docs ended their dinner having grappled with semantics and concluded that the word *professionalism* defines the essence of what doctors can do to make life more full for individuals and society. As they left the table and said their good-byes, there was a sense that the exchange was no mere exercise in splitting hairs, that the future of the health care profession really did depend on such explorations: doctors realigning their compasses to true north.

The Social Contract for Children's Health

How do these issues about professionalism play out in child health? Are the child health professions also taking a serious look at themselves? Yes. Slowly but surely. In part because they are bumping up against so many impediments to getting their job done.

In the earlier chapters of this book, we point to some of the barriers to professional work that impede individual practitioners and the field of child health as a whole. Pediatric physician scientists are stopped in their tracks by lack of funds or by federal interdictions on particular types of scientific inquiry, such as stem cell research. Primary care physicians stumble over seemingly endless constraints as they attempt to offer comprehensive care. Specialists are held back from employing life-saving technologies. International medical missionaries are fettered by financial, political, and military realities. When there are more locked doors than open gates, where does the leadership come from to march forward, to carry on, to advocate for the right of professionals to act professionally?

Through the Hippocratic oath, medical professionals verbally enter into a social contract with patients. In contemporary terms, child health clinicians promise to prevent illness, cure disease, and care for those who are chronically afflicted. That is a tall order, one that no individual clinician can fill on his own. The entire profession needs to organize itself to get up each morning, check the daily task list, and make sure each task is covered. This involves individuals putting themselves and their needs forward, an action child health professionals find uncomfortable, even occasionally distasteful. Child health clinicians find discussions of the ends far easier than considerations of the means. So before talking about how professional advocates make the case for what they need, let us review the core components of the child health social contract.

Prevention

It may be self-evident that prevention should be highly valued and that efforts to enhance preventive strategies should be supported, but prevention is generally regarded as a stepsister or poor cousin in medicine. There is something uncompelling about a problem that is not there. Complacency slips in when there hasn't been a case of smallpox for more than two decades. The general public just does not recognize the critical part that preventive strategies play in keeping the nation's people healthy.

Despite the fact that prevention remains low on the national list of priorities, evaluation data show how effective well-implemented prevention efforts can be (see table 7.2; also see chapter 3). Unfortunately, despite these data, prevention gets far too little attention within and outside the child health profession. One advocacy strategy that has not been employed optimally is cost-benefit analyses. The dollars saved by preventive work accrue over the lifespan of children and can add up to very substantial societal savings. For instance, several studies argue that $1 spent on prenatal care saves up to $3 by preventing low birth weight. Careful economic assessments show that folic acid intake by young women is highly efficient and cost effective in the prevention of neural tube defects.[5] Clinical advocacy involves a full embrace and implementation of preventive strategies despite a lack of enthusiasm for these activities by the general public, policymakers in Washington, and the local health insurance company administrator.

Cure

The next best thing to prevention is cure. Total cure and a child's return to full functioning is the highest accomplishment in medicine. In childhood, many acute conditions (such as most infectious diseases, many injuries, and some congenital anomalies) can be cured completely. Professional advocacy for these situations consists of ensuring that physicians can get to the children and youth who need to receive the appropriate medicines or surgical intervention in a timely fashion under optimal conditions. In Washington State, physicians and nurses of the Washing-

Table 7.2. Prevention Works: Infancy, Early Childhood, School Age, and Adolescence

Age	Strategy	Supporting data	Impact
Newborn	Newborn hearing screen	Increased early detection of hearing loss; improved language outcomes	Less need for specialized service; improved life chances and function
	Back-to-Sleep campaign	SIDS rate declined from 1.2/1,000 to 0.7/1,000	Saved lives
	Newborn metabolic screen	Increased detection and treatment of PKU, hypothyroidism, and other metabolic diseases	Improved survival, decreases in mental retardation
	AIDS prevention	75 percent decline in perinatally acquired HIV since the institution of PACTG 076 in 1994	Saved lives; improved outcomes for mothers and babies
Early Childhood	Vaccine use	See table 3.2, this volume	Saved lives; decreased hospitalization; decreased disability from viral and bacterial illness
	Literacy	Increases in parents reading to children	Potential for improving preschool and school performance
	Children Can't Fly program	Window falls reduced by 75 percent and fatalities by 80 percent	Saved lives; decreased hospital and ICU admissions; decreased traumatic brain injury
	Lead screening	Mean blood levels decreased; screening in Boston led to 51 percent reduction in blood lead levels over 5 years	Decreased hospitalization; decreased need for chelation; improved cognition; improved school performance; 1 to 5 IQ points for every 10 microgm/dL of blood Pb
	Anemia prevention	Prevalence of anemia in low-income children dropped from 15–30 percent to 5 percent since the institution of WIC in 1960s	Improved physical and mental performance; improved attention
School age	Bicycle helmet use program	50 percent decrease in head injury	Saved lives; decreased traumatic brain injury; decreased hospital and ICU stays
	Pedestrian safety program	43 percent decline in pedestrian fatalities among children 0–14	Saved lives; decreased disability; decreased hospital and ICU stays
Adolescence	Violence prevention program	Decrease in homicide among adolescents	Saved lives; improvements for both the victim and aggressor
	Condom use program	Condom use increased	HIV/AIDS and STD prevention as well as teen pregnancy reduction
	Reduction in teen pregnancy program	Birth control and abstinence	Improved life chances for mothers and infants; reduction in child abuse
	Smoking prevention program	Minimal but detectable decreases; see figure 3.8 this volume	Decreased risk for lung disease, cancer, blindness, small-for-gestational-age infants

Table 7.2. continued

Source: Kennedy C, McCann D, Campbell MJ, Kimm L, and Thornton R, Universal Newborn Screening for Permanent Childhood Hearing Impairment: An 8-Year Follow-Up of a Controlled Trial, *Lancet* 366 (2005):660–62; Keren R, Helfand M, Homer C, McPhillips H, and Lieu TA, Projected Cost-Effectiveness of Statewide Universal Newborn Hearing Screening, *Pediatrics* 110 (2002):855–64; Downs MP and Yoshinage-Itano C, The Efficacy of Early Identification and Intervention for Children with Hearing Impairment, *Pediatric Clinics of North America* 4b (1999):79–87; Moon RY, Oden RP, and Grady KC, Back to Sleep: An Education Intervention with Women, Infants, and Children Program Clients, *Pediatrics* 113 (2004):542–47; National Institutes of Health, Consensus Development Panel, Phenylketonuria: Screening and Management, *Pediatrics* 108 (2001):972 82; Section on Endocrinology and Committee on Genetics and American Thyroid Association Committee on Public Health, Newborn Screening for Congenital Hypothyroidism: Recommended Guidelines; *Pediatrics* 91 (1993):1203–9; Fisher DA, Effectiveness of Newborn Screening Programs for Congenital Hypothyroidism: Prevalence of Missed Cases, *Pediatric Clinics of North America* 34 (1987):881–90; Connor EM, Sperling RS, Gelber R, et al., Reduction of Maternal-Infant Transmission of Human Immunodeficiency Virus Type 1 with Zidovudine Treatment, Pediatric AIDS Clinical Trials Group Protocol 076 Study Group, *New England Journal of Medicine* 331 (1994):1173–80; Achievements in Public Health, 1900–1999: Impact of Vaccines Universally Recommended for Children, United States, 1990–1998, *Morbidity and Mortality Weekly Review,* April 2, 1999, pp. 243–48; Weitzman CC, Roy L, Walls T, and Tomlin R, More Evidence for Reach Out and Read: A Home-Based Study, *Pediatrics* 113 (2004):1248–53; Silverstein M, Iverson L, and Lozano P, An English-Language Clinic-Based Literacy Program Is Effective for a Multilingual Population, *Pediatrics* 109 (2002):76; Spiegel CN and Lindaman FC, Children Can't Fly: A Program to Prevent Childhood Morbidity and Mortality from Window Falls, *American Journal of Public Health* 67 (1977):1143–47; Needleman H, Lead Poisoning, *Annual Review of Medicine* 55 (2004):209–22; Centers for Disease Control, Trends in Blood Lead Levels among Children: Boston, Massachusetts, 1994–1999, *Morbidity and Mortality Weekly Review,* May 2001, pp. 337–39; Sherry B, Mei Z, and Yip R, Continuation of the Decline in Prevalence of Anemia in Low-Income Infants and Children in Five States, *Pediatrics* 107 (2001): 677–82; Centers for Disease Control, *Injury Fact Book 2001–2002*; bicycle-related injuries available at www.cdc.gov/ncipc/fact_book/11_Bicycle_Related_Injuuries.htm; Wesson D, Spence L, Hu X, and Parkin P, Trends in Bicycling-Related Head Injuries in Children after Implementation of a Community-Based Bike Helmet Campaign, *Journal of Pediatric Surgery* 35 (2000): 688–89; Traffic Facts 2001, available at www.nhtsa.dot.gov; Access Safety City, available at www.nhtsa.dot.gov/people/outreach/safedige/spring2003/spr03:w10?NY.htm; www.childstats.gov/americaschildren/hea8.asp (accessed September 21, 2005); www.childrendsdatabank.org/PDF/Violence.pdf (accessed September 21, 2005); www.childrendsdatabank.org/indicators/28CondomUse.cfm (accessed November 2, 2005); Adolescent Birth Rates, by Age and Race of the Mother, 2001, *Child Health, USA* 2002, p. 35; Monitoring the Future (Institute for Social Research, University of Michigan, 2004).

ton Alaska Montana Idaho (WAMI) Corps transport children and youth from all over the Northwest so that the 5-year-old with osteomyelitis can be treated with intravenous antibiotics, and the 19-year-old can receive surgery for her inflamed dermoid cyst. On the international front, through the auspices of Project Smile, plastic surgeons travel around the world on month-long missions to operate on and cure children with cleft lip and palate.

Disappointingly, total cure is not possible for many chronic problems of childhood. The best that families and children can expect is what the physician essayist Lewis Thomas ironically terms "half-way technology."[6] Endocrinologists, for instance, use half-way technology for diabetes: to keep the blood glucose of a young boy with diabetes in the 90–130 range, the child must test his blood three or four times a day and inject himself three times a day with the calculated amount of insulin, and he must to this every day without fail. As long as the child complies with each technical step, he will achieve a normal sugar level and the absence of symptoms.

Much of child health service is composed of maintaining children in these partial cure states. Professional advocacy opportunities to do this present themselves in many forms. Physicians and nurses at the Judith M. Power Clinic, a dialysis center at the Cleveland Clinic, have pushed the professional envelope to redefine holistic care. They have advocated for special funding to enable them to work with the families in establishing routine regimens, to arrange visiting nurse services to assist the family, and to ensure access to medicines and supplies not covered by the child's insurance companies. These child health advocates consider special community and sports outings key components of the health care they provide to their patients. Bolstering the children's self-esteem seems to help keep their blood pressure in a healthy range and their electrolytes in better balance.[7]

Care

When a condition can be neither prevented nor cured, what is left is the art of medicine: the bedside presence and the cooling sponge on the feverish forehead. Lacking the efficacy of prevention or the drama of cure, care in medicine is frequently underappreciated and almost always underfunded. For children in poverty and for children with severe chronic conditions, advocacy around care must be a constant drumbeat, kept up against the changing times, the exigencies of budget cuts, and the skepticism of administrators. Such advocacy is hard but not impossible. The physicians and nurses of the Coordinated Care Service at Children's Hospital in Boston, who tend children with complex medical conditions and disabilities, have learned from long experience which home care company administrator to insist on speaking to. They have figured out just how to make the most persuasive case to obtain the needed equipment or services.

Three Requirements for Professionalism

Julius Richmond is mentor to countless professionals. He is the sounding board for pediatricians, public health professionals, nurses, psychiatrists, sociologists, and on and on. When his protégés—baffled, discouraged, or tired—come to ask for advice about life and work, he says, "Unless something is getting in your way, just keep doing what you are doing." Most of the time, what is getting in the way is more imagined than real; the only adversary is self-doubt. But there are also forces that conspire against professionals. Some are subtle, such as the downstream effects of market forces. Some are overt, such as the competing demands for limited dollars. When professionals are stopped in their tracks, they should speak out.

Whether the health care arena is primary or specialty and whether the focus is prevention, cure, or care, professional advocacy at the most basic level calls for (1) up-to-date knowledge and technology, (2) space and time, and (3) adequate funds to reimburse themselves and their support staff and to pay for resources for patients.

Knowledge and Technology

In the United States the availability of training, continuing medical education, and access to both cognitive and technical resources is generally a given. Nonetheless, the exigencies of time and the press of patient care sometimes limit the ability of practitioners to keep current with the pace of knowledge breakthroughs. The professional organizations in pediatrics do an extraordinary job of offering continuing education in live forums and through the Internet, but these offerings are expensive and involve the commitment of time away from the clinical setting. Individual physicians frequently find themselves standing up to their bosses (in managed care or even in academic institutions) just to be granted the funding and necessary time to keep their knowledge base up-to-date.

For the most part, American doctors do have access to reliable clinical laboratory technology. Access to such technology is certainly not a given in many parts of the world. The "brain drain" from Africa, India, the Middle East, Eastern Europe, and South America is largely driven by the fact that doctors literally cannot doctor in many countries. Without basic clinical laboratories, standard X-ray equipment, sterilization capability, clean needles, antibiotics, and vaccines, they cannot practice the medicine they know. Professional advocacy is needed to see that the precious resource of these skilled individuals is not wasted because they do not have the tools they need to do their job. Something is really getting in their way.

American physicians can readily send their patients for the latest blood level of protocadmiumIL-2zincoxidealuminum or an enhanced MRI (magnetic resonance imaging) of the left fifth metatarsal. Oddly enough, getting the results back from those laboratory and radiological studies can often be a formidable chore. Most child health practices are behind the times in communication technology. Despite huge national investments in informatics, there are still no universally accepted child health electronic records. Physicians working in multiple health maintenance organizations and hospital groups face huge dilemmas in getting hold of simple test results on their patients. Each morning they log on to the screens of three or four affiliated hospitals, each with its unique password and specialized identity card. Professional advocacy for more uniform approaches to medical data management has been painstakingly slow because of technical, financial, and political issues. The confidentiality concerns embodied in the Health Insurance Portability and Assurances Act (HIPAA) have added an additional layer of complexity to information sharing.[8]

The built-in inefficiencies in medicine are astounding. Parents surely expect that there is an established process for monitoring data on their children's immunization status. There is not. Across the United States, with huge support from the Centers for Disease Control, there are demonstration projects trying to find the best way to track shot records.[9] The fact that families in the United States move so often and that employers change medical insurance coverage (and therefore providers) confounds the problem. Professional advocacy by many physicians in primary care, infectious diseases, and community medicine is directed at improving the technology available to medical practices, health centers, hospitals, and schools to facilitate the monitoring of this information. In one small attempt to conquer this problem, Ronald Samuels at the Primary Care Center at Children's Hospital in Boston is borrowing a commercial technology, bar codes, for use on medicines. If Samuels can render this aspect of health care delivery half as efficient as grocery checkout, he will have advocated well for the profession.

Space and Time

The issue of space is a constant problem in some settings. Physicians in crowded university facilities often juggle their multiple responsibilities under adverse physical circumstances. To dramatize the problem, for their annual skit the fellows of the Division of General Pediatrics at Children's Hospital in Boston dressed up like the wandering Jews searching the Sinai Desert for somewhere to see a patient or to jot a note. In many academic health centers, the term *laptop* has taken on a new meaning, with two or three physicians forced to share one desk. It is not unusual for one examination room to serve three or four doctors. Private practitioners can be plagued by the same problems, particularly when their practices are located in urban or dense suburban areas, where rent is high. The more suburban or rural a practice is, the less that space is a problem, but in that case distance causes its own professional dilemmas.

There never is enough time. In chapter 4 we discuss time management at considerable length because the wise use of time is a form of clinical advocacy. Professional time is the "commodity" of medicine. It is what is bought and sold. Clinical session work is reimbursed based on large blocks of time, but there is no such metric for the rest of a physician's time. Medical administrative minutes are not measured in stopwatch aliquots the way legal professional time is. Pediatrics is unlikely ever to go to such a system, but certain child health professionals might benefit greatly from this methodology. In pediatrics, subspecialists in infectious diseases, genetics, and metabolism struggle financially because little of their time is billable, and their valued consultation is frequently given free. Which brings us to the third requirement, adequate pay.

Adequate Pay

An infectious disease consultant may spend a large amount of time providing detailed information to a pediatric orthopedist about the appropriate antibiotic coverage for a 5-year-old child with an invasive bone infection. He may fill out the three excessively detailed pharmacy forms required to clear the restricted antibiotic and, then spend a half hour on hold trying to get in touch with the state lab to report the rare infection. He will do all of this without a penny's compensation because the work was not face-to-face with the patient and the patient had already quite properly been charged for physician's services by the orthopedic surgeon.

In thinking about the above example as professional advocates, we might ask, Whose problem is this? Is it the patient's problem? The insurance company's problem? Is it a concern for the doctor that asked for the infectious disease consultation? The consultant himself? In the long run, the infectious diseases department or the hospital will end up subsidizing the cost, somehow, some way. But, what way? Professional advocacy is needed to get to the bottom of complex problems like this one. It takes poring through charts and billing sheets, profit-and-loss spreadsheets, just to define and explain the problem—let alone find a reasonable solution. This is why hours and hours of professional time are spent in meetings of physicians' organizations and hospital-physician organizations.

Sometimes we can see a problem better when it is depicted in stark terms. The following story from the Philippines points to the brave efforts of a group of child health providers who refused to let illogical payment structures stand in the way of offering high-standard services to children in the greatest need. In the Philippines the infant mortality rate is 27 per 1,000, the under-5-year-old death rate is 36 per 1,000, and child sexual abuse is rampant. Unfortunately, there is no government or insurance funding available to doctors to address these medical and social issues. Private practice is the only viable source of reimbursement.

To address these problems, a group of pediatricians formed the Philippine Ambulatory Pediatric Association (PAPA). Members are well trained in pediatrics and in developmental and behavioral interventions and are committed to dealing with the complex medical and social problems they encounter. When the doctors get together at their annual PAPA meetings, they decry their inability to attack the devastating problems of the majority of children in their country. They drive through the Manila streets filled with 4- and-5-year-olds playing in the gutters with matches, the only "toys" they have. They are mindful of the high rates of infectious diseases, the high levels of parental smoking, and the poor nutrition that make these children vulnerable to ill health. They worry about children with chronic illness and disability. But to put bread on the table for their own children, they take private patients from among the wealthy and spend their time on children who are, perhaps, already well cared for.

In the late 1990s Bernadette Madrid, a young physician, realized that what stood in her way from doing the job she wanted to do was literally the source of her salary: if she was earning money from private patients, her contract was with them. Determined to work on the problem of child abuse, she was fortunate to find that David Bradley, the president of the Advisory Board Foundation, and Vicki Herrera, an American pediatric cardiologist with family ties in the Philippines, were eager to create a program to address child abuse. They established the Child Protection Center in conjunction with the Philippine General Hospital and provided funding to Madrid so that she could concentrate her efforts on building the program. Over time, the highly successful pilot effort in Manila has evolved into a comprehensive medical and psychosocial program for abused children; it is staffed by pediatricians, nurses, and social workers. Through a memorandum of agreement between the University of the Philippines and the Departments of Health and Social Welfare, there is now a referral and management system and a network of twenty-one child protection units throughout the country. The original investment in Madrid's professional salary has demonstrated that, with adequate reimbursement, programs can flourish, grow, and effect change.

All over the developing world, physicians confront the same dilemma as Bernadette Madrid's. They struggle to find support for the work that they believe needs to be done. In the United States, the problem is the same, but the dimensions are more subtle and the constraints less obvious. Perhaps the nearest parallel is in the area of mental and behavioral health. The Surgeon General's task force reported that only 20 percent of children with mental health concerns were receiving mental health care, suggesting a great shortage of trained mental health practitioners.[10] But the problem is not so much a shortage of providers as a poor reimbursement system. Since psychologists, psychiatrists, social workers, and nurse clinicians cannot afford to offer their services for the meager fees that private and public insurance pay, they often use their office hours to care for patients who are willing to pay outside of any formal health system. A quick perusal of the Los Angeles Japanese Yellow Pages reveals ads for twenty-six clinical psychiatry and psychology groups primed and ready to care for Japanese children as long as the families are willing to pay directly out of their pocket.

Wanting to get paid for a day's work is not unreasonable. Physicians who care for children in poverty and children with chronic conditions find that they often cannot count on health insurance payers to pay them. Medicaid rates for children in some states are so low that doctors who want to care for poor children in their communities simply cannot afford to do so; Medicaid doesn't even pay at the scale as Medicare. There is probably no bigger issue crying out for professional advocacy than that of adequate reimbursement. Although child health professionals are shy about speaking of money, worried that they will appear self-serving and greedy, the truth is, when the doctor cannot pay the office bills, there is no office and there are no patients.

Tapping the Power

To fulfill the social contract with children and families, the child health profession needs a radical reorientation. This entails an exploration of all the pragmatic details reviewed above—and more. Professional self-assessment must involve a difficult (perhaps wrenchingly difficult) look into the topic of power.[11] Many of the discussions fostered by groups such as the Anne E. Dyson Community Pediatrics Training Initiative, the Soros Professions in Medicine, the Joint Federal Commission on Interprofessional Education, and the Gold Foundation delicately approach this topic. Generally, the conversations skirt a full-blown examination of what gives professionals power, why sharing that power is so hard, and what the benefits of shared power might be. It is time for an open and forthright exploration.

Child health professionals do have power. They rarely label it. They use power every day—often effectively, rarely hurtfully, but never maximally. Because the power of the profession is seldom acknowledged, the power dynamic is not identified, not utilized, and often undermines the professionals' stated objectives.

Let's think about the child health profession from the beginning. It may be helpful to consider the process through which a person is transformed into a professional and given the charge, the trust, and the respect that attend that role. During that process, young people acquire the stupendous gifts of new information, new skills, and new abilities. Two other less recognized things happen: they become isolated and they stop questioning the status quo.

In general, young people choose the child health professions because they want to alleviate suffering, care for children and families, and promote health within society. Students often choose the field of pediatrics explicitly because they want to work in concert with communities. But then whammo, something happens. The very knowledge, skills, abilities, and experiences that make a professional useful to society and the community render the individual different, isolated, removed.

The trip through the doors of the medical school classroom into the lab and the hospital is long and arduous. Problem sets, the Krebs cycle, lab experiments, learning which gene codes for which disease, tests and more tests, papers and board examinations absorb the students' attention. They find they have less time for dinner out, for a movie, to volunteer at the homeless shelter, or to visit with a friend. When the students start on clinical rotations, they spend their days with very sick people. They are present at the bedside as a patient dies. They are in the emergency room when the ambulance sirens announce the arrival of three car crash victims.

The clinical experiences move and change them. The students no longer think the way their parents, their roommates, and their spouses think. They see life and death in stark new terms. It can be hard for their loved ones to appreciate the toll of the daily experiences. The students become lonely and seek the comfort of others who understand. The unforeseen consequence of all this is that some of the everyday self (the part that can tie professionals to patients and friends) literally gets lost in translation. The health-professionals-to-be enter a nether sphere where even their language separates them from everyone else. A cold becomes an upper respiratory infection; fever is hyperpyrexia; a scrape is an abrasion, and a rash is an exanthem. Professionalism cuts professionals off.

The health professions are hierarchical, and for good reason. Supervision and oversight are critical to ensure patient safety. The veteran surgeon who has removed more than 5,000 gallbladders guides the second-year resident through his first case. The staff nurse with a lifetime of experience oversees the new hire as she prepares the 2 a.m. medicines for the boy on renal dialysis. The rules of hierarchy are explicit. The chief of staff of the hospital determines the protocol for admitting patients. The head nurse decides the procedures for the floor and assigns staff roles. Interns are taught, monitored, and evaluated by senior residents. Senior residents in turn report to the chief resident, who reports to the chief of service.

As young people put on their new professional identity, they become acutely aware of the pecking order. Pleasing the attending physician and not sounding stupid in front of the senior resident on rounds are all-important. To stay in school, to meet the expectations of the daily grind, they find the groove, follow the unwritten curriculum, and walk in the footsteps of those in front of them.[12] Without necessarily meaning to, they merge with the status quo. Firmly on the medical track, they have less and less meaningful interaction with colleagues outside health care. Within the child health structure, with so much to know and so much to do, it is hard to reach out to work with community agencies, families, and other professional groups. Most health care institutions have rigid traditions. If the institution does not routinely reach out to other partners in the community, young medical professionals will be reticent to try. Inertia is a very strong force.

Unfortunately, health care professionals find it hard to shift gears when they move out of the familiar territory of the clinic, the office, and the ward. Accustomed to the hierarchy—to being in charge and giving orders—health professionals often assume that they are the natural leaders of any given child health effort. This attitude is not terribly helpful. The so-called medical model is not always viewed positively by families, community agencies, and other professionals.[13] In fact, when child health professionals lay exclusive claim to expertise on children's health, they are undercutting other professional and grassroots groups with valuable knowledge, skills, and talents.

True professionalism means shared power. Child health professionals who are not constrained by notions of hierarchy but embrace the observations, skills, and talents of parents and community-based workers multiply their own effectiveness many times. Bron Anders, a pediatrician in Southern California, uses her leadership skills and the power of her medical knowledge and position to assist the Sequan Indian tribe in their quest for healthy children and families. Never abrasive or forceful, Anders respects the leadership of the tribe and shows up at meetings only when asked. She brings the authoritative information that the tribal leaders need to design their health clinic, to create their outreach programs, and to support their sister tribes across the border in Northern Mexico. She knows what power is about and how to make it work for the health of children and families.[14]

Speaking Out

Professional advocacy is also needed to get the facts about prevention and care coordination across to those who hold the purse strings. Insurers and governmental authorities must be convinced that making good on children's health care is fiscally possible. They also must be brought up to speed on the recent dramatic shift in the contours of child health care utilization that dictate a parallel shift in financing.

Prevention works. The Centers for Disease Control estimate that the cost of cardiovascular disease and stroke each year is more than $352 billion and that 33 percent of deaths each year are attributable to three preventable behaviors: tobacco use, lack of physical activity, and poor eating habits. Child health preventive activities also save money. Data on screening for metabolic, sensory, and development problems; on promotion of breast-feeding, immunizations, car seat use, and bicycle helmet use; on programs addressing violence and obesity; and on home visiting programs all show a positive impact on both child outcome and cost. Professional advocacy is needed to get the resources for these programs.

Comprehensive care for children with complex disorders also works. Good evidence is now mounting that child health providers working with families and communities can make inroads into each of these, but insurers rarely pay for the preventive interventions that address these concerns. Moreover, each additional $400 invested in coordination of care activities for children with special health care needs (CSHCN) has the potential of reducing health care costs for emergency visits and hospitalizations.[15] Probably more important, dollars spent in this way keep parents at work and ensure a consistent employee force for business.

Part of the problem is communication. Health care advocates and health care financers get caught up in an unproductive clash, with neither group listening to the other's goals and constraints. Doctors and nurses argue for a long-term perspective: a healthy body today means a stronger and brighter future. Insurers tend not to hear these concerns, not because they do not see the relevance but because they are concerned with patient volume, the so-called throughput. Insurers are eager to realize the payoff for their investment in the current fiscal year. When health professionals and business people compare notes, startling differences become apparent. Health care profession: long term, new knowledge, societal effect, no profit motive. Health care industry: short term, present knowledge, focus on today's outcomes, profit motive.

Business is business. Insurers answer to their stockholders, not to children and families. Professional health advocates interested in removing barriers have started to walk in the shoes of the business people, to ask what makes the economy tick, and to speed up the timetable of health care impact. The masters at this are the health care professionals at the Institute for Health Improvement. They have made it their business to understand business.[16] They translate between insurers and health care deliverers. Business people speak in terms of productivity, wise time use, quality outcomes, and saving money. They examine systems carefully to find how to improve throughput and cut waste and redundancy. Coupled with health care goals, such approaches can foster significant improvements in clinical operating systems. Unfortunately, without such translation, the business approach may only pick up on process inefficiencies and miss the ultimate goal of improved health outcomes.

Within the Institute for Health Improvement, the National Initiative for Child Health Quality (NICHQ) focuses specifically on children's issues. Directed by pediatrician Charles Homer, NICHQ uses the lens of quality improvement to reengineer pediatric clinical practice.[17] The NICHQ approach abhors waste and values outcomes. As the NICHQ team examines practice patterns, they uncover the natural drift into the regular routine of doing things the way we have always done them (the status quo all over again). Routine is an essential element of practice, but just as too little routine can confound, too much routine stagnates. The NICHQ model builds a conscious mechanism for evaluating and adjusting the practice routine to avoid drift and to champion mastery.

The NICHQ team teaches practitioners how to use models for improvement to incorporate nationally standardized guidelines into their clinical care.[18] Pediatricians know that they should take advantage of the National Heart, Blood, Lung Institute's asthma treatment protocols but are not sure how to fit the required patient teaching into their already packed day. One model, however, emphasizes the use of small tests of change, termed the plan-do-study-act cycle. This approach allows pediatricians to make small changes, evaluate how a new form is working, add a handout, see the effect, buy some new teaching materials, check how the clinical specialists like them, and so on. Successes from small changes in behavior lead to huge changes in attitude and to systems that optimize practice patterns and improve clinical outcomes. NICHQ has developed approaches to immunizations, asthma, ADHD, and special health care needs and is beginning a venture on preventive care. Here are health care professionals doing their best to come half way toward business, to be self-critical, to change. An unanswered question is whether business will return the courtesy and come the other half of the way. If they see a fiscal benefit, they may.

To engage with the powerhouses of business and government, professional advocates should be familiar with a few pertinent facts. First, children don't cost much. Whereas children and youth represent 25 percent of the population, child health expenditures are only a tenth of the national health care dollar. The proportion has actually declined over the 1990s and early 2000s with fewer and fewer children being hospitalized and emergency room visits cut in half.[19]

But that is only part of the story. Share the above facts with any doctor struggling to get through the day and night on an inpatient ward in one of the nations children's hospitals and he will be incredulous, as will the head nurse of the babies' intensive care unit and the emergency room physician. Never have hospital teams worked so hard. Where is the disconnect? The answer is that there has been a significant shift in child health epidemiology and in the types, intensity, and complexity of child health service.

If what is presented in chapter 3 is correct, then we can square the facts and the impressions. Fewer children are going to the hospital for care because preventive services (immunizations, rapid detection of treatable disease, and injury, child abuse, and domestic violence interventions) are working. Children are not going to the emergency room as often because common infectious diseases are better controlled and the local systems are working overtime to provide care and intervention. But the children and youth who are going to the emergency room and being admitted to the hospital and the intensive care unit (ICUs) have much more complicated conditions than the average child admitted to the hospital in the past.

The health care needs of children with these complex conditions are driving health care utilization and cost. A rational system of care for these children is possible, but it will depend on the use of better epidemiological models to predict how many pediatric ICU beds a given region needs. It will involve the painful closing of facilities whose low volume means inadequate experience. And it will entail an exploration of coordination of care, so as to decrease hospital costs and promote community inclusion. Decisions of this kind should not be made without child health professionals weighing in. As important are the voices of families.

Sharing the Power

We speak about professional responsibility and a social contract. Who is the contract with? Sometimes, it seems as if the contract is with insurance companies and government agencies, but they are third parties. The contract is with all children. It is with families: workers in unions, employees at McDonalds, professors at law schools, teenage mothers on welfare. Mothers and fathers and children rarely have a voice in decisions about health care. They sign up for health insurance as an employee benefit, but their choice is limited after that. Fortunately, some families of children with special health care needs have become progressively more sophisticated in their understanding of health care financing. Not only are they learning about health care insurance policies, they also are learning to flex some muscle in getting insurance companies to expand coverage for their children. The families identify waste in the system that can be fixed with a little common sense. Why rent an IV pole for home use for $50 a month when the purchase price is only $150? Why pay a registered nurse $35 an hour for home care when the child's aunt would be thrilled to help out for a $15-an-hour stipend?

The families also call for help with the coordination of a nonexistent "system" of health care. When parents describe their experiences with the fragmentation of services, the gaps, the duplication, the paperwork, and the red-tape that bars their children from access to therapies and specialty care, there is a special authority in their voices. Professional-family partnerships make sense. Who better to get the information across to employers and to the general public about the priorities for child health?

When parents and professionals approach employers in an attempt to align incentives, there are facts they need to keep in mind. Employers want to keep health care costs down, they want a healthy and productive workforce, they don't want to lose trusted employees and have to recruit new staff. So they need to be made aware of the toll that family ill health takes on their workforce. When a factory employee is exhausted from being up all night with her 15-year-old daughter with cerebral palsy and pneumonia, she is unlikely to fully engage in making today's quota of widgets. When the executive vice president has to be out for two weeks because his 3-year-old with autism has graduated from an early intervention program and the family is in a battle with the school system to continue her in another program, the whole company suffers. These facts need to be communicated better.

Making a Difference

The publication of the American Council on Graduate Medical Education's core competencies has spurred medical schools, hospitals, and professional organizations to look squarely at what professionalism is. In child health, true compliance with the new standards requires at least three things: (1) a hard look at the question of responsibility, (2) family-community collaboration as an ethical bellwether, and (3) sustained commitment to a diverse professional workforce. Professional advocacy entails speaking up at the right times and places to make sure that these things happen, not only to enhance professional effectiveness but also to keep true to the social contract professionals have made with children and families.

Responsibility and Power

As pointed out in earlier chapters, the story of responsibility for children's health in the United States is an odd tale. It is an unfinished saga unfolding in the context of a disconnect between child health care delivery and child health outcomes. It is the silence that resounds in answer to the question, What will it take to meet all our children's health needs, now and in the future? Child health professionals do their best to take responsibility for the individual children who come to their offices and clinics. They often expend tremendous energy railing against system barriers that block them from doing their job responsibly for specific children in their practice. When the issue of responsibility for children in general comes up, professionalism is stretched to the limit. I do what I can for my own patients; isn't it someone else's role to look out for all the rest? Won't public health take that on? Shouldn't the professional organizations that we pay all those dues to fight those battles? Of course, the answers are yes, yes, and yes.

But there is a problem with the assignment of all the responsibility to the government, to public health, or to organized medicine and nursing. None of those groups can actually get the job done. None of them can fully implement the rhetoric, the political platforms, or the lofty recommendations of commissions and committees. For one thing, the government, public health, and the organizations are not really in the business of delivering care. They largely depend on health professionals in the private sector and the academic environment to do this. In a few circumstances, the government does fill in some gaps through programs like the Indian Health Service and the National Health Service Corps. But this approach has limited opportunity for the development of sustained systems of community-based, family-centered health care delivery. If the government could fill in the gaps, then the persistent questions about the responsibility would be muted. This is where professional advocacy is desperately needed. Professionals know best what will draw them to underserved areas and what will keep them there. They also have the clout and power to call on the government and public health for increased funding and support for professionals who are willing to take the responsibility for extending care to all children, including those in urban centers, those in remote areas, and those whose families are just entering the United States.

And what about the responsibility of the professional organizations? They do not have an easy task. They must balance competing demands within the child health profession. For example, what do the elected officials of the American Academy of Pediatrics do when the federal government and the national philanthropies are allocating only so many dollars to children and some academy members think those funds should be divided for *prevention*/cure/care while other members believe the best distribution will be prevention/*cure*/care and still another group makes equally compelling arguments for prevention/cure/*care*? The leaders of the child health professional organizations face this dilemma every year, with more difficult choices in the lean years.

The other challenge that the organizations face is that they are not only advocates for children and families, they are also the designated advocates and ombudsmen for professionals. Each organization has a particular allegiance to one specific professional constituency, be they generalists, subspecialists, nurses, nurse practitioners, adolescent medicine doctors, or family practitioners. The organization was created in large part to detect and fend off threats to that group. This sometimes means fighting unfortunate turf battles with like-minded professionals.

Defining responsibility is especially hard in child health because responsibility is a moving target. Professional responsibility is the reaction to a transforming, changing, never still, never same set of concerns. Children's health is determined by external forces that are in constant motion: the markets, public opinion, demographic shifts, political winds. The nutrients that children eat are more and less available. The schools that children attend are more and less tuned in to the children's needs. The bacteria that live in the air and soil are more and less susceptible to the antibiotics on the pharmacy shelf. The threats of bioterrorism and natural disasters are more and less present. The surgical techniques to improve gait of children with cerebral palsy or to enhance the stroke volume of a child in heart failure are more and less in vogue. The constant motion of the opportunities and challenges to health, the swirl of political commitment to and abandonment of children's programs, means that at least child health professionals themselves need to agree on a common vision about child health and child health service. The principles delineated in the Bright Futures Charter, the 2010 Healthy People Goals, and the American Academy of Pediatrics Medical Home Statement are a start.

Where does that leave the individual professional as she contemplates professionalism and the notion of responsibility? Back to basics, with a slight twist or two. As always, professional responsibility means the maintenance of the highest quality standards and commitment to providing the best possible care (even if that means fighting the good fight against irrational systems impediments). In addition, responsibility means resisting the status quo. A core element of professionalism is dissatisfaction with what is; a fear of creeping mediocrity. Even when his practice is very good or excellent, a professional has the nagging notion that excellent is just not good enough. Responsible professionals never rest on their laurels. Finally, responsibility in professionalism involves an openness to new relationships, new power dynamics. If what matters is the health of children, then professional responsibility says, Let's try something different. That may mean changing traditional practices and questioning long-standing professional assumptions.

Family-Community Collaboration

The reevaluation of professional conduct grows out of a concern that the ethics of the profession are in jeopardy. What better way to protect professional integrity than by having the input of families and communities? There are many benefits to expanded professional partnerships with families and communities. Among other things, families are in a strong position to help set agendas for children's health.

Family-community collaboration can keep child health professionals on an ethical course through setting priorities for the allocation of resources, counteracting professional isolation and elitism, and protecting against profit motivation. Additionally, families and community groups can translate to the larger public the concepts of professionalism and ethics that may not ring as clear when health professionals speak them.

When it comes to setting priorities, parents are the authorities on child health needs. They are the ones who experience the compromised breathing of the 2-year-old with bronchiolitis. They are the ones who call drug store after drug store searching for the special formula the doctor ordered for their daughter with malabsorption syndrome. They are the ones who go to town meetings trying to get someone to understand that their kids are the prey of gangs and drug pushers. How hard can it be for the selectmen to vote funds for after-school sports and tutoring? It might save some lives. Parents know.

Community groups also know. Increasingly, there are models of parent and community involvement in making decisions about how public moneys will be spent. For example, federal agencies and National Institutes of Health study sections frequently include parents and community members on panels reviewing research grant applications. This model ensures the vetting of professional ideas through the eyes of those who are most affected both by the study protocols and by the results of the studies. With the appreciation of racial disparities in health, more emphasis is now being placed on racial and ethnic factors in research. A racially and ethnically balanced review panel will approach the research questions looking for bias in the conduct of the study. Representative panels will also caution researchers about the potential for backlash from the improper interpretation or reporting of data.

Of course, there are tricky issues in the involvement of nonprofessionals in professional business. What if parent representatives vote no on a topic of great relevance to the profession? What if they cannot see the promise of a potentially revolutionary technique or are opposed on ethical grounds to the risks of a particular study? Before the widespread use of institutional review boards, professionals would often take amazing risks, exposing themselves, their students, and even their own children to new medicines, vaccines, and other interventions. Should scientific advancement be slowed because less-informed, less-visionary people are deliberating on the conduct and safety of the scientific enterprise? There are no easy answers to this one. Institutional review boards with community representatives require that the investigators make their case in plain English so that reasonable people can understand the request and ask questions. If the research is so esoteric or hazardous that it cannot pass this test, then maybe the scientists would benefit from reworking their project both in technical and in ethical terms. Some professionals see this as unnecessary. Others welcome the opportunity to put their work into a social and temporal context.

Earlier in this chapter, we discuss professional parochialism, the potential for an elite class to cut itself off from the larger society by its own rites, rituals, and rules. Parent and community partnerships are a way to counteract isolationism. Child health professionals who practice in smaller communities are less likely to spend their days in the exclusive company of other health professionals, but in cities and particularly in academic health centers, the only other people waiting in line for lunch or to pick up their car at the garage may be musing about the same problems, seeing things from the same point of view, and wondering about the same benefits and liabilities. These professionals benefit enormously from opportunities to exchange ideas more broadly.

If partnership with families and communities is factored into the ultimate view of professionalism, then the making of a professional profits from experience in the community and the home. Child health professionals go out to where the injuries are prevented, where the curative medicines are delivered, teaspoon by teaspoon, where the caring hands hang the gastrostomy feedings for the 6-year-old who has never eaten a peanut butter and jelly sandwich, where caring eyes watch the 15-year-old boy as he labors for every breath. With such grounding, professionals gain knowledge about resources, the strengths in families, clever ways to accomplish health care goals; learn that the schoolteacher can be part of the asthma care plan, that the scout leader can reinforce a message about healthy snacks, that one mother has figured out a way to limit TV watching, that Johnny can play tag in his wheelchair, and that Auntie Sarah is on top of the family dynamic.

What about the ethical concern that market forces are making it more and more possible for professionals to earn high profits from their work? Is there a way that parent and community liaisons can modulate these forces or make them more rational? Probably. And what of the rush of large pharmaceutical companies to get their latest medicines into the market? Could the Cox-2 safety concerns have been detected earlier with a more obvious family and community presence in the licensing and monitoring? Perhaps.

When professionals profit from their innovation and entrepreneurial interactions with business and industry, what are the mechanisms for plowing some of the monetary gain back into aspects of child health that have no hope of ever being profitable? A partnership of professionals with communities and families allows for some creative thinking on this. Some professionals who have benefited financially from product or drug development have arrangements with their university base about the sharing of royalties and feeding the monies back into the same area of inquiry or service. Other professionals direct the profits of medical and scientific entrepreneurship to start family and community ventures. The Howard Hughes Institute (HHI) has an active recruitment program to provide training and jobs to youth in the communities where HHI has its centers. Similarly, Columbia University entered into a partnership with the Washington Heights community to rebuild the Audubon Ballroom as a museum in honor of Malcolm X as part of the construction of Columbia's expanding laboratory facilities. As part of the package, there are scholarships for community high school students to work with research scientists in the labs, with the ultimate goal of improving the science knowledge of the community and the professional opportunities for community young people.

Family centered, community based: good words, good concepts. They may even promote what Howard Gardner calls Good Work.[20] Professionals are not impartial when they speak out about themselves and what they are trying to accomplish. Even the most ethical professional has a vested interest in ensuring that his favorite project finds favor with the public, the media, or the funding agency. Professionals benefit enormously when families and communities translate to the general public what the professionals are trying to accomplish. Family and community alignment with the work of child health professionals fosters a more general impact.

Diversity

In a democracy, the chance to become a professional cannot be an exclusive privilege. And yet in the United States the ranks of professionals do not mirror the national distribution of races or ethnic, religious, and cultural groups.[21] The Accreditation Council for Graduate Medical Education specifically charges academic institutions to grapple with this problem because only through so-called pipeline strategies can the imbalance possibly be redressed. Many educators, policymakers, and professional groups are also dissatisfied with the ineffectiveness of strategies that attempt to provide professional care to underrepresented and underserved groups. Assigning young professionals just out of training to spend a few years in communities that they will never call home misses the mark.

As bleak as the current distribution picture is, positive things are happening with regard to the diversity of the child health workforce. You may not see that at the Old Docs Club, but you do at faculty meetings and in the executive councils of the professional organizations. At the grand rounds in many hospitals you may see a only hint of change. But pop into the anatomy lecture or the microbiology lab at the local medical school, and there the story is different. Talented students from all classes of society and all racial, ethnic, and cultural backgrounds are preparing to enter the profession. Twenty years from now, the professional child health community will be far more representative of the general population. Professional advocacy has played a huge role in accomplishing this.

Angela Diaz, the chief of Adolescent Medicine at Mount Sinai in New York City and the head of the President's Commission on Bioterrorism, tells her story.[22] Born in the Dominican Republic, she moved with her mother to New York City when she was in elementary school. She spoke no English but was blessed with a remarkable natural ability in mathematics. Her 9th-grade teacher picked up on her abilities and, using the language of numbers, mathematical sets, algebraic formulas, and proofs, guided and encouraged Angela.

Diaz dropped out of school in the 12th grade. She rarely saw her mother, who worked two jobs. But Diaz wanted to make things better for her family, worked hard, and went back to school. Toward the end of her college years, on an impulse, she took the A Train to 168th Street and walked into the admissions office of the medical school at Columbia. She had no idea about due dates, testing, screening; something just told her it was time to direct her talents to important work.

At the reception desk sat the person who would change her life. She was a by-the-books university administrator who had put generations of aspiring premedical students through their paces. She knew all the reasons why Angela Diaz should not be an applicant. She could recite them, chapter and verse. But she didn't. Instead, she took a good, long, hard look at the young woman standing in front of her and saw the future. Here was a doctor-to-be born in the same country as 70–80 percent of the families whose homes flanked the medical center along Broadway and Fort Washington Avenues. She handed an application to Diaz, who sat down, then and there, answered all the questions, and handed the form right back. That September, Angela would be back as a first-year medical student.

This story is emblematic of the big and little deeds, the risks and uncertainties that administrators, government officials, deans, philanthropists, and many others have been taking for the past thirty to forty years. At first these were isolated acts, a commitment by one or two individuals in a nursing school or an urban hospital. But each success has strengthened the argument for the next step, opened the door of opportunity a little wider. The effectiveness of the voice of advocacy for a strong and diverse workforce can be appreciated by a review of the federal programs of loan repayment, fellowships, and scholarships available to scientists and physicians from underrepresented minority backgrounds.[23]

Pioneering child health professionals who break race and cultural barriers know from personal experience how the process of becoming professionals transforms them. Many of these professionals have been the first in their family to finish high school, or to graduate from college, or to move away from family and community, or sign a mortgage application. Or the first of their race to publish an article in *Science,* to open a free clinic in Johannesburg. And now who are they? Where do they fit? When they return home, the distance they have traveled may have made a gulf between them and their family and community. Some will find themselves unable to communicate their new life to their family. They may have learned the language of science but lost their Mandarin or Portuguese. If they show interest in working with families in poverty, they may hear, Why in the world would you want to plunge back into the misery we just came from? Or there may be another message from the neighborhood pastor: How can you think of going into the lab when you know that so many of our brothers and sisters in the church are suffering in poverty?

That is where groups like the Partnership in Boston come in.[24] Whether anyone acknowledges it or not, professionals derive enormous benefits from whom they know and whom they meet. They work systems; they network; they pick up on opportunities from being in the right place at the right time. Programs like the Partnership make this explicit. Through outreach and yearlong fellowships, professionals of color are introduced to notions of power and powerful connections. They get an inside track in the race for prestige in their greater community.

Caught in a no-man's land between where they were and where they are going, professionals from underrepresented minorities face one other challenge: resentment and backlash from antiaffirmative action groups who question preferential treatment from granting agencies, loan forgiveness programs, and professional outreach. Are such practices fair? The question of fairness is a hard one, but turned on its head it asks, How does a society counteract the entrenched unfairness of centuries? Where do we find the professional leadership to start turning things around? Without the explicit initiatives, not only might the future professional leaders from diverse backgrounds not get the inside track, they might not even get to the field.

Katie Plax at the Washington University Department of Pediatrics in St. Louis has begun a training program in advocacy, teaching medical students and residents the distinction between selfish, selfless, and self-interest. She defines *self-interest* as being relational.

Professional advocates who work from a relational position not only fight against unreasonable constraints but also have a host of allies who stand alongside them. Parents, community-based organizations, and other child-oriented professionals confirm that the work the child health professionals do is part of a larger scheme, one that is neither selfish nor selfless. It is the fulfillment of the social contract that the child health professional has made with colleagues and with children and families.

Political Will   8

CHAPTER 1 ENDS WITH a description of Julius Richmond's model of
advocacy, which places equal importance on three components: knowledge base, social strategy, and political will. Chapter 3 reviews the *knowledge base* in some detail, and chapters 4 through 7 delineate *social strategies*
for child health advocacy in clinical care, group programming, legisla-
tive/systems reform, and professional activities. The last and perhaps the
hardest concept is *political will*. What is political will as it relates to children and their health? How does it operate? And how do advocates lasso
enough of it to make a difference for children and families?

Citizens express political will by making choices about how they want
to be governed. On election day, the Millers and the Jawalskis and the
Ngs go to the local elementary school, draw the yellow curtain behind
them, and mark X's at the names of the people they want to represent
them. They choose their aldermen and councilwomen, their senators
and presidents, based on notions of what a government is for and how it
should operate. People also express their political will at the cash register
by how they spend their money and by how they direct their representatives to use other people's money.

Political will is attitude. It is what a group of people wants and cares
about. It is the energy that fuels movement and change. For political
will to be harnessed, there has to be clarity of purpose and a fundamental agreement among the general populace that they are for the movement or change. There can be no shilly-shallying. That is where the child
health dilemma is stuck. Political will around children's issues has never
galvanized. Let us explore why that is and what child health advocates
might do about it.

Little Kids, Little Import

Americans have a profound ambivalence about children. Yes, there is a
youth culture and the perennial search for Ponce de León's fountain. But
our individual and collective actions demonstrate day in and day out that
Americans do not put a high value on childhood. The early years are to

be passed through as rapidly as possible on the way to a good-paying job and real life as an adult. The ambivalence toward youth is tied in with the American values of independence, individual rights, and getting ahead. Kids are by their very nature dependent. They do move ahead but on a schedule that has stops for toddling, potty training, singing the ABCs, learning right from wrong, dying their hair blue, trying on the most fab dress, and taking on the latest persona. Each of the stops has its own value, but Americans are driven to reach the final destination. What will Johnny be doing in fifteen years? they ask, rather than, What is Johnny doing now?

No citizen would ever say, Young people do not deserve a fair shake. In fact when the topic of child health advocacy comes up, most people say, Who could be against children? Few people consider that they are *against* children, but the fact is that few people are actually *for* children. Small kids, small issues, small dollars, small impact. Advocates have to fight continuously for child health dollars, for schoolbooks, for children to be considered as subjects in federal health studies. Why else did it take a huge task force to approve the increased surgical fee for sewing the tiny heart vessels of premature infants?[1]

America's hesitancy about children is worse than most people would like to admit. Many American policies are blatantly child unfriendly. Even the Grinch who stole Christmas would find a way to sponsor gym and recess in school. What sense does it make that in some neighborhoods there are more cheap handguns than playground swing sets? Why do our maternity units push baby formula rather than support breastfeeding? How can a nation tolerate having twenty children spend their afternoon cramped in one small room because there is nowhere else for them to go? These problems are what families endure every single day. But somehow there is no political will to change them.

Children's issues have never taken a central place in American political thought. A comparison of the U.S. Constitution with the constitutions of other nations is telling. The words *child, children, youth, mother, father, family, education,* and *health* do not appear in the U.S. Constitution or in the Bill of Rights. The Irish Constitution includes language on family and home life: "The state must ensure that economic circumstances do not oblige a mother to work outside of the home. The provision also guarantees that in the event of divorce adequate financial provision must be made for any children and for both spouses." Article 26 of the Japanese Constitution guarantees that "all people shall have the right to receive an equal education correspondent to their ability." The Constitution of the Republic of South Africa spells out in great detail the rights of children with regard to their personhood, their protection, and their rights to decent housing and education. The South African Constitution actually guarantees health care as a right for children.

Because the United States vests so much authority in the states, each state has the responsibility for domestic issues.[2] The various state laws and regulations set out the provisions for children and families. American children generally do find their way to school. In fact, in most states their parents can be prosecuted if their children don't attend school. U.S. children mostly are housed and clothed and fed, certainly better than in countries like South Africa. And for the most part they do get their immunization shots, though not at the uniform rates as in countries where central authorities pride themselves on public health accomplishments. What is different is that there is no collective expression of children's rights in the United States. There is no public statement or celebration of the uniqueness of children, their special gifts, and their special needs. Without such a declaration, there is no moral imperative driving the protection of children. There is no accountability.

The United States is one of only two countries that have not ratified the United Nations Convention on the Rights of the Child.[3] The other is Somalia. The United States does not like to sign any international commitment. Is it because we have done so well on our own that we do not need to be bound by any other authority? Or is it because the convention interdicts military conscription of anyone under age 18 and our armed forces depend on being able to sign up 17-year-olds? Does our reticence relate to the language about capital punishment of minors or about the possibility that some pro-life factions will not be satisfied with the convention? The United Nation's language is pointed in indicating that no country is so wealthy or so endowed that it should aspire to remain outside the convention. "Some people assume that the rights of children born in wealthy nations—where schools, hospitals, and juvenile justice systems are in place—are never violated, that these children have no need for the protection and care called for in the Convention. But that is far from the truth. To varying degrees, at least *some* children in *all* nations face unemployment, homelessness, violence, poverty, and other issues that dramatically affect their lives."[4]

American noncompliance with the Convention on the Rights of the Child has potential negative consequence beyond the U.S. borders. The country's economic interests are so enmeshed in multinational enterprise that decisions made in government and corporate conference rooms determine global conditions for children and youth. Without a political will around children's issues at home, there is little hope that Americans will stand up for the rights of children and youth around the world. Without the United States as a partner in the convention, many of its most important provisions remain essentially moot.

Children's Place

If children are not in the center of American public debate, where is their place? What meaning does the presence of children have? What would a world be like with an empty niche where children are supposed to be? To think about these questions, let's examine the physical, societal, and spiritual implications of childhood.

Physical Implications

Humans are physical beings, no different from all other physical life. Human genes are made of nucleic acids, and our growing cells and bodies are dependent on air, water, and nutrients. Like all other animals, humans have an innate desire to reproduce and to continue the species. There is a natural predisposition to nurture and safeguard our young. Intense feelings well up as birth approaches, anxieties about how to keep the baby from harm. Even the sloppiest of housekeepers may find herself cleaning every corner of the apartment. Like a little mother titmouse, she is "nesting," preparing a safe, clean, and comfortable place for her young. The distinct infant aroma or cry stimulates an urge to feed, to nurture, and to cuddle.

Human children are dependent on adult protection for a very long time, much longer than most other species. We need only think of the newborn foal that unwinds from the birth canal to stand on spindly legs, to totter briefly, and within days to dance deftly away from the mare's side. Contrast that picture with the newborn human baby whose coarse movements qualify as little more than uncoordinated kicks. Even at age 2 or 3 years, human children cannot be left on their own to find food, to distinguish edible items from poison, to find shelter, to make their way from one safe place to another. Children's state of total dependence requires an external environment that understands dependency and is prepared to support it. Not such a hard concept but one that rarely finds salience in American discourse. Otherwise, the protection of the environment and the celebration of the early family years would hold more weight.

For Americans, physical resources have not been limited until recently. With the wide frontiers, there has always been the potential of moving farther out. Children have been part of that expansion. In settlers' families, more young strong hands and backs meant more rocks that could be lifted and more trees that could be felled. Have we not readjusted from that thinking? Do we still consider that there is no limit of physical resource and that the environment will be forever forgiving of the use we make of it? The Environmental Protection Agency periodically explores the impact of industrial and residential development on children.[5] Environmentalists raise questions about topics like global warming, waste management, mercury poisoning of fish. But the voice of the environmentalists is still relatively weak, and the pairing of environmental and children's issues is like putting Tweety Bird and Elmo together to take on Godzilla.

American child unfriendliness shows itself most clearly in the paltry national response to support for young families. The call for family leave and for the promotion of parental-child interaction has been far less successful in the United States than in Europe. Sweden guarantees fifteen months of paid parental leave after the birth of each baby. In France parents receive sixteen weeks of paid parental leave plus the assurance of paid child care for their young children. In the United States the Family and Medical Leave Act of 1993 allows twelve weeks of unpaid leave, a limited benefit at best. The eligibility requirements and practicality of going without pay make this option open to only a modest proportion of American working parents.[6]

Unlike the topics of the environment and family leave, issues around sexuality and reproduction have generated enormous political attention in the early twenty-first century. Perhaps the United States is just now realizing that the sexual revolution is fact and that it has profound implications for children. The sexual revolution derived in large part from the wide availability and social acceptability of birth control technology. Birth control technology uncoupled, for the most part, sexuality and reproduction. This uncoupling has changed the size and shape of families and has profoundly altered how relationships are formed in adolescence and young adulthood.

American families are dramatically smaller at the beginning of the twenty-first century than they were at the beginning of the twentieth. The U.S. birth rate (births per 1,000 women ages 15–44) dropped from a baby boom high in 1957 of 123 per 1,000, to 70 per 1,000 in 1980, to an all-time low of 65 per 1,000 in 2000.[7] This change occurred in a typically American way. There were no edicts from on high about the need for zero population growth, as in Europe. Nor were there government-enforced measures like the one-child-family law in China. Rather, in U.S. fashion, market forces and the availability of contraceptives led to this widespread change in lifestyle over two to three decades.

The change in the world of adolescents and young adults is most apparent in the public expression of acceptable sexual behavior. In the 1950s, the crooner Frank Sinatra was all the rage with the hit song "Love and Marriage," whose take-home message was "you can't have one without the other." Television rarely showed anything more sensual than a kiss between lovers, and movies did not carry R ratings because there was no explicit sexuality to rate. Innuendo would fly over the heads of the young, and only those in the know would get the point. By the 1980s and 1990s prime-time television was portraying the sexual entanglements and ever-changing attachments of six young people (*Friends*); and in the late 1990s *Sex and the City* raked in popularity awards. Lots of love. Not much marriage.

Of course, birth control methodology has not completely severed the link between sexuality and reproduction. Major sexual decisions are still driven by the human desire for life partnership and family formation. Concerns about what a family is, who constitutes a married couple, and who can bear and raise children emerged in national debate during the 2004 presidential campaign. The election exposed a deep rift in thinking about these issues in the United States.

Generating political will about the physical needs and place of children means grappling with hard topics: the environment, family protection, and family rights. To come to grips with fundamental concerns, people (all people/the people) will have to confront essential questions and engage in difficult conversations. What does it mean to be a physical being? What is our relationship to other species? Are humans dominant or are we interdependent with other life forms? What is precious about an unborn human life? What is precious about a life half lived? What commitment should sexual relationship entail? What constitutes a family? These are questions no one likes to confront because they are so basic and so difficult. But not confronting them allows politics rather than political will to prevail.

Societal Implications

There is an argument that children are a binding societal force. The home and the hearth create a center, where family life exists primarily (although certainly not exclusively) for the nurturance of the next generation. The ties that bind families and promote tradition create the cohesion and predictability that all people (and especially children) need. In the clinical world, physicians, psychologists, and social workers urge families to maintain continuity and to set boundaries and routines for children so they know what to expect and how to behave; so that they understand their place in the family order. Children learn from their parents and from family tradition; expectations and experiences pass down from parents to children. In the ideal world, the family is always there when any member is in need. They slay the fatted calf for the prodigal son, the pregnant teenage daughter, the school-failing nephew, the war-shattered cousin. Loyalty to one's own. Home is where it is always safe. Home is where you matter.

But here comes trouble. Family identity and the placing of one's own children and lineage above all creates the clans, tribes, and family allegiances that drive conflict and division. Hatfields hate McCoys simply because they are McCoys; and McCoys hate Hatfields simply because they are Hatfields. Identity is formed around the attribute of sameness, of continuity, of inflexibility. We always have broken our eggs on the big end, we always will break our eggs on the big end, and we are right. The definition of self and family is frequently cast as our difference from others. The problem of how to preserve what is right and good and true about family loyalty without buying into an associated intolerance is the central theme of countless books and movies. Many, like the New Zealand film *Whale Rider*, end with sentimental music and the children returning to the old ways to please their elders and to keep tight hold of meaning in their lives. But why is it that when the tribe rides out into the sunset it is in a war canoe?

Family cohesion and loyalty also contributes to another serious societal problem. Those who have resources naturally invest them in their own families and children. There is nothing wrong with that. The trouble is that investment in private health care, private child care, and private education undermines public health care, public child care, and public education. A major challenge for parents, communities, and advocates, then, is to find ways that children and children's issues can be a binding force for all families and communities.

The idea of the binding force of children is being tested in the United States, where they make up a smaller and smaller proportion of society. And according to the 2000 census, more adults are living by themselves than ever before.[8] For some, the single lifestyle means freedom to pursue personal dreams and aspirations, free hours that can translate into business, academic, or creative production. But isn't something missing? In a childless world, what serves as the binding force? Institutions such as communal living facilities and universities are becoming a new kind of social aggregator. Urban centers are attracting unmarried young couples and empty nesters to easy-maintenance townhouses. Is this good, bad, or just different? Wouldn't a child-friendly society provide multigenerational ways to live?

Spiritual Implications

Interaction with children reaffirms fundamental truths, untainted by complex experience, because children express the basics of being. In them the life force displays itself to its fullest and unfolds the possibilities of all humanity.

The newborn takes the first breath in, and there is a completely new life. Act one, scene one, curtain up—with all hopes and possibilities. The 3-month-old coos and smiles; she signals her longing for connection. Alert, aware, and active, children are all about movement. The runaway Sweet Pea scoots across the kitchen floor. The toddler flops on his back to sculpt angel wings in the winter's first snow. The 3-year-old covers her face in chocolate brownie batter. Basic being.

The presence of children reminds us of the value of innocence and purity. Little children do not know what it means to be mean, what it is to hate and to hurt. They do not come into the world with notions of bad guys and good guys. When they first discover sport, they love the bats and the balls, the sliding into base, the hotdogs and the green grass. They don't get it that there is another team that is trying to outdo them, that wants our team to lose, to have a bad day, to fail. Little children do not know anything about getting ahead or staying behind or being passed over. They know only the essence, the basics. They see and hear and feel the pure.

Troubling Issues: It's about Time to Talk

Political will around children has not galvanized, but the failure is not because people don't agree on children's issues. It is because people do not bring children's concerns to a high enough level of public discourse. Open discussion about children's physical, societal, and spiritual place is painful and potentially divisive. Nonetheless, such public conversation is far more constructive than political ennui and disengagement about basic questions of human rights. Naming and discussing issues gives them value, priority, and weight. It matters that there are families, children, health care, and education. Congressmen have to read legislative summaries with these words in them. The briefs in lawyers' briefcases have language about what a child can and cannot have, a youth may or may not do, a family does or does not need.

To understand political will is to understand the pushes and pulls that form it. Rather than try to tease some of the issues apart and insist on resolution, child health advocates occasionally need to acknowledge the multiple knots and nodes of the problems and to work within the web of complexity. Below are four dichotomies to be grappled with, and not necessarily untangled, in order to garner political will for children: investment/development, child/family, simple/complex, and family/society.

The Investment Case versus the Development Case

One of the conceptual complexities of childhood is its evolving nature. Children are always in a state of flux, growth, and forward movement. A conceptual grasp of this nature requires an understanding of differential calculus, not simple arithmetic. The present and future are twisted together. What happens for or to a 3-year-old predicts a lot about what kind of adolescent and young adult he will be. When policymakers and the public turn a blind eye to the connection between early influences and later outcomes, good policy is at hazard. The advocate's stance is to link present and future, and there are two concrete ways to do this: the investment case and the development case.

The Investment Case

When that average American citizen views young people in economic, or investment, terms, a dramatic tension is evident. Every newborn represents years of fiscal dependency on the family, community, and society. Money keeps flowing into a bottomless pit to pay for rice cereal, disposable diapers, cute little teddy bears, and the salaries of an army of day care workers, elementary school teachers, pediatricians, and karate masters. On the other hand, there is growth potential and return on investment. Yes, children start as a burden on society, but they eventually become the answer for its long-term viability. Although infants and little children must be provided for, youth prepare to be providers, and young adults stride out into a world ready to hit the production lines.[9]

Another way of looking at the economic argument is to consider what happens in the absence of an adequate investment plan. Longitudinal studies like the Perry Preschool Program make it abundantly obvious that children need consistent input and nurture for their long-term development as productive citizens.[10] Nothing can be left to chance. When insufficient fiscal, emotional, cognitive, and health investments are made in early childhood, the study shows that children grow up devoid of personal resources. As adults, their cognitive, emotional, and even moral bank accounts are low. Lacking personal reserves, they turn against their neighbors, and in their anger and sadness they may lash out in dangerous ways. They become a new generation of dependents, often behind bars and drawing far more of society's dollars than it would have cost to support them during the early childhood years. Not only does lack of investment in children harm them, it harms society. The Perry Preschool study demonstrates that early developmental services can save society $7.16 for every $1.00 invested through increased productivity and decreased school retention, crime, and welfare-related costs.

The Development Case

If the public is concerned that children not be a drain on society, it makes sense for families, communities, and society at large to foster the development of citizenship in children from a very early age. One example is the feeding program at the St. James Episcopal Cathedral Church in Chicago. On Sunday mornings, a group of parishioners meets in a sunny, upper room of the parish hall to prepare a meal for the homeless men and women who sleep in the alleyways and passages of the streets that surround the church. There are boxes and boxes of bread and bananas and fruit roll-ups. On Sandwich Sundays, one finds an assembly doling out the food. The workers include children as young as 3 smearing peanut butter on bread, or counting paper bags, or marking the bags with H for ham and PB for peanut butter.[11]

As children grow, the ratio of dependence to production shifts. School-age children can help with work in the house, on the farm, in the community. Teenagers make up a substantial part of the service workforce from McDonald's to Baghdad. But this productivity of children and youth is almost never appreciated, valued, or celebrated. At the beginning of the twentieth century, children were exploited so badly that Progressive reformers fought to prohibit child labor; their campaign protected little children from terrible abuses. Now, although children are no longer exploited as workers, they are exploited as consumers. The highly profitable child market foists unhealthy food products, morally devoid and sexually explicit entertainment, and useless products on children from the time they can teeter up to the family television set. Children are viewed by society as takers not givers, learners not teachers, depen-

dents not independents. At least some of the increase in obesity, poor fitness, depression, and suicidal ideation among children may have roots in
the way adolescents and young adults are viewed by adults. In the complex U.S. economy, with an increasingly healthy and longer-living adult
population, youth are competitors for jobs and for security. There is an
enormous irony in the fact that Americans are in such a rush to see children grow up but then have not quite figured out how to welcome youth
into the grown-up world. There is a disconnect between young people's
physical status and fiscal dependency. Ready and able to contribute to
society, older children and youth may feel only a sense of worthlessness.
When that sense is combined with severely limited opportunities, youth
will seek excitement and purpose anywhere they can find it.

Some positive stories: As president of the W. T. Grant Foundation,
Karen Hein created a campaign for public awareness of the strengths
and assets of young people. In radio spots on National Public Radio she
called on the nation to give youth a chance to write, to perform, to com-
pete, to contribute; invited the nation to value the ideas and viewpoints
of youth and to invite their voices into the political arena. John Palfrey,
the director of the Berkman Center on Internet and Society, has also been
watching what could happen if youth began to have a political voice. He
argues that youth are increasingly learning to create networks and organizations through the Internet: that these digital tools offer an unparal-
leled opportunity for the empowerment of youth as a strong democratic
force.[12] John Chen, a high school teacher at Cambridge Rindge and Latin,
brings eight to ten of his civics class students to prepare the Friday evening meal at the University Lutheran Church homeless shelter. Together
in the kitchen with hip-hop music blaring, they prepare dinner, wash the
dishes, and learn about giving back to the community—while the community learns something about them.

The fact is that children will be productive citizens and that investment needs to be made in their health, their education, their moral and
spiritual development in as planned a way as one would invest in an
individual retirement account (IRA). But unlike an IRA, investors get
a return on the dollar at the time of the investment: the smiling 7-year-
old jumping rope on an Astroturf play surface rather than on an uneven
pavement strewn with glass shards, a teenager reciting lines from a speech
by Nelson Mandela rather than shouting obscenities at his girlfriend, a
10-year-old asking if he and two friends can take the cookies they have
just baked to share with their friends at the senior center. Young people
exercising citizenship now.

Child-Centered versus Family-Centered Approaches

Health care and other services (educational, day care, and so on) for children are generally oriented toward the individual child, but often clinicians discover that the child's situation is an expression of a more deep-seated family problem. All the adult members of the family smoke cigarettes, and the child suffers asthma attacks and periodic bouts of pneumonia as a consequence. The schoolteacher cannot understand why the 3d grader never completes his homework assignments. Then she learns that his mother and father cannot read and so have never understood that the child had homework. One child wheezes, one child gets unsatisfactory marks—these problems cannot be solved by a political will that focuses only on the child. Unless a family-centered approach is taken, the problems will persist.

Child-centered approaches can be helpful at some level to whip up sympathy for children. In fact that is much of the tone of this chapter. Nonetheless, there can be a downside of that strategy. The child is shown as a victim, the parents and the community as scoundrels. The child-centered approach is what the Bush administration took in 2002 in attempting to change the State Child Health Insurance Program (SCHIP) eligibility rulings in order to save some money. While the original SCHIP insurance coverage afforded health insurance to pregnant women, the 2002 change made the health insurance recipient only the unborn child.[13] This meant that the mother could receive only the care that was directly related to her obstetric condition, not care that might in the long run have an impact on both herself and the baby. For instance, the mother would not have health insurance coverage for a sprained ankle or broken arm. No, that is not directly related to fetal development, but think of what the stress might be for the mother if she had two other children, had to spend hours finding an orthopedist to take on her free care, and had to get the house ready for Dad and the children by 6 p.m. That type of physical and emotional stress has an effect on the whole family. A rational child and family orientation would take all of the factors into account, and there would be a political will that cherished families as much as it did unborn fetuses.

Simplicity versus Complexity

Children may be small and kids may be kids, but children's concerns are not always simple. Garnering political will involves a recognition that the steps toward solutions may be simple, but they are often best car-

Table 8.1. Yes, It Is Rocket Science

Characteristic	Rocket science	Brain surgery	Community child health
Discipline	Astronomy, physics, fuel dynamics, etc.	Anatomy, physiology, etc.	Medicine, public health, sociology, urban design, etc.
Importance	Life or death	Precision of intervention (life or death)	Delicacy of interventions to do no harm; balance "goods"
Timing	External factors often determine timing	Careful timing of components	Timing is often everything
Personnel	Teamwork; multidisciplinary	Teamwork	Multidisciplinary
Urgency	Politically determined urgency	Urgency	Longer time frame—but lack of urgency is a problem
Visibility	High visibility of novel events	High visibility of single cases	Low visibility of single cases
Ultimate goal	Flight surgeons' role well defined	Surgeons' role well defined	Needs better definitions of role

ried out in the context of an overall plan that acknowledges the complex world. Toward the end of the chapter, we return to the importance of an advocate's attitude that constructs, implements, and celebrates small simple steps. For now, let us think about how to conceptualize children's concerns in their fullness. Too often, the public and the policymakers trivialize children's issues. Child health advocacy is about refusing to accept such putdowns. They insult the intelligence.

So often we hear child-focused work treated as simple and unsophisticated: It's not rocket science; or, It doesn't take a brain surgeon to figure this out. The fact is that children's problems are just as challenging as astrophysics and neurosurgery, maybe more so. The child advocate's answer is to approach the problems with the same rigorous steps as the rocket scientist and the neurosurgeon do. Table 8.1 displays how similar child health advocacy, rocket science, and neurosurgery are. A big difference is that those other fields articulate their missions in terms that the general public can understand easily. That is an important difference.

NASA succeeded in getting a man to the moon and yet the United States cannot succeed in teaching all our children their sums and times tables nor ensure that young children will have adequate health insurance coverage and responsive health care. NASA's mission was unequivocal—so direct, so simple. We want to put a man on the moon before the Russians do. Goal clear, urgency apparent. The system and steps to accomplish the mission were anything but simple. Scientists, industrialists, politicians would all need to cooperate to get the job done. They would translate to one another from their different technical jargon in terms that all could understand. They would break down turf barriers because turf is silly. They would send a man to the moon, and they would all rejoice with the entire country when the mission was accomplished. Political will was garnered, galvanized, and used to the utmost.

Besides not articulating the goals, another trap that people who care about children fall into is feeling overwhelmed by how intractable the problem seems to be. Anyone who takes the time to delve into children's issues feels a headache coming on as she sorts through the relationships between child outcomes and all the possible inputs. Look at the question of financing for education. It would make sense that the more money a state devoted to educating children and youth the better the academic outcomes would be. It should be a linear relationship. It is not. The Heritage Foundation argues that putting more money into education is not the answer because they find no simple cause-effect relationship.[14] States like Massachusetts and Connecticut have high investment and high achievement, but this relationship is offset by the statistics of Washington, D.C., and Delaware, where there is low achievement despite high investment. The Heritage Foundation also shows the relationship of achievement and investment in states where the expenditure is low. Achievement in Mississippi and New Mexico, with their low investment, is low; but achievement in Montana and Colorado, also states where investment is low, is high. Sticky trap. Does the advocate give up? Or does she probe deeper to understand the details of how Montana and Colorado support its families and children. Where are the other subsidies coming from? Does it matter that the average class size in Montana is thirteen to one and that over half of elementary schoolchildren attend schools that have fewer than 350 students?[15] Could be.

Ferreting out the relationships, understanding the vulnerabilities of some communities and the assets of others, takes time and energy, but it can and should be done. Child outcomes depend on the complex interplay of family factors, community factors, and ethnic, racial, religious, cultural, and historical influences. There is no one-size-fits-all model, no streamlined interaction; and there is the constant pressure of change. But instead of overwhelming those interested in children, these complexities should draw in those who like conundrums and puzzles, who enjoy looking for clues and common denominators. If the same attention were devoted to understanding how children grow and develop as the scientific world devotes to understanding the human genome, directions for action would be made clear. The National Institute of Child Health and Human Development has proposed a multibillion-dollar national children's study to do such a careful analysis.[16] If this major study is funded, it will be a signal that Congress and others have an interest in the complexity of children's lives and that there is a political will to take children's issues seriously, to move beyond simplistic generalizations about child health and development.

Family Responsibility versus Societal Responsibility

Whose kids are these anyway? If children are living in poverty, whose problem is it? If an affluent 8th grader shoplifts, whose concern is it? If a teenager is turned away from a doctor's office for lack of health insurance, whose fault is it? If a third of the children in Miss Soto's 6th-grade class cannot write a sentence, who should take the blame?

The closer that we look at the complexity issues discussed above, the clearer it is that children have the best health and educational outcomes when they are supported by families and by communities with shared values. Fiscal resources are definitely needed, but they are not sufficient to ensure children's health, safety, and welfare. Children who live in communities that are rich in human capital and social resources thrive. Without family and community supports, all the money in the world is not enough to ensure a safe passage through childhood and adolescence. Further, some children have innate vulnerabilities (physical or mental health disorders, behavioral concerns) that demand even higher levels of societal, community, and family support.

The real concern is how a society provides families and communities with the fiscal building blocks, the human construction materials, and the moral foundation to create a nurturing structure for children and youth. When families and communities are themselves under attack, it is hard for them to pull themselves together to do what children and youth need. In Boston the so-called Boston Miracle virtually eliminated youth homicide because the entire community—families, churches, police, and the media—assembled a multipronged plan to get gun-toting offenders into jail and to reach out to young people before they got swept up into gangs and drug selling.[17] But in the summer of 2004, when the offenders returned to the streets at the end of their jail terms, the community was again overtaken, and the shooting and deaths began again. This negative tipping point comes when individual families and individual neighborhoods cannot do it alone. It is time for a larger societal responsibility. Surely an answer will come in Boston. But will it be after another and another son is buried? The families' tears call out for a society that takes responsibility before the tragedy, not because of it.

Why doesn't society take responsibility for its children? Through national opinion polling, Bob Blendon has found that the problem is largely one of we/they thinking.[18] We will care for our own, but other people's children are their business. If only they had behaved well, their children would be fine. We want to be sure our kids get the very best of everything; that's what good parents do for their children. So it follows that, if parents cannot provide "everything" for their children, they are not good parents. Children's issues get distorted and confused with concerns about poverty and fears of a welfare state. The old Puritan ethic and Horatio Alger myths come into play. When policymakers finally do decide to make commitments to children, there is a tendency simply to shore up a bad situation, patch the gaping hole, to please the naysayers. This response reflects the low national value placed on children.

The we/they dichotomy also breaks down as majority/minority, middle class/lower class, mainstream/marginalized, white/nonwhite, well-off/poor. Policymakers, social reformers, conservative think tank mavens, and do-gooders easily conflate childhood issues with poverty. And then the concept of poverty gets tied in with race and ethnicity. In analytic terms, such connections make sense. No question: the census, the National Health Interview Survey, and the National Center for Educational Statistics document that the children most likely to be in adverse circumstances are the children of poor families (see chapter 3). Statistical chances are high that they are also black or Hispanic. Race drives a wedge, separates societal groups, and causes Americans to treat each other's families as "other," "different," "not our own." To treat all children well and fairly, the United States must tussle with racism head on. This is uncomfortable. The civil rights accomplishments of the twentieth century changed the laws and guaranteed protections, but as long as some of the fundamental inequities of attitude and circumstance remain, children will continue to suffer. Political will is the attitude, the tone, that says there is no we and they; all children are our children.

That is not to say that a diverse group of people standing in a circle singing "We Shall Overcome" will change anything for children. Confronting racism and poverty means really engaging those problems. One could wish that the Government Accountability Office would look at how racism and poverty affect child health and development and that a great Aha would sound from Washington. It was just such a careful assessment of the issue of poverty in the 1950s and 1960s that energized the Congress to do something for the elderly. When it became apparent that the escalating costs of medical care were driving large numbers of the elderly into poverty, Congress created Medicare. Unfortunately, it is unlikely that there will be such a dramatic impetus to care for children:

they are only children, after all. Instead, children's advocacy will rest on the painstaking, deliberate, block-by-block, group-by-group, situation-by-situation struggle with the daily realities. It will take the courage of families to break out of old modes of operating. The poor and marginalized will have to speak up. The mainstream will have to listen. If child health advocates can set the stage for that conversation to happen, it will be a first, an enormous, big step. Without such work, children and children's issues will remain some one else's problem: them, not us.

Who Takes the Lead?

Political will is the collective attitude of a group, a community, or a nation. It is the sense of the people. But political will has no power until it is gathered and named. Some one or some group must sense the attitude—the mood of the public—and articulate it. Making use of political will depends on the skilled leadership of those who know how to read the hopes and desires of the people and their readiness for change. Leaders then mix that political will with the brainstorms of dreamers and the designs of planners. Leaders fashion a substantial agenda that can stand the test of time. As we ask questions about the slow pace of a children's agenda in the United States, one of the answers is that leadership for children has been spotty at best. At every level—governmental, professional, philanthropic, and community—there is a leadership void. Children's health and welfare concerns have far too few champions.

Presidents

Few American presidents have placed children's issues high on their list of executive priorities. And when they have, they have rarely generated a national political will around those concerns. Under pressure from the Progressive social reformers, Theodore Roosevelt called the first White House Conference on Children in 1909 just as he was leaving the presidency. Herbert Hoover endorsed the Children's Charter in 1930.[19] While Franklin Roosevelt's New Deal had sweeping implications for children, the history books record few quotable quotes from FDR about children and youth.

John Kennedy's administration demonstrated how presidential leadership could focus on a particular age group and capture the nation's imagination. Kennedy's inaugural assertion that young adults should ask what they can do for their country was followed up with creative programming and bold action. With this example of an age-oriented agenda, is it unreasonable to ask whether a similar political will could ever be generated around children and youth? As Lyndon Johnson proposed to build the Great Society, he and his team found that *fighting* generates more political will than *building;* as part of the War on Poverty, poor children were the recipients of substantial presidential attention. With the Civil Rights movement in full gear, there was forceful political will aligned with a carefully articulated social strategy to alleviate the suffering of poor children and to right the years of wrong to black children. Children benefited from LBJ's leadership, but his main targets were poverty and racism.

Jimmy Carter learned the hard way that the public views sentimentality about children and childhood with disdain. When he mentioned in a speech on nuclear weapons that he had discussed national policy with his daughter, he was held up to scorn by the press and by other politicians. With that cautionary experience, presidents in the future thought twice about the wisdom of consulting the young. After all, presidents must be serious, worldly, and tough. The Reagan-Bush years were filled with seriousness, worldliness, and toughness. Presidents should be spending their time with heads of state and attending to world affairs, not with little children. The federal government should stay out of a citizen's business, out of family lives, and certainly out of their living rooms, backyards, and neighborhood school.

Many child advocates expected a change in attitude about children and families with the Clinton administration. Hillary Clinton spoke often about her years as a member of the board of the Children's Defense Fund, the large, vocal national child advocacy organization headed by Marian Wright Edelman, an attorney who had been active in civil rights litigation during the 1960s. As discussed in chapter 6, Bill Clinton did fall back to a child-health-at-all-costs position once his major health care initiative failed. But his administration will be best remembered for the passage of the largest federal welfare cutback in history. Only time will tell whether this was pro- or anti-child legislation.

The 1996 Clinton-Dole presidential election opened up national dialogue about children in ways that had never happened before. Hilary Clinton used the African proverb, It takes a village to raise a child, in her book, *It Takes a Village.*[20] The phrase resonated with much of the public, especially those feeling isolated in their attempts to do the best for their children against great odds. When Robert Dole belittled the concept of societal responsibility for children, he compromised his presidential chances. There was clearly an untapped political will around children and families.

Recognizing the political capital in children's issues, George W. Bush has made children (and particularly their education) a cornerstone of his domestic policy. Unapologetically, he co-opted Marian Wright Edelman's slogan, Leave No Child Behind, changing it to No Child Left Behind. Isn't it said that imitation is the highest form of flattery? Bush must have thought that Edelman was on to something. Not so: the president's bill is just the reauthorization of the Elementary and Secondary Education Act of 1965. By contrast, Edelman's legislation, the Dodd-Miller bill, is comprehensive in nature and has a timetable for improving conditions for children across the board. Edelman has called Bush a "deceptive weasel" for his bait-and-switch use of her original notion.[21]

At best, the No Child Left Behind legislation has been a mixed blessing for children and families. There has been only a small increase in federal money added to state budgets for children's education, but those moneys are long overdue. From 1990 to 1996 there were only the tiniest annual increases in per pupil expenditures. In 1991 and 1992 there were actually decreases.[22] The total amount of state and federal dollars spent on education during 2001–2 was $400 billion, or roughly 5 percent of the gross national product. The 2005 presidential budget recommended $38.7 billion for K–12 education, less than one-tenth of national education expenditures. A real commitment by the government would require it to provide full funding for the Elementary and Secondary Education Act (ESEA) and Individuals with Disabilities Education Act (IDEA). It must also ensure equity across school districts in quality of education. Average per pupil expenditure is only $7,000, with a wide range from district to district and state to state.

The No Child Left Behind Act places heavy burdens of academic accountability on the schools. This is not necessarily a bad thing, particularly in light of the fact that American children rank low academically in comparison to children in other parts of the world. The United States ranks twenty-fourth in math literacy in comparison with countries like Korea, Japan, Poland, Hungary, and the Slovak Republic and are no better than average on the OCED comparison for literacy, despite the second-highest expenditures on education.[23] Unfortunately, the price tag for all the new testing and monitoring requirements eats up many of the new No Child Left Behind dollars.

The one thing that can be said about the No Child Left Behind legislation is that the topic of children and their educational and developmental needs are deemed important enough to be addressed by the U.S. president. Some of the 3 million votes that kept George W. Bush in office no doubt came as a result of a political will for leadership and direction on children's issues.

Other Leaders

Government policy around families and children is, of course, more of a state and local issue than it is a federal one, and the main children's issue is education. Leaders at the state legislature and in the governor's mansion are likely to be preoccupied with children's concerns at budget time. States and localities share the bulk of educational expenditure. In 2002 states paid 46 percent and localities paid 37 percent of the K–12 budget.[24] The distribution formulas for federal-state-local monies vary state to state, region to region, and county to county. The federal government has never insisted on regional distribution of tax assets to smooth out within-region differences. Many states have developed elaborate methodologies for factoring in the neediness of local school districts and adjusting for this in the state matches.

Governors like James Hunt of North Carolina and Howard Dean of Vermont have put children front and center with outspoken commitment to early childhood programs and universal health care, while there are many examples of heroic leadership for children at the mayoral level: Thomas Menino in Boston, Richard Daly in Chicago, Jerry Brown in Oakland, Charles Royer in Seattle, George Lattimer in St. Paul. Such leadership is often a personal matter, however, with little carryover from one mayoral administration to another. Big city mayors often feel left out in the cold by state and federal leaders, even though they are by default the major governmental leadership for many children and families.

As for leaders at the nongovernmental level, anyone who has ever tried to raise money for children's issues from philanthropic organizations can attest that children are low on their priority lists and that only a handful of corporations primarily support children's causes. The many community child-helping agencies and organizations have enough trouble getting their assigned work done on their shoestring budgets and their own good hearts without having any resources left to drum up political will.

Professionals and professional organizations are like such agency workers. They have full plates and generally feel that by fulfilling their contracts with the public they are responding to political will. Why should they do anything more? They do not necessarily believe it is the business of professionals to stimulate political will beyond the professions themselves. Even though groups such as the American Academy of Pediatrics, the National Education Association, and the National Bar

Association take responsive positions on legislative agendas, weighing in with professional experience and judgment, they are more hesitant about being proactive in the generation of political will. Certainly individual professionals do take a lead on children's issues. Chapter 2 tells the stories of a number of child health professionals who have made a difference because they learned how to capture the imagination of the public (or a segment of the public).

Leadership to garner political will often comes from the grass roots, from the community of affected individuals. The civil rights movements for minorities and for people with disabilities are testament to the powerful political wills that communities can ignite. The community of children is a complex entity. Half of the members cannot speak for themselves and the half who can are rarely taken seriously by the larger public. Youth leadership has the potential to be quite a force, particularly with the emergence of the worldwide Internet communication system.

But leadership is perhaps really a group affair. In the mid-1990s Ruby Hearn, Paul Jellinek, and Rush Russell of the Robert Wood Johnson Foundation built the Urban Health Initiative on the premise that making a difference at the systems level is what matters.[25] They proposed granting $1 million a year for ten years to five large cities to improve child services. To compete successfully for the funds, the cities had to demonstrate that they could combine leadership at the mayoral level with that of agencies, professionals, and the community at large. Everybody mattered. Lots of arms to hammer the nails. To amplify the political will of those in the urban centers, they challenged the city leaders to try to leverage the assets of the wealthier communities in their regions. The initiative was largely unsuccessful at this last endeavor, but otherwise there have been stunning accomplishments in the five cities, demonstrating that leaders and constituents of all sectors can create a common political will that can accomplish effective social change for children.

Recognizing how important the issue of leadership is in marshaling political will for action, the Urban Health Initiative sponsors urban fellowships for newspaper editors, civic leaders, businessmen, academics, and clergy to learn about children's concerns, to see in action how best practice can work, but most important to act as champions in their various societal sectors, to upgrade the importance of children and youth, and to counteract the ambivalent feelings Americans hold about children and youth.

The National Scientific Council on the Developing Child, chaired by Jack Shonkoff, is also working on the issue of political will.[26] Building on the landmark Institute of Medicine publication, *From Neurons to Neighborhoods*, the council has been using its scientific leadership position to argue for policy change based on cutting-edge research. The council, recognizing that political will can best be created through mutual engagement with policy and business leaders, has invested heavily in communication research methodology. Like the Urban Health Initiative and Institute for Health Innovation (discussed in chapter 7), the National Scientific Council works to learn the language and needs of the business community, because without the power and influence of that community, the fight for a larger political agenda for children will continue to be an uphill battle.

One Coherent Vision

Leaders can only do so much. Even leaders with extraordinary charisma, wonderful ideas, and productive staffs need the larger political will to be with them. Engaging that political will is a dynamic affair. There is an aching in the community to do better by our children, but the longing is poorly documented and poorly articulated, and few public citizens know what to do about it. Leaders pick up on the general mood and tenor, they express the public's yearning in ways that make sense. Once the leaders have carried out their analysis, the ideas must be turned back to the public for action. It is a dance. It takes two to tango and eight to do the Virginia reel.

Part of child health advocacy involves deciding who needs to be invited to the party and making sure that there are reasons why they should want to come. In the dance of political will, there are all sorts of partners, some willing, some coy, some outright resistant. For child health advocacy, the public partners may be a group as small as the staff of the local neighborhood health clinic or as large as the citizenry of the state of North Dakota. The public may be as homogeneous as the congregation of the downtown mosque or as diverse as all Americans. Within these larger groups, there are always at least three subgroups: those who are inclined to support the child health advocacy, those who are not sure what they think, and those who would just as soon scuttle any initiative.

No matter who they are, public invitees all want music and choreography and look to leaders for that. Before the public will invest their political will in an idea, they ask for at least three things: (1) a coherent vision, (2) a stepwise plan for getting from here to there, and (3) a set of goals to measure there progress against.

Child health advocacy has struggled to come up with a coherent vision of child health and development, but too often the message to the public has been garbled. Advocates have not made the connections between early and late inputs, between family and individual, between a healthy society and healthy children. Child health advocacy needs to wrestle with this problem until it is solved. Not with sound bytes and catch phrases (although in the end the best vision can be captured in a few words). To make its case forcefully, the child health community needs to articulate for the public the most profound and meaningful vision possible. A vision of children's health tied into the general well-being of all.

The American public definitely wants health. They talk about it constantly, spend their hard-earned cash on health products, and eagerly follow the health advice offered on television, radio, and Internet chat rooms. Signaling the high value that twenty-first-century America places on health, massive laboratories, medical research campuses, and hospital complexes dot the landscape of most large U.S. cities. Recognizing how fast the medical industry is growing, wise mayors and governors vie to attract biotechnology and pharmaceutical enterprises. In cities like New York and Boston, the health care industry is one of the main employers.

With health as a value, advocates for children need to do a better job of getting across to the public the fact that a society is only as healthy as its least healthy infant. It is only as educated as the least educated child, and only as secure as its least peaceful neighborhood. The interconnections between health, education, and neighborhood stability must be boldly drawn. The message needs to be repeated over and over until it is incorporated into the thoughts and actions of every American. If the *Daily Newsbit* reporter asks the man in the street about child health, the man should respond without a second's hesitation that the United States ensures the healthy growth and development of every child. That is how the richest country becomes the greatest country.

Knowing that we are far from a time when the man in the street would ever say that, child health advocates need to find the best way to foster that response. As a bare minimum, the public deserves a clear description of what is meant by the words *the healthy growth and development of every child.* Some people can readily understand language that sets the goal of reducing the number of teen births from A to B by the year 2010, and they can understand the direction of the advocacy. For others, the vision may be better expressed as a metaphor.

An example: Barbara Barlow describes a dynamic vision of healthy growth and development that relies on individual, family, and community interdependence. She asks her public to envision a neighborhood vegetable garden. Imagine neighbors, families, the local community agencies, and town authorities have received a small grant from one of the business interests in town. That the mayor has declared that the vacant lot on 10th St. is available to the group. Mothers and fathers, little children and teenagers, grandparents and maiden aunts are in the garden in the spring planting and weeding. One youngster arrives in his electric wheelchair. Some days they all come to tend the garden. Some days, just the teenagers show up. Sometimes the garden just grows. In the fall, the time for harvest, the children are all a little older. Maybe a grandparent has died. There is a new baby in the Smith's baby stroller. A summer has passed, and the neighbors are closer and there is food to harvest.

In Barlow's vision, there is no room for drug pushers, for AK-47s, or oversexualized commercial advertising. The children are outside, in the fresh air. Hoed, seeded, and tended, the earth is producing healthy food for the families. The families themselves are growing and developing. The teenagers' independence is recognized. The reality that life moves from health to death to rebirth is captured. Productivity and meaning and caring are all essential parts of the picture of health. Is this Eden? Hillary Clinton's village? Brook Farm? No—it is Harlem, Miami, Des Moines. These gardens really exist. They are sponsored by business interests who have decided that it is in their best interest to have lively, healthy, vibrant communities. Healthy families are good customers. Healthy neighborhoods attract and keep healthy families; they foster business and growth.

This is a vision that realizes that the true constituents for a children's health agenda are all citizens. Cities and towns that care about families and children care about themselves. They want what every American wants—life, liberty, and the pursuit of happiness. They want to be able to provide decent circumstances for their families. Children mean so much to adults because the cycle of life is interdependent. Children bred from parents breathe new life back into family and adult life. The beauty of human development lies not in one moment in time. It is a complex unfolding. With each stage of each child's life and then with each stage of multiple children's lives, parents have to readjust: to be ever the same and ever different.

As adults parent, they revisit their own growing up in a new context. As parents, they need to be creative in reshaping lives, both their own and their families'. Some people are capable of doing this because they have the constitutional, financial, and physical resources to do so. Other people have difficulty dealing with children's developing nature.

Some are even incapable. Because of limited intelligence or emotional disability, they cannot understand place and change. They get entangled and enmeshed in their children's lives. Lovingly, they try to parent, but they cannot see themselves as separate from their children. They huddle over or run away. Nothing moves or resolves. Many child health concerns arise from parental confusion about how to guide children through their natural stages of development. Clinicians who work with runaway youth, teen pregnant girls, adolescents with mental health and substance abuse problems can often pinpoint the ways that a deeper parental understanding of child development could have prevented some of these problems.

Some families lack the fiscal resources and settings to let the children's lives unfold. They do their best to provide for their children but simply cannot win with the cards life has dealt them. There is no quality time for the mother and father who are forced to work two full-time jobs at minimum wages simply to cover the rent and the food bills. When they come home, exhausted, all they can do is cook a meal and crawl into bed. The alarm clock will be going off again in less than six hours. There is no time for roughhousing, building Legos and castles in the air, setting up a blanket fort in the living room, reading *Amazing Grace.* Time is all these families want and need, and time is what American society has taken away.

All American families—rich, poor, black, white, native born, foreign born, suburban, urban, ex-urban—could benefit from the chance to slow down. Families hear too late the wise words of the elderly, who say, I don't miss a single day at the factory, but what I would give for another chance to bake sugar cookies with Sally. They are not talking about the daughter who is first in her class in law school. They are talking about 7-year-old Sally who just came home from 2d grade with a special Haiku she wanted to read to her family.

Celebrating children's health and development and preserving what is good in family life does not de facto mean an Ozzie and Harriet existence. That world never existed, or if it did only a few families fit the mold. That world depended on gender inequities that harmed little Sally too. The early twenty-first-century family does not look like the family of the 1950s; and the family of the 2050s will look different still. A deep appreciation of child development recognizes that, within families, all of the members have needs, ever-changing ones. Families need community and societal supports to balance those needs. And to have the time and the capacity to glory in the here and now.

Fulfilling the Vision: Action Plans

Fulfilling the vision requires an action plan to give the public specifics that they can get their mind around. The action plan starts with an outline of the problem and then describes the population of children and youth involved in the plan (all the students in a classroom, all the teenagers in a neighborhood, all 0- to 5-year-olds in a town, or all the children and youth in an entire state). A needs assessment then depicts how far the affected children and youth are from attaining good health and development. What conditions are putting them at risk? What resources are there in the area that can be used to improve the situation? How much money will the plan require? What is the time line? Who else can help?

Action plans are of two kinds: (1) short-term, incremental strategies such as the homeless health van in Miami or the Pediatric Alliance for Coordinated Care described in chapter 5; and (2) longer term planning such as the development of the medical home or a program like Medicaid as described in chapters 4 and 7. All of these strategies require chipping away at the problems that interfere with children's health and well-being. Strategic plans have to be flexible enough to adapt to changing forces and newly emerging threats, but they need to have enough staying power to create permanent systems for children and youth.

The success of all child health planning involves capturing the political will of an invested public. Because the public is made up of many different types of people, advocates reach out to different segments of the public in a variety of ways with a variety of expectations of how the public will interact with the plan. In some cases, the plan will involve the actions of the public. In others, the plan calls for endorsement and possible investment by the public. In still others, a tacit agreement by the public not to interfere with the plan is all that is hoped for or needed.

Engaging the public who are already inclined toward the child health plan is often described as preaching to the choir, but the choir has a lot to offer. Part of any child health advocacy plan should involve specific actions that the public can do: writing letters to the school board about the importance of gym and recess for children's health, voting for a ballot initiative to improve the food in the county elementary schools, attending a hearing to comment on the special education bill that is up for reauthorization this year.

Political will as endorsement is critically important when the action plan calls for funding. The town meeting or the PTA or the state voters have to agree to expend the dollars for the child health plan. For too many years, local areas, the states, and the nation have had too little money for health care, child care, education, after-school programs, and housing. The bottom line on the bottom line is that we will never achieve the nation's child health goals until dollars shift—in the private sector, at the local level, and at the state and federal levels.

Over the past decade, a variety of commissions and groups have created funding formulas that allot money to child-friendly services and emphasize prevention.[27] These recommendations aim at support for activities that will have a long-term payoff. To decrease health care costs, the recommendations call for funding efforts that reduce conditions such as prematurity, teen births, obesity, injury, and violence. They recognize that child health outcomes are affected also by what happens at school and in the community. The best estimates are that the additional costs to improve the health and developmental status of children are

- Health care: $10 billion to $20 billion
- Child care and after-school programs: $20 billion to $25 billion
- Education: $35 billion to $40 billion

These are large numbers, but when they are divided by fifty (the number of states) or by 190 (the number of corporations with annual budgets over $10 billion),[28] or by 70 million (the number of children in the United States), they come down to manageable sums. Adding these dollars to the system will require specific legislative initiatives to ensure universal health insurance, to ensure comprehensive care planning for children with disabilities, to fund elementary and secondary school and special education, and to increase child care and after-school slots. These initiatives will combine funding mechanisms such as parental tax credits, incentives for industries that sponsor child and family programs, and tax increases for those who do not—as well as mandates for a universal buy-in to health insurance and local, state, and federal increases in fees and special revenue-generating programs (such as license plates that support child-oriented service projects).

The shift to prevention will generate some dollars to offset some of the additional costs. A good deal of the needed money is already in the system but being used in inefficient ways. For instance, prenatal care prevents premature births and saves dollars for lifelong health costs. It costs twice as much to house and feed a prisoner a year than it does to provide high-quality early childhood education.[29] Every time a child does not become a criminal, society saves all along the line. More preventive efforts in school and after school have the potential of improving the health, fitness, and function of children, cutting down on physical and mental health care costs.

Child health advocacy has frequently floundered because the public has not understood the connection between child health and societal welfare. Child health advocates are wise to call on enlightened self-interest, pointing out the ways in which the long-term viability of the nation rests on the strength and promise of the next generation. The past twenty or so years have been extraordinary ones in the amount of change that has occurred for the average American. Everyday life is different in every way in 2006 from the way that it was in 1980, and the rate of change is speeding up so that we cannot anticipate the world of 2030. We can only imagine that life spans will be even longer than they are at present, that humans will depend increasingly on technology, that the world's ecosystem will be tested increasingly to support the world's population, and that the global community will be ever tighter. What will America's place be in the world order?

At the beginning of the millennium, the United States is still the richest nation but is struggling in the race for a well-prepared workforce. India, China, and Brazil are nipping at our ankles—and surpassing us in technological education. And our child health outcomes lag behind those of other nations. How can we claim leadership when we cannot guarantee our children adequate health care?

Americans are competitive. We like to see ourselves as strong, as ahead, as accomplished, and as right. To engage political will on a large scale, advocates may want to appeal to American self-interest and pride. How can we be behind Italy in education? Less effective in delivering immunizations than many Eastern European countries? Have more teen pregnancies than any other developed country? Every child health plan should include information about how the success of the child health intervention will improve the status of the general population now and in the future.

And what of the responsibility of the richest country in the world to the nations whose child health care status is worse than ours? While we can be embarrassed that the United States does not provide its own children with the best in health care, there may be an even greater condemnation that we are so lax in helping the poorest nations as they struggle to provide their children with the most basic nutrition, shelter, hygiene, and preventive measures. Close to 10 million children die each year of causes that are largely preventable. The U.S. fiscal and moral commitment to the improvement of health conditions on a global scale would provide a huge lift to the effort, and yet America continues an arrogant stance with regard to mechanisms such as the United Nations Convention on the Rights of the Child.

It is time for some bold steps. It is time for us to ask questions about children in the United States and in the world. Where do Americans stand? Do we care about children? Are we willing to mark our X's and spend our dollars for children? No real change will come until advocates push the issue. For too long, children's issues have been flying below the radar. The implicit needs to be made explicit.

The United States needs to ratify the UN Convention on the Rights of the Child. This will commit the country to a rights focus for children and their families. It will also mean that the United States will take a positive role in global health concerns. The United States also should pass either a Children's Rights Bill akin to the Civil Rights Bill or a constitutional amendment ensuring health, education, and housing to children as fundamental rights. Without this national assurance, there will continue to be states and localities where some children suffer because of lack of health care, decent schooling, and housing. Finally, there needs to be a cabinet-level official in the federal government (and a comparable person in each state) who is responsible for the rights of children and youth.

The lack of accountability for children's issues has been a serious flaw in the American system. In the dance of political will, leadership is critical. Children need champions at all levels. Having a member of the cabinet who wakes up every morning worrying about children's health and development will greatly improve the status of children and increase the likelihood that children's issues will be kept in front of the public, will be a part of serious public discourse, and will be addressed as if the present and the future depended on it. Which they do.

Bright Futures

Advocacy is about success. It is about setting attainable goals and marching forward toward them. The group of child health providers and families who drew up the Bright Futures Children's Health Charter did so to create a road map, to declare some achievable ends. Nothing they suggest is beyond reach. The knowledge base delineates the scope of the problem, social strategies set the solutions in motion, and political will sustains the effort. Here is a restatement of the charter's goals, with the outcome checkpoints of successful child health advocacy. We will know when we have arrived when all children have the chance:

To be born well. Every baby will be born into a family that celebrates its arrival and has the physical, emotional, and fiscal resources to embrace the new life fully and to enjoy what the child brings. No baby will be born with a preventable disability, and the children who are born with chronic problems will be welcomed with the same enthusiasm and love as all other children.

To be physically fit. The nation will be expressing its political will for children when there are safe play spaces in every neighborhood and when children can run as freely as birds fly. All schools will offer daily exercise, and their gyms will have proper equipment in working order. Well-trained, decently paid gym teachers will teach the children the exercises that they will use for the lifelong care of their bodies.

To achieve self-responsibility for good health habits. Adults will value good health and will share with children the importance of taking personal responsibility for physical, oral, and mental health. Effective school and college wellness programs will help adolescents and young adults to make healthy decisions about tobacco, alcohol, drugs, and sexual experiences. Information and materials (abstinence pledges, safe-driving contracts, nicotine patches, condoms, birth control) will be available for young people so that they can follow through on their personal health commitments.

To have access to coordinated, comprehensive, health-promoting, therapeutic, and rehabilitative medical, mental health, and dental care. The nation will have made the commitment to full health insurance benefits for all mothers, infants, children and adolescents. That insurance will adequately cover all expenses for physical, mental, and dental health care. Health care will be a declared right of all children and youth.

To have nurturing families and supportive relationships. A child's health begins with the health of his parents. Family policy in the United States will support all families, and particular attention will be paid to foster families to ensure that they have the adequate physical, fiscal, and mental health backup they need to heal the wounds of the children they have taken in. Health care will also be a right of all Americans; the interdependence of child and family health will mean that if a child health provider detects a health problem in a family member (e.g., depression, smoking, victimization), the child health provider will have access to adult services for that parent.

To grow in physically and psychologically safe homes and school environment, free of injury, abuse, violence, and exposure to environmental toxins. The nation will invest in the infrastructure of the schools and community environments where children learn and play. Schools and communities will not tolerate intimidation or violence. There will be adequate monitoring of the air, water, and soil to detect hazardous substances. Environmental impact will be assessed and the environment protected whenever there is substantial industrial or residential growth. New building will incorporate green methodology to the greatest extent possible.

To have satisfactory housing, good nutrition, a quality education, an adequate family income, a supportive social network, and access to community resources. The richest nation in the world will no longer tolerate homelessness or hunger for any family or child. All American children will have educational opportunities tailored to meet their needs. In some cases this will mean that the nation will have to invest far more in schools than it has done in the past to make up for the poor quality of instruction, the lack of resources and books, and the "you will never succeed anyway" attitudes that have kept so many of our children down. All workers will receive a living wage so they can pay their rent, buy groceries, and have the opportunity to spend waking hours with their families. Community centers will have resources that support the positive development of families.

To have quality child care when parents are working outside the home. All day care slots will meet national standards for quality and safety. Child care providers will be paid at least a living wage, with full benefits, and there will be a career ladder for advancement to retain experienced child care workers in the field. Child care workers will work in partnership with health care providers to promote the health of the children in their care.

To learn how to cope with stressful life experiences. Community centers, faith-based organizations, and schools will provide skills-based learning programs for children and youth that teach social interaction skills so they can handle disappointment and confront life's challenges. When possible, these programs will offer opportunities for peer leadership.

To develop positive values and become responsible citizens. Parents, faith-based organizations, schools, and community agencies will actively seek the participation of children (from as young as 3 and 4 years) in helping others—the elderly, the sick, the bereaved, the poor. Whenever possible, community agencies will have board positions for youth representatives or sponsor junior boards that are composed of youth leadership.

To experience joy, have high self-esteem, have friends, acquire a sense of efficacy, and believe they can succeed in life. There will be adequate time in family and community life for celebration. All children will have hope about a future that waits for them, wants them, and needs them.

Appendix: Resources Online

Administration for Children and Families
www.acf.hhs.gov

American Academy of Pediatrics
www.aap.org

Annie E. Casey Foundation
www.aecf.org

Annie E. Casey Foundation, KIDSCOUNT
www. aecf.org/kidscount

Centers for Disease Control and Prevention (searchable by health topic)
www.cdc.gov

Children's Defense Fund
www.childrensdefense.org

Child Trends
www.childtrends.org

Commonwealth Fund
www.cmwf.org

Future of Children
www.futureofchildren.org

Healthy People 2010
www.healthypeople.gov

Institute of Medicine
www.iom.edu

Maternal and Child Health Bureau
www.mchb.hrsa.gov

National Institute of Child Health and Human Development
www.nichd.nih.gov

National Institutes of Health (searchable by health topic)
www.nih.gov

UNICEF
www.unicef.org

Notes

Chapter One. Child Health Advocacy

1. National Center for Health Statistics, *Health, United States, 2004* (Hyattsville, Md., 2004), p. 14.

2. The World Health Organization defines health as "a state of complete physical, mental, and social well-being and not merely the absence of disease or infirmity." Health "is a fundamental human right, and . . . the attainment of the highest possible level of health is a most important worldwide social goal, whose realization requires the action of many other social and economic sectors in addition to the health sector." See www.who.int/hpr/NPH/docs/declaration_almaata.pdf (accessed September 29, 2005).

3. Palfrey JS, *Community Child Health: An Action Plan for Today* (Westport, Conn.: Praeger, 1994); Duncan GJ and Brooks-Gunn J, *The Consequences of Growing Up Poor* (New York: Russell Sage, 1997), abstracted at www.jcpr.org/conferences/povinfo_dunc2.html (accessed September 20, 2005).

4. Green M and Palfrey JS, eds., *Bright Futures: Guidelines for Health Supervision of Infants, Children, and Adolescents,* 2d ed. (National Center for Education in Maternal and Child Health, 2000). Other documents lay out similar goals; see U.S. Department of Health and Human Services, *Healthy People 2000* (1990); U.S. Department of Health and Human Services, *Healthy People 2010* (2000); U.S. National Commission on Children, *Beyond Rhetoric: A New American Agenda for Children and Families* (Government Printing Office, 1991); Vanderpol NA and Richmond JB, Child Health in the United States: Prospects for the 1990s, *American Review of Public Health* 11 (1990):185–205.

5. U.S. Department of Health and Human Services, *Healthy Children 2000,* p. 62.

6. Ogden CL and others, Prevalence and Trends in Overweight among Children and Adolescents, 1999–2000, *Journal of the American Medical Association* 288 (2002):1728–32.

7. Centers for Disease Control, School Health Policies and Programs Study (SHPSS), *Journal of School Health* 71 (2001), available at www.cdc.gov/HealthyYouth/shpps/factsheets/pdf/pe.pdf (accessed September 20, 2005). See also Pate RR and others, School Physical Education, *Journal of School Health* 65 (1995):339–43, available at www.kidsource.com/kidsource/content4/promote.phyed.html (accessed September 20, 2005).

8. Centers for Disease Control, School Health Policies and Programs Study.

9. People without Health Insurance for the Entire Year by Selected Characteristics, 2001 and 2002, table 1, available at www.census.gov/prod/2003pubs/p60-223.pdf (accessed September 29, 2005); Burns BJ and others, Data Watch: Children's Mental Health Service Use across Service Sectors, *Health Affairs* 14 (1995):147–59; also see www.surgeongeneral.gov/topics/cmh/childreport.htm#sum (accessed November 29, 2005); Child Health Insurance Research Initiative (CHIRI), Issue Brief 2, *Children's Dental Care Access in Medicaid: The Role of Medical Care Use and Dentist Participation,* AHRQ publication 03-0032, June 2003; American Dental Association, *Increasing Access to Medicaid Dental Services for Children through Collaborative Partnerships,* March 2004, available at www.ada.org/prof/advocacy/issues/medicaid_introduction .pdf (accessed September 20, 2005).

10.   See www.acf.hhs.gov/programs/cb/publications/afcars/report8.htm (accessed September 20, 2005); children in foster care tend to be moved from home to home, often suffering new emotional trauma from the multiple placements. Of great concern are the high death rates (one in a thousand) among children in foster care.

11.   Nearly 9 percent of students were threatened or injured with a weapon at school in 2001; see U.S. Department of Health and Human Services, *Healthy Children 2000*, p. 41.

12.   Needleman H and Landrigan P, *Raising Children Toxic-Free* (New York: Farrar, Straus, and Giroux, 1994); Stein J and others, In Harm's Way: Toxic Threats to Child Development, *Journal of Developmental Behavior Pediatrics* 1 supp. (2002):13–22.

13.   The National Mental Health Association reports that 40 percent of the homeless are children; see www.nmha.org/homeless/childrenhomelessnessfacts.cfm (accessed September 20, 2005).

14.   The 2004 poverty threshold for a family of four was $19,307 in annual income; see www.census.gov/hhes/www/poverty/threshld/thresh04.html (accessed September 20, 2005); rates of poverty are reported as Indicator ECON1.A in *America's Children: Key Indicators of Well-Being, 2003 Forum* (Government Printing Office, 2003), p. 16. A comprehensive analysis of the impact of poverty on child health, educational, and behavioral outcomes is in Duncan and Brooks-Gunn, *The Consequences of Growing Up Poor*.

15.   See http://nces.ed.gov/nationsreportcard/reading/results2002/districtachieve.asp (accessed September 20, 2005); also see Centers for Disease Control, *CDC Fact Book 2000/2001: Profile of the Nation's Health*, p. 25. The overall high school dropout rate was 12 percent in 1998, but the rate for Hispanic youth was close to 30 percent.

16.   Carnegie Corporation, *Starting Points: Meeting the Needs of Our Youngest Children* (New York: Carnegie Corporation, 1994), available at http://childrensdefense.org/earlychildhood/childcare/child_care_basics_2005.pdf (accessed September 20, 2005). Also see National Institute of Child Health and Human Development, *Study of Early Child Care and Youth Development: A National Day Care Study*, available at http://secc.rti.org/ (accessed September 20, 2005).

17.   Selman R, *The Promotion of Social Awareness* (New York: Russell Sage, 2003).

18.   Benson P, *A Fragile Foundation: The State of Developmental Assets among American Youth* (Minneapolis: Search Institute, 1998).

19.   Neighborhood Health Plan and New England SERVE, *Shared Responsibilities Project: Summary of Neighborhood Health Plan's Family Survey Results* (Boston: New England SERVE, 2000).

20.   See www.familyvoices.org (accessed October 22, 2005).

21.   See http://projecthealth.org (accessed September 20, 2005).

22.   For instance the Harvard Medical School established a Division of Service Learning in the early 2000s.

23.   Weitzman CC and others, Care to Underserved Children: Residents Attitudes and Experiences, *Pediatrics* 106 (2000):1022–27.

24.   In the early 1990s the resident section of the AAP began a grassroots initiative to increase community and advocacy activity. Their efforts resulted in commitment of funds for small CATCH grants for residents as well other activities at the AAP.

25.   Rothman D, Medical Professionalism: Focusing on the Real Issues, *New England Journal of Medicine* 342 (2000):1284–86.

26.   Graduates of the Dyson advocacy program have continued in advocacy and community-based medicine, serving on local and state boards and commissions, addressing health care access concerns, and directing programs for high-risk youth.

27.   Maternal and Child Health Bureau advocacy programs aim to widen the access to health care and specialized programming to all citizens by breaking down barriers of race, language, culture, ethnicity, and disability.

28.   The AAP's advocacy efforts strive for full insurance coverage for children and access

to health care within a medical home model; see www.aap.org (accessed September 20, 2005). Also see chapter 4 for further discussion.

29. Genel M, Public Policy Activities of the American Pediatric Society (1974–1988), in Pearson H, ed., *The Centennial History of the American Pediatric Society, 1888–1988* (New Haven, Conn.: American Pediatric Society, 1988).

30. Rothman D, speech, Professions in Medicine, Soros Foundation, New York, 2003.

Chapter Two. A History of Child Health Advocacy

1. Viner R, Abraham Jacobi and the Origin of Scientific Pediatrics, in Stern AM and Markel H, eds., *American in Formative Years: Children's Health in the United States, 1880–2000* (Ann Arbor: University of Michigan Press, 2004).

2. Ibid., pp. 34–35. Also see Viner R, Abraham Jacobi and German Medical Radicalism in Antebellum New York, *Bulletin of the History of Medicine* 72 (1998):434–63. Jacobi lost six newborn children. Viner writes, "Medicine for children became for Jacobi the foremost part of a Virchovian social medicine that combined reform of the provision of care to the individual poor with socialist political activism designed to remove the conditions that produced disease" (pp. 456–57).

3. Faber HK, Job Lewis Smith, Forgotten Pioneer, *Journal of Pediatrics* 63 (1963):794–802.

4. Faber reports that Austin Flint was the inventor of the binaural stethoscope and the bedside teaching method.

5. This description, reported in Faber, is originally from Smith JL, The Etiology of Tetanus Neonatorum, *Archives of Pediatrics* 11 (1894):876.

6. Viner, Abraham Jacobi and the Origin of Scientific Pediatrics, p. 36, comments that "these simple nine rules are the first known public health initiatives specifically targeted at the preservation of infant lives in America."

7. Pearson HA, *The Centennial History of the American Pediatric Society, 1888–1988* (New Haven, Conn.: Yale University Press, 1988).

8. Ibid.

9. Addams J, *Twenty Years at Hull House* (New York: Penguin, 1998); Richmond JB, The Hull House Era: Vintage Years for Children, *American Journal of Orthopsychiatry* 65 (1995):10–20.

10. Addams, *Twenty Years at Hull House*, p. 113.

11. Alice Hamilton (1869–1970) at www.distinguishedwomen.com/biographies/hamilton-a.html (accessed September 20, 2005). Also see *Morbidity and Mortality Weekly Report*, June 11, 1999, available at www.cdc.gov/mmwr/preview/mmwrhtml/MM4822bx.HTM (accessed September 20, 2005).

12. Addams, *Twenty Years at Hull House*, p. 196.

13. Richmond describes the predicament Alice Hamilton ran into when she was accused of cruelty to animals because of her laboratory investigations into the effects of cocaine. See Richmond, The Hull House Era, p. 13.

14. Hamilton A, Industrial Diseases: With Special Reference to the Trades in which Women are Employed, *Charities and the Commons* 20 (1908):655–58.

15. See www.lead.org.au/bblp/sld016.htm (accessed September 20, 2005). Gingival lead lines are considered a marker of lead of more than seventy micrograms per deciliter and an indication of a medical emergency.

16. Addams, *Twenty Years at Hull House.*

17. See www.distinguishedwomen.com/biographies/hamilton-a.html (accessed September 20, 2005).

18. The correspondence between Franklin and Baker can be found in Kovarik W and Hermes ME, *Fuels and Society*, available at http://chemcases.com/tel/tel-16.htm (accessed September 20, 2005).

19. Centers for Disease Control, *CDC Fact Book 2000/2001: Profile of the Nation's Health.*

The proportion of children with blood lead levels of more than ten micrograms per deciliter in 1976–80 was 88.2 percent, as opposed to 4.4 percent in 1991–94.

20.   For a photograph of Taussig examining a baby's heart (showing only her hands and the baby holding the stethoscope), see Baldwin J, *To Heal the Heart of a Child, Helen Taussig, M.D.* (New York: Walker and Company, 1992), p. 41.

21.   Ibid. See also www.nlm.nih.gov/changingthefaceofmedicine/physicians/biography _316.html and www.whonamedit.com/doctor.cfm/2034.html (both accessed September 20, 2005).

22.   The Johns Hopkins School of Medicine was built on a tradition that women had something to offer, and women were responsible for the lion's share of the $500,000 original endowment. Mary Elizabeth Garrett, heir to the B&O fortune, gave $354,764, and another $100,000 was raised by local women. The Garrett sisters' story is chronicled in Nancy McCall, Hopkins History: Mary Elizabeth Garrett, Founding Benefactor of the School of Medicine Special to the *Johns Hopkins Gazette*. The *Gazette* is available at www.jhu.edu/~gazette/2001/feb1201/12garret.html (accessed September 20, 2005).

23.   Taussig H, *Congenital Malformations of the Heart*, 2 vols. (New York: Commonwealth Fund, 1947; rev. ed., 1960–61).

24.   Blalock A and Taussig HB, The Surgical Treatment of Malformations of the Heart, *Journal of the American Medical Association* 128 (1945):189–202.

25.   Public Broadcasting System, *Partners of the Heart: The American Experience*, available at www.pbs.org/wgbh/amex/partners/ (accessed September 20, 2005).

26.   Blalock's surgical note for the first blue baby operation can be read at www .whonamedit.com/synd.cfm/2290.html (accessed September 20, 2005).

27.   Markowitz M and Gordis L, *Rheumatic Fever* (Philadelphia: W.B. Saunders, 1972); Markowitz M, Rheumatic Fever: A Half-Century Perspective, *Pediatrics* 102 supp. (1998):272–74.

28.   Parrott RH and Jenkins M, Howland Award Presentation to Roland B. Scott, *Pediatric Research* 30 (1991):626. Also, Pochedly C, Dr. Roland B. Scott: Crusader for Sickle Cell Disease and Children, *American Journal of Pediatric Hematology/Oncology* 7 (1985):265–69.

29.   National Medical Association, Dr. Roland B. Scott, Distinguished Service Medalist for 1966, *Journal of the National Medical Association* 58 (1966):468–69.

30.   Parrott and Jenkins Howland Award Presentation to Roland B. Scott.

31.   Savitt TL and Goldberg MF, Herrick's 1910 Case Report of Sickle Cell Anemia: The Rest of the Story, *Journal of the American Medical Association* 261 (1989):266–71; Fixler J and Styles L, Sickle Cell Disease, *Pediatric Clinics of North America* 49 (2002):1193–210.

32.   Scott RB and others, Studies in Sickle Cell Anemia. II: Clinical Manifestations of Sickle-Cell Anemia in Children (an analysis of thirty-seven cases with observation on the use of ACTH and cortisone in two additional cases), *Journal of Pediatrics* 39 (1951):460–71; Banks LO, Scott RB, and Simmons J, Studies in Sickle Cell Anemia: Inheritance Factor, Including Effect of Interaction of Genes for Sicklemia and Thalassemia, *American Journal of Disabled Children* 84 (1952):601–8.

33.   Parrott and Jenkins, Howland Award Presentation to Roland B. Scott.

34.   The Sickle Cell Act of 1971 established centers in Augusta, Boston, Cincinnati, Chicago, Indianapolis, Los Angeles, Memphis, New York, Pittsburgh, and Washington, D.C.

35.   Watson JD, *The Double Helix* (New York: Touchstone, 1968). Also see http:// yourgenesyourhealth.org/sickle/whatisit.htm (accessed September 20, 2005).

36.   Bernstein A, Roland Scott Dies, Sickle Cell Researcher, *Washington Post*, December 12, 2002, p. B6.

37.   Ibid.

38.   Strong Memorial Hospital, Medical Pioneer Honored Near and Far for Advancing

Pediatric Care, *Strong Health,* October 20, 2004, available at www.stronghealth.com/news/article.cfm?art_ID=673 (accessed September 20, 2005).

39. Meyer RJ and Haggerty RJ, Streptococcal Infections in Families: Factors Affecting Individual Susceptibility, *Pediatrics* 29 (1962):539–49.

40. Haggerty RJ, Roghmann KJ, and Pless IB, *Child Health and the Community* (New York: John Wiley and Sons, 1975).

41. Alpert JJ and Charney E, *The Education of Physicians for Primary Care* (Government Printing Office, 1974).

42. Alpert JJ and others, Delivery of Health Care for Children: Report of an Experiment, *Pediatrics* 57 (1976):917–30.

43. J. J. Alpert, personal communication with author.

44. Weitzman CC and others, More Evidence for Reach Out and Read: A Home-Based Study, *Pediatrics* 113 (2004):1248–53; Minkovitz CS and others, A Practice-Based Intervention to Enhance Quality of Care in the First 3 Years of Life: The Healthy Steps for Young Children Program, *Journal of the American Medical Association* 290 (2003):3136–38, available at www.projecthealth.org and www.familyadvocacyprogram.org (accessed September 20, 2005).

45. Richmond JB, Stipek DJ, and Zigler E, A Decade of Head Start, in Zigler E and Valentine J, eds., *Project Head Start: A Legacy of the War on Poverty* (New York: Free Press, 1979); Office of the Surgeon General, Julius B. Richmond (1977–1981), at www.surgeongeneral.gov/library/history/biorichmond.htm (accessed July 30, 2004).

46. Lipton EL, Steinschneider A, and Richmond JB, The Autonomic Nervous System in Early Life, *New England Journal of Medicine* 273 (1965):147–53.

47. Stossel S, *Sarge, The Life and Times of Sargent Shriver* (Washington, D.C.: Smithsonian Books, 2004).

48. Lyndon Johnson's War on Poverty and Great Society speeches are available at www.npr.org/templates/story/story.php?storyId=1589660 (accessed January 15, 2005).

49. Richmond JB and Palfrey JS, Keeping Head Start strong and successful, letter to the editor, *Boston Globe,* July 12, 3003.

50. J. B. Richmond, personal communication with author. Richmond and David Satcher are the only two individuals who have held both positions.

51. Health Services and Centers Act of 1978 (P.L. 95-626), available at www.nachc.com/about/aboutcenters.asp (accessed September 20, 2005). The Bureau of Health Professions reports that these centers (more than 3,000) provide care for more than 15 million people. Also see Dailard C, *Guttmacher Report on Public Policy,* October 2001, available at www.agi-usa.org/pubs/ib_6-01.html (accessed September 20, 2005).

52. See Richmond J, *Healthy People: The Surgeon General's Report on Health Promotion and Disease Prevention* (Government Printing Office, 1979); to monitor the impact of the Healthy People 2000, see www.cdc.gov/nchs/about/otheract/hp2000/childhlt/chdcharts.htm (accessed September 20, 2005).

53. Koop CE and Kessler D, *Final Report of the Advisory Committee on Tobacco and Public Health,* available at http://ash.org/report2.html (accessed September 20, 2005).

54. Watson K, Dr. Margaret Heagarty: Advocate for Harlem's Children, *P&S Journal* 18 (1998), archives of the Columbia *P&S Journal* (at www.cumc.columbia.edu [accessed September 20, 2005]).

55. For information on the Injury Free Coalition for Children, see www.injuryfree.org/ (accessed September 20, 2005).

56. Laraque D and others, The Central Harlem Playground Injury Prevention Project: A Model for Change, *American Journal of Public Health* 84 (1994):1691–92; Laraque D and others, Injury Prevention in an Urban Setting: Challenges and Successes, *Bulletin of the New York Academy of Medicine* 72 (1995):16–30.

57. See www.injuryfree.org/ (accessed September 20, 2005).

58. C. Sia, personal communication with author; Altonn H, The Godfather and the

Grandfather, *Honolulu Star-Bulletin,* available at http://starbulletin.com/96/10/30/news/story2.html (accessed September 20, 2005).

59.   The Medical Home, *Pediatrics* 110 (2002):184–86.

60.   The Future of Pediatric Education II: Organizing Pediatric Education to Meet the Needs of Infants, Children, Adolescents, and Young Adults in the 21st Century: A Collaborative Project of the Pediatric Community, *Pediatrics* 105 supp. (2000):163–70.

61.   For biographical details about Phillip Porter, see Robert Wood Johnson Foundation, *Healthy Children Program,* Special Report 2 (1989).

62.   Porter PJ and others, Municipal Child Health Services: A Ten-Year Reorganization, *Pediatrics* 58 (1976):704–12.

63.   AAP Committee on Community Health Services, The Pediatrician's Role in Community Pediatrics, *Pediatrics* 103 supp. (1999):1304–6; Hutchins VL, Grason H, and Aliza B, CATCH in the Historical Context of Community Pediatrics, *Pediatrics* 103 supp. (1999):1373–83; Alpert JJ, History of Community Pediatrics, *Pediatrics* 103 supp. (1999):1420–21; Minkovitz C and others, Evaluation of the Community Access to Child Health Program, *Pediatrics* 103 supp. (1999):1384–93.

64.   Tonniges T, Reflection from the Department of Community Pediatrics, *Pediatrics* 103 supp. (1999):1430–31; Tom Tonniges, personal communication with author.

65.   Erenberg A and others, Newborn and Infant Hearing Loss: Detection and Intervention, *Pediatrics* 103 supp. (1999):527–30.

66.   See www.aap.org/commpeds/ (accessed September 20, 2005).

67.   Anne Dyson, personal communication with author.

68.   Smith J, *Giving Back: The Dyson Foundation;* see www.chronogram.com/issue/2002/12/communitynotebook/notebook_2.html; also see http://webpage.pace.edu/mweigold/dyson.html (both accessed September 20, 2005).

69.   The Hole in the Wall Gang Camp provides camperships for children with HIV and with cancer. The first camp, outside New Haven, Connecticut, served as the model for camps throughout the world; see www.holeinthewallgang.org/ (accessed September 20, 2005).

70.   The Anne E. Dyson Community Pediatrics Training Initiative has funded residency programs to experiment with training that emphasizes community pediatrics and advocacy. For reports on the program, see www.aap.org/commpeds/cpti.cptihistory.htm (accessed April 9, 2006).

71.   Dyson AE, speech at the Inaugural Symposium, Anne E. Dyson Community Pediatrics Training Initiative, New York City, 2000.

Chapter Three. The Current Status of Child Health

1.   Characteristics of Children under 18 Years, by Age, Race, and Hispanic or Latino Origin; Characteristics of Children under 18 Years, by Age, Regions, States, and Puerto Rico, tables in *Census 2000,* series PHC-T-30. See also Centers for Disease Control, *CDC Fact Book 2000/2001: Profile of the Nation's Health,* p. 5.

2.   U.S. Bureau of the Census, *Census 1975,* series A 29-42, Annual Estimates of the Population by Age, 1900 to 1970; Historical Statistics of the United States, Colonial Times to 1970. The total population of the United States in 1960, at the height of the baby boom, was 180,671,000, with 64,528,000 children and youth under the age of 18.

3.   *Child Trends,* Estimated Life Expectancy of Newborns by Year of Birth, Race, and Gender, Selected Years 1970–2001, available at www.childtrendsdatabank.org/figures/78-Figure-2.gif (accessed September 20, 2005). For life expectancy figures for 1900, see National Center for Health Statistics, *Health, United States, 2004,* available at www.cdc.gov/nchs/data/hus/hus04trend.pdf#027 (accessed September 20, 2005).

4.   Annie E. Casey Foundation, *The Right Start,* available at www.aecf.org (accessed September 20, 2005). Also see Meyer J, *Brief* (U.S. Census Bureau, October 2001).

5.   Four percent of American children are foreign-born; see www.childstats.gov/ americaschildren/pop4.asp (accessed September 20, 2005).

6.   Child Poverty, table in *America's Key Indicators of Child Well-Being, 2005*, available at www.childstats.gov/americaschildren/eco1.asp (accessed September 30, 2005).

7.   The poverty threshold is based on money income and family size and composition. It is calculated each year and adjusted using the consumer price index. In 2004 the poverty threshold for a family of four was $19,307.

8.   Information on high and very high incomes is also based on a family of four; see *America's Key Indicators of Child Well-Being 2005*, available at www.childstats.gov/ americaschildren/xls/econ1b.xls (accessed September 20, 2005).

9.   Percent of Total Population Living in Metropolitan Areas and in Their Central Cities and Suburbs: 1910 to 2000, table in Hobbs F and Stoops N, *Demographic Trends in the 20th Century* (Government Printing Office, 2002).

10.   Hobbs and Stoops, *Demographic Trends in the 20th Century*, figures 1-15 and 1-17, compare population density in central cities of 2,716 people per square mile in 2000 to 7,517 in 1950. The percent of the total population living in central cities has remained relatively steady since 1930 (30.8), while the percent of the population living in suburbs had increased to 50.0 percent from 23.3 percent in 1950; 80.3 percent of the population lives in central cities and their suburbs. Urban sprawl has implications for health services delivery.

11.   Small cities like Brockton and Fall River, Massachusetts, experience high rates of problems as poor families move away from Boston, Worcester, and Springfield. Homicide, domestic violence, and child abuse and neglect are disproportionately represented. See Massachusetts data on child abuse and neglect at www.mass.gov/ Eeohhs2/docs/dss/annual_report_cy2004.pdf (accessed September 15, 2005).

12.   Meyer, *Brief.*

13.   Family Structure and Child Living Arrangements, figure in *America's Key Indicators of Child Well-Being, 2005*, available at www.childstats.gov/americaschildren/pop6.asp (accessed September 28, 2005).

14.   The divorce rate is difficult to pin down. *Statistical Abstract of the United States, 2003*, sec. 2, table 83, cites 2001 rates of four divorces per 1,000 population; see www.census .gov/prod/2004pubs/03statab/vitstat.pdf (accessed September 20, 2005), which suggests a divorce rate of 40–50 percent. But Wallerstein J, The Consequences of Divorce, in Cosby A and others, eds., *About Children: An Authoritative Resourced on the Status of Children Today* (Elk Grove Village, Ill.: American Academy of Pediatrics, 2005), reports that the divorce rate is about 45 percent for first marriages and 60 percent for second marriages.

15.   Living Arrangements of Children under 18 Years Old Living with One or Both Parents, table 69 in *Statistical Abstract of the United States, 2000*.

16.   According to Hobbs and Stoops, *Demographic Trends in the 20th Century*, table 15, the number of families with a male householder with children and no spouse present was 2,190,989 in 2000, up a huge amount from 256,347 in 1950. Children Living in the Home of Their Grandparents, table 71 in *Statistical Abstract of the United States, 2000*, reports that in 1998, 1,417,000 children under the age of 18 lived in the home of their grandparents without a parent or parents present, an increase from the 1980 number of 988,000 children. Additionally, in 1998 about 2.5 million children lived in their grandparents' home with a parent or parents present; of these, 1,827,000 lived with their grandparents and mother only.

17.   Twenty percent of children under the age of 18 have no siblings; see www.census.gov/ population/socdemo/hh-fam/cps2002/tabC4-all.xls (accessed September 20, 2005).

18.   Average Household Size, 1900 and 1930 to 2000, figure 5-3 in Hobbs and Stoops, *Demographic Trends in the 20th Century*. Small households are now the norm, with an average household size of 2.59 persons in 2000, compared with 4.6 persons in 1900.

In 2000, 11.4 percent of households had 5 or more people; see figure 5-1, Households by Size: 1900 and 1940 to 2000.

19.   Administration for Children and Families, available at www.acf.hhs.gov/programs/cb/dis/afcars/publications/afcars_trends.pdf (accessed September 20, 2005).

20.   The institutionalized population includes children and youth in correctional institutions, nursing homes, hospitals and hospices for chronically ill, mental hospitals and wards, and juvenile institutions. Data are from the Census 2000 Summary File (SF 1) 100-Percent Data.

21.   See www.csun.edu/~vceed002/health/docs/tv&health.html (accessed September 20, 2005). The average American child, by the time she finishes elementary school, watches 1,680 minutes of television a week and every year sees 20,000 thirty-second TV commercials and 8,000 murders.

22.   Annie E. Casey Foundation, *Kids Count 2003*, p. 58 (Washington, D.C.: Center for the Study of Social Policy, 2003).

23.   Ibid.

24.   Robert Bateman says in his introduction to Peterson RT and Marie V, *Peterson's Birds of Eastern and Central North America*, 5th ed. (Boston: Houghton Mifflin, 2002), "For most of human history, our species has lived close to nature and therefore has been familiar with the names of their neighbors of other species. Even today, the few remaining tribes of hunter gatherers can name thousands of kinds of plants and animals and what they do through the seasons. In our modern society, it has been said that the average person knows only 10 wild plants but can recognize 1,000 corporate logos," p. xiii.

25.   National Center for Educational Statistics, *The Nation's Report Card,* at nces.ed.gov/nationsreportcard/pubs/dst2003/2004459.asp (accessed September 21, 2005). (In major cities in 2003, the percent of children scoring below basic at 4th-grade reading were as follows: Houston 52%, New York City 47%, Atlanta 63%, Chicago 60%, Los Angeles 65%, and Washington, D.C., 69%.)

26.   See www.childstats.gov/americaschildren/edu5.asp (accessed September 20, 2005); Centers for Disease Control, *CDC Fact Book 2000/2001,* p. 25.

27.   Infant mortality rate consists of two components, neonatal mortality and postneonatal mortality. Neonatal mortality refers to infant deaths occurring in the first 28 days of life; these constitute two-thirds of the deaths and generally are related to complications around birth, prematurity, and low birth weight. Complex congenital anomalies can also contribute to neonatal mortality. Postneonatal mortality refers to infant deaths occurring between 28 days old to 1 year old. Causes include congenital anomalies, SIDS, and accidents.

28.   The infant mortality rate for the turn of the century is for Massachusetts; see *Historical Statistics of the United States: Colonial Times to 1970* (Bureau of the Census, 1975), pt. 1, series B 148, p. 57, Infant Mortality Rate for Massachusetts 1851 to 1970. The infant mortality figure for 2002 is 7 per 1,000. See Kochanek KD and Martin JA, Supplemental Analysis of Recent Trends in Infant Mortality, in National Center for Health Statistics, *Monitoring the Nation's Health,* available at www.cdc.gov/nchs/products/pubs/pubd/hestats/infantmort/infantmort.htm (accessed September 20, 2005).

29.   Markel H, For the Welfare of Children, in Stern AM and Markel H, eds., *Formative Years: Children's Health in the United States, 1880–2000* (Ann Arbor: University of Michigan Press, 2002).

30.   The international comparison figures for infant mortality rates are from Maternal and Child Health Bureau, Comparison of National Infant Mortality Rates, 2000, in *Child Health USA 2002* (U.S. Department of Health and Human Services, 2002), p. 24, available at www.mchb.hrsa.gov/mchirc/chusa_04/_pdf/c04.pdf (accessed September 21, 2005).

31.   Racial and Ethnic Disparities in Infant Mortality Rates, 60 Largest Cities, 1995–1998, *Morbidity and Mortality Weekly Report,* April 19, 2002, p. 342. International compara-

tive data are available at www.marchofdimes.com/professionals/871_14450.asp (accessed September 21, 2005). Total health expenditure as a percent of gross domestic product is 6.9 for Barbados, 9.3 for Costa Rica, and 14.6 for the United States. Per capita health expenditures are Barbados, $1,018; Costa Rica, $743; and United States, $5,274. Data from World Health Organization for each country are available at three websites: www.who.int/countries/brb/en/; www.who.int/countries/cri/en/; www.who .int/country/usa/en/ (all accessed September 1, 2005).

32. Maternal and Child Health Bureau, Low Birth Weight and Very Low Birth Weight, in *Child Health USA 2002*, pp. 20–21, available at www.mchb.hrsa.gov/mchirc/chusa _04/_pdf/c04.pdf (accessed September 21, 2005).

33. Deaths and Percentage of Total Deaths for the 10 Leading Causes of Infant Death: United States, 2000–2001, table G in *National Vital Statistics Reports*, November 7, 2003, p. 11. For a detailed discussion of the reasons for persistently high rates of low birth weight and premature deaths in the United States, see Office of Technology Assessment, *Infant Mortality*, available at www.wws.princeton.edu/cgi.bin/byteserve .prl/~ota/disk1/1994/9418/ (accessed September 21, 2005).

34. Deal LW and others, Unintentional Injuries in Childhood: Analysis and Recommendations, *Future of Children* 10 (2000): 4–22.

35. HIV first appeared on the top ten list in 1987, its prevalence increasing until by 1996 it was the sixth leading cause of death for children 1–4 years; by 1998 it was off the chart. The two websites are www.cdc.gov/nchs/data/mvsr/supp/mv37; www.cdc.gov/ nchs/data/nvsr/nvsr48/nvs48_11.pdf.

36. AIDS Clinical Trials Group 076 shows that the drug AZT reduces maternal infant transmission. See Connor and others, Reduction of Maternal Infant Transmission of Human Immunodeficiency Virus Type 1 with Zidovudine Treatment, *New England Journal of Medicine* 133 (1994):1173–79.

37. Maternal and Child Health Bureau, Childhood Deaths Due to External Cause, by Cause and Age, 2000, table in *Child Health USA 2002*, p. 33, available at www.mchb .hrsa.gov/mchirc/chusa_04/_pdf/c04.pdf (accessed September 21, 2005).

38. SEER national cancer surveillance system available at http://seer.cancer.gov (accessed September 21, 2005).

39. The five-year survival rates for childhood acute leukemia are available at www .leukemia-lymphoma.org/ (accessed September 21, 2005).

40. For this statistic and the following statistics, see Maternal and Child Health Bureau, Adolescent Mortality, in *Child Health USA 2004*, available at www.mchb.hrsa .gov/mchirc/chusa_04 (accessed March 31, 2006). See also Annie E. Casey Foundation, *Kids Count 2003*, p. 44; Deaths and Percentage of Total Deaths for the 10 Leading Causes of Death, Selected Age Groups, by Age and Sex, United States, 2000–2001, table 1 in *National Vital Statistics Reports*, November 7, 2003.

41. Decline in Adolescent Death Rate, figure 4 in Annie E. Casey Foundation, *Kids Count 2003*, pp. 43–44. Note the comment: "The declining number of teen deaths is even more impressive in light of the fact that the number of 15–19-year-olds increased from 17.8 million in 1990 to 20.2 million in 2000."

42. Williams, AF, The Compelling Case for Graduated Licensing, *Journal of Safety Research* 34 (2003):3–4; Adger H Jr, Macdonald DI, and Wenger S, Core Competencies for Involvement of Health Care Providers in the Care of Children and Adolescents in Families Affected by Substance Abuse, *Pediatrics* 103 (1999):1083; Adger H and others, Helping Children in Families Hurt by Substance Abuse, *Contemporary Pediatrics*, December 2004; Palinkas LA, Prussing E, Landsverk J, and Reznik V, Youth Violence Prevention in the Aftermath of the San Diego East County School Shootings: A Qualitative Assessment of Community Explanatory Models, *Ambulatory Pediatrics* 5 (2003):246–52.

43. Information on illness is much more difficult to obtain than mortality data. There are major definitional problems around morbidity data. Moreover, states and localities

often do not have systems for collecting morbidity data; collection varies in terms of validity and reliability. Perhaps the most challenging problem is the lack of comparability among levels of severity, and there is no national system for this kind of information gathering. Nonetheless, we do know a good deal about childhood morbidity, and the availability of databases has greatly improved over the past two decades.

44.   Schwartz B and others, Respiratory Infection in Day Care, *Pediatrics* 6 (1994):1018–20.

45.   Visits to Hospital Emergency Departments by Diagnosis, 1998, table in *Statistical Abstract of the United States, 2000*, p. 126.

46.   See American Academy of Pediatrics, Committee on Infectious Diseases, Recommendations for the Prevention of Pneumococcal Infection, Including the Use of the Pneumococcal Conjugate Vaccine (Prevnar), Pneumococcal Polysaccharide Vaccine, and Antibiotic Prophylaxis, *Pediatrics* 106 (2000):362–66; Lin PL and others, Incidence of Invasive Pneumococcal Disease in Children 3 to 36 Months of Age at a Tertiary Care Pediatric Center 2 Years after Licensure of the Pneumococcal Conjugate Vaccine, *Pediatrics* 111 (2003):896–99.

47.   Baskin MN, O'Rourke EJ, and Fleisher G, Outpatient Treatment of Febrile Infants 28 to 89 Days of Age with Intramuscularly Administration of Ceftriaxone, *Journal of Pediatrics* 120 (1992):22–27.

48.   Wise PH, Clinical Innovation, Social Change, and the Dichotomization of Pediatrics, paper prepared for the conference The Future of Pediatrics, the Josiah Macy Foundation, June 2003. Wise reports on the changes from 1962 to 2000 in hospitalization rates for children younger than 17 years using data from the National Hospital Discharge Survey.

49.   Institute of Medicine, The Prospects for Immunizing against Respiratory Syncytial Virus, *New Vaccine Development: Establishing Priorities* (Washington D.C.: National Academy Press, 1986); Shay DK and others, Bronchiolitis-Associated Mortality and Estimates of Respiratory Syncytial Virus–Associated Deaths among US Children, 1979–1997, *Journal of Infectious Diseases* 183 (2001):16–22; National Center for Infectious Diseases, *Fact Sheet on Rotavirus*, available at www.cdc.gov/ncidod/dvrd/revb/gastro/rotavirus.htm (accessed September 21, 2005).

50.   Polack FP and Karron R, The Future of Respiratory Syncytial Virus Vaccine Development, *Pediatric Infectious Disease Journal* 23 supp. (2004):65–73; Kneyber MC and Kimpen JL, Advances in Respiratory Syncytial Virus Vaccine Development, *Current Opinion in Investigational Drugs* 5 (2004):163–70; De Quadros CA and Santos JI, Rotavirus: The Search for the Next-Generation Vaccine, *Pediatric Infectious Disease Journal* 23 supp. (2004):147–48.

51.   Gray JW, MRSA: The Problem Reaches Paediatrics, *Archives of Disease in Childhood* 89 (2004):297–98.

52.   Dietrich DW, Auld DB, and Mermel LA, Community-Acquired Methicillin-Resistant Staphylococcus Aureus in Southern New England Children, *Pediatrics* 113 (2004):347–52; Naimi TS and others, Comparison of Community-and-Health-Care-Associated Methicillin-Resistant Staphylococcus Aureus Infection, *Journal of the American Medical Association* 290 (2003):2976–84.

53.   Whitney CG and others, Increasing Prevalence of Multidrug-Resistant Streptococcus Pneumoniae in the United States, *New England Journal of Medicine* 343 (2000):1917–24.

54.   Dowell SF and others, Principles of Judicious Use of Microbial Agents for Pediatric Upper-Respiratory Tract Infections, *Pediatrics* 101 (1998):163–65.

55.   Finkelstein JA and others, Reduction in Antibiotic Use among US Children, 1996–2000, *Pediatrics* 112 (2003):620–27.

56.   Kemper K, *The Holistic Pediatrician: A Parent's Comprehensive Guide to Safe and Effective Therapies for the 25 Most Common Childhood Ailments* (New York: Harper Perennial, 1996); Kemper, KJ, Complementary and Alternative Medicine for Children: Does It Work? *Western Journal of Medicine* 174 (2001):272–76.

57. For more discussion on Hepatitis B and MMR vaccines, see chapter 6.

58. Blaschke GS and Lynch J, Terrorism: Its Impact on Pediatrics, *Pediatric Annals* 2003, three-part series, February, March, and April.

59. Ferguson LE, Parks DK, and Yetman RJ, Health Care Issues for Families Traveling Internationally with Children, *Journal of Pediatric Health Care* 16 (2002):51–59.

60. McPherson M and others, A New Definition of Children with Special Healthcare Needs, *Pediatrics* 102 (1998):137–40.

61. The CSHCN screener asked the following five questions:

    1. Does your child currently need or use medicine prescribed by a doctor (other than vitamins)?

    2. Does your child need or use more medical care, mental health, or educational services than is usual for most children?

    3. Is your child limited or prevented in any way in his or her ability to do most of the things that children of the same age can do?

    4. Does your child get special therapy, such as physical, occupational, or speech therapy?

    5. Does your child have any kind of emotional, developmental, or behavioral problem for which he or she needs or gets treatment or counseling?

    See Blumberg SJ, Comparing States Using Survey Data on Health Care Services for Children with Special Health Care Needs (CSHCN), available at www.cdc.gov/nchs/data/slaits/Comparing_States_CSHCNA.pdf (accessed September 21, 2005); also see www.cdc.gov/nchs/slaits.htm; Bethell CD and others, Identifying Children with Special Health Care Needs: Development and Evaluation of a Short Screening Instrument, *Ambulatory Pediatrics* 2 (2002):38–47.

62. The following review articles document some of the major therapeutic advances of the late twentieth century: Puntis JW, Home Parental Nutrition, *Archives of Disease in Childhood* 72 (1995):186–90; Rowe MI and Rowe SA, The Last Fifty Years of Neonatal Surgical Management, *American Journal of Surgery* 180 (2000):345–52; Karl TR, Cochrane AD, and Brizard CP, Advances in Pediatric Cardiac Surgery, *Current Opinion in Pediatrics* 11 (1999):419–24; Chan KW, Acute Lymphoblastic Leukemia, *Current Problems in Pediatric Adolescent Health Care* 32 (2002):40–49; Laufer M and Scott GB, Medical Management of HIV Disease in Children, *Pediatric Clinics of North America* 479 (2000):127–53; Beris AE, Soucacos PN, and Malikoz KN, Microsurgery in Children, *Clinical Orthopedics* 314 (1995):112–21; Liou TG and others, Predictive 5-Year Survivorship Model of Cystic Fibrosis, *American Journal of Epidemiology* 345 (2001):345–51.

63. Palfrey JS and others, Technology's Children: Report of a Statewide Census of Children Dependent on Medical Supports, *Pediatrics* 87 (1991):611–18.

64. Williams TV and others, A National Assessment of Children with Special Health Care Needs: Prevalence of Special Needs and Use of Health Care Services among Children in the Military Health System, *Pediatrics* 114 (2004):384–93; Mayer ML, Skinner AC, and Slifkin RT, Unmet Need for Routine and Specialty Care: Data from the National Survey of Children with Special Health Care Needs, *Pediatrics* 113 (2004):109–15; Szilagyi PG and others, Children with Special Health Care Needs Enrolled in the State Children's Health Insurance Program (SCHIP): Patient Characteristics and Health Care Needs, *Pediatrics* 112 (2003):508; Canty-Mitchell J and others, Behavioral and Mental Health Problems in Low-Income Children with Special Health Care Needs, *Archives of Psychiatric Nursing* 18 (2004):79–87.

65. Children's Health Care Needs Are Different: Why One Size Won't Fit All, briefing paper (Alexandria, Va.: NACHRI, 1993); Vertrees JC and Pollatsek JS, *Paying for Pediatric Inpatient Care*, Final Report of the Universal Access for Children Reimbursement Study Project conducted for NACHRI (Alexandria, Va.: Solon Consulting Group, 1993).

66. Kohn LT, Corrigan JM, and Donaldson MS, eds., To Err Is Human: Building a Safer Health Care System (Washington, D.C.: National Academy Press, 2000).

67.   Porter S and others, *Children and Youth Assisted by Medical Technology in Educational Settings: Guidelines for Care,* 2d ed. (Baltimore: Brookes, 1997).

68.   Reisman J and others, Diabetes Mellitus in Patients with Cystic Fibrosis: Effect on Survival, *Pediatrics* 86 (1990):374–77.

69.   Harman D. Alzheimer's Disease: Role of Aging in Pathogenesis, *Annals of the New York Academy of Science* 959 (2002):384–95; Pearlson GD and others, MRI Brain Changes in Subjects with Down Syndrome with and without Dementia, *Developmental Medicine and Child Neurology* 40 (1998):326–34.

70.   See for instance Gissen AS, CoQ10 Helps the Immune System and Brain Function, available at www.immunesupport.com/95sum096.htm (accessed September 21, 2005).

71.   Smith M, McCaffrey R, and Karf J, The Secondary Leukemias: Challenges and Research Directions, *Journal of the National Cancer Institute* 88 (1996):407–18.

72.   Wertlieb D, Converging Trends in Family Research and Pediatrics: Recent Findings for the AAP Task Force on the Family, *Pediatrics* 111 (2003):1572–87; Sullivan-Bolyai S and others, Great Expectations: A Position Description for Parents as Caregivers, pts. 1 and 2, *Pediatric Nursing* 29 (2003):457–61, and *Pediatric Nursing* 30 (2004):52–56.

73.   Williams PD, Siblings and Pediatric Chronic Illness: A Review of the Literature, *International Journal of Nursing Students* 34 (1997):312–23.

74.   Shilts, R, *And the Band Played On: Politics, People, and the AIDS Epidemic* (New York: St. Martin's, 2000).

75.   Karon JM and others, HIV in the United States at the Turn of the Century: An Epidemic in Transition, available at www.cdc.gov/hiv/pubs/ovid/epidemic-in-transition.pdf.

76.   Robbins KE and others, U.S. Human Immunodeficiency Virus Type 1 Epidemic: Date of Origin, Population History, and Characteristics of Early Strains, *Journal of Virology* 77 (2003):6359–66.

77.   Connor EM and others, Reduction of Maternal Infant Transmission of Human Immunodeficiency Virus Type 1with Zidovudine Treatment, *New England Journal of Medicine* 331 (1994):1173–79.

78.   Meyers A, Natural History of Congenital HIV Infection, *Journal of School Health* 64 (1994):9–10.

79.   HIV/AIDS among US Women: Minority and Young Women at Continuing Risk, available at www.cdc.gov/hiv/pubs/facts/women.pdf (accessed September 21, 2005).

80.   Centers for Disease Control, *CDC Fact Book 2000/2001,* p. 19.

81.   Malveaux FJ and Fletcher-Vincent SA, Environmental Risk Factors of Childhood Asthma in Urban Centers, *Environment Health Perspectives* 103 (1995):59–62.

82.   Asthma Mortality and Hospitalizations among Children and Young Adults, United States, 1980–1993, *Morbidity and Mortality Weekly Report,* May 3, 1996, pp. 350–53.

83.   The New England Asthma Regional Council reports asthma costs for direct health care at $12.7 billion a year for adults and children; see www.asthmaregionalcouncil.org/about/aboutarc.html (accessed September 21, 2005).

84.   Kuczmarski RJ and others, 2000 CDC Growth Charts for the United States: Methods and Development, *Vital Health Statistics* 246 (2002):1–190. The growth charts are available at www.cdc.gov/nchs/about/major/nhanes/growthcharts/charts.htm (accessed September 21, 2005).

85.   See www.cdc.gov/nccd hp/dnpa/obesity/trend/maps/index.htm (accessed September 21, 2005).

86.   Overweight in children is defined as at or above the 95th percentile for body mass index (BMI) for age. BMI is the child's weight in kilograms divided by the square of the child's height in meters for age. See Ogden CL and others, Prevalence and Trends in Overweight among U.S. Children and Adolescents, 1999–2000, table 4, Trends in Overweight for Children Birth through 19 Years, by Sex and Age Group, *Journal of the American Medical Association* 288 (2002):1731.

87. Datar A, Sturm R, and Magnabosco JL, Childhood Overweight and Academic Performance: National Study of Kindergartners and First-Graders, *Obesity Research* 12 (2004):58–68.

88. Rosenberg TJ and others, Prepregnancy Weight and Adverse Perinatal Outcomes in an Ethnically Diverse Population, *Obstetrics and Gynecology* 102 (2003):1022–27.

89. Aye T and Levitsky LL, Type 2 Diabetes: An Epidemic Disease in Childhood, *Current Opinions in Pediatrics* 15 (2003):411–15; American Diabetes Association, Type 2 Diabetes in Children and Adolescents, *Diabetes Care* 23 (2000):381–89; McConnaughey J, Lifestyle Puts 1 in 3 Kids at Diabetes Risk, speech at the American Diabetes Association annual meeting, New Orleans, June 14, 2003, available at www.drwoolard.com/peinnews/warning_4_children.htm (accessed September 21, 2005).

90. U.S. Department of Education, *Special Education Report for School Year 1999–2000*, table AA12, Number of Children Served under IDEA by Disability and Age Group during School Years 1990–1991 through 1999–2000, available at www.ed.gov/about/reports/annual/osep/2001/appendix-a-pt1.pdf (accessed September 21, 2005).

91. Autistic spectrum disorder consists of qualitative impairment in social interaction and communication; restricted, repetitive, and stereotyped patterns of behavior, interests, and activities; and (with onset before the age of 3) delays or abnormal functioning in social interaction, language used in social communication, or symbolic or imaginative play. For the full definition, see American Psychiatric Association, *Diagnostic and Statistical Manual of Mental Disorders (DSM-IV)*, 4th ed. (Washington, D.C.: APA, 1997).

92. Yeargin-Allsopp M and others, Prevalence of Autism in a US Metropolitan Area, *Journal of the American Medical Association JAMA* 289 (2003):49–55; Bryson SE and Smith IM, Epidemiology of Autism: Prevalence, Associated Characteristics, and Service Delivery, *Mental Retardation and Developmental Disabilities Research Review* 4 (1998):97–103.

93. DeStefano F and Thompson WW, MMR Vaccine and Autism: An Update on the Scientific Evidence, *Expert Review of Vaccines* 3 (2004):19–22. Also see Murch SH and others, Retraction of an Interpretation, *Lancet* 363 (2004):750.

94. Fombonne E, The Prevalence of Autism, *Journal of the American Medical Association* 289 (2003):87–88; Barbaresi WJ and others, The Incidence of Autism in Olmsted County, Minnesota, 1976–1997: Results from a Population-Based Study, *Archives of Pediatrics and Adolescent Medicine* 159 (2005):37–44.

95. AAP, Clinical Practice Guideline: Diagnosis and Evaluation of the Child with Attention-Deficit/Hyperactivity Disorder, *Pediatrics* 105 (2000):1158–70. The NIMH website (www.nimh.nih.gov; accessed September 21, 2005) quotes a 4 per 100 (or 40 per 1,000) figure, referencing Shaffer D and others, The NIMH Diagnostic Interview Schedule for Children Version 2.3 (DISC-2.3): Description, Acceptability, Prevalence Rates, and Performance in the MECA Study: Methods for the Epidemiology of Child and Adolescent Mental Disorders Study, *Journal of the American Academy of Child and Adolescent Psychiatry* 35 (1996): 865–77; Wolraich ML and others, Examination of DSM-IV Criteria for Attention Deficit/Hyperactivity Disorder in a Countywide Sample, *Journal of Developmental and Behavioral Pediatrics* 19 (1998):162–68; the 7 percent figure is from www.ahrq.gov/clinic/epcsums/adhdsutr.htm (accessed September 21, 2005).

96. The Surgeon General's office has reported that approximately 20 percent of children and adolescents have mental disorders with some functional impairment and 5–9 percent are considered to have severe emotional disorder (SED). See www.surgeon general.gov/library/mentalhealth/pdfs/c3.pdf (accessed September 21, 2005).

97. Mrazek PJ and Haggerty RJ, *Reducing Risks for Mental Disorders: Report of the Committee on the Prevention of Mental Disorders of the IOM* (Washington, D.C.: National Academy Press, 1994).

98. Martin A and Leslie D, Trends in Psychotropic Medication Costs for Children and Adolescents, 1997–2000, *Archives of Pediatrics and Adolescent Medicine* 157

(2003):997–1004; Zito JM and others, Psychotropic Practice Patterns for Youth: A 10-Year Perspective, *Archives of Pediatrics and Adolescent Medicine* 157 (2003):17–25, found a 6-percentage-point prevalence in 1996 in youth under 20. Calculating from this, Steven Hyman, the former director of NIMH, estimates that by young adulthood one quarter of people may have been on a psychotropic medication (personal communication with author). See also Vitiello B and Jensen PS, Medication Development and Testing in Children and Adolescents: Current Problems, Future Directions, *Archives of General Psychiatry* 54 (1997):871–76.

99. CDC, *Healthy Youth 2003*, reports on the biannual Youth Risk and Behavior Survey (the YRBSS): http//apps.nccd.cdc.gov/yrbss/index.asp (accessed September 21, 2005).

100. Action on Smoking and Health, Smoking and Cancer, Factsheet 4, available at www .ash.org.uk/html/factsheets/html/fact04.html (accessed September 21, 2005).

101. National Institute on Drug Abuse, Monitoring the Future Survey,2000, available at www.nida.nih.gov/Newsroom/02/NR12-16.html (accessed September 21, 2005).

102. The NHSDA Report: School Experiences and Substance Use among Youths, available at www.oas.samhsa.gov/nhsda.htm (accessed September 21, 2005). Also see www .drugabusestatistics.samhsa.gov/2k3/school/school.cfm (accessed September 20, 2005).

103. John Knight, David Holder, and Lon Sherritt at Children's Hospital in Boston are working on a study of spirituality and substance abuse. Early results suggests correlations of responsible behavior with a strong understanding of the concept of forgiveness. Personal communication with author.

104. See CDC, *Healthy Youth 2003*, available at http//apps.nccd.cdc.gov/yrbss/index.asp (accessed September 21, 2005).

105. Maternal and Child Health Bureau, Adolescent Birth Rates by the Race of the Mother, *Child Health USA 2002*, p. 35.

106. Maternal and Child Health Bureau, Prenatal Care, *Child Health USA 2002*, p. 60.

107. The information on teen pregnancy, international comparisons, and the declines in abortions are found at the website of the Alan Gutmacher Institute, www.agi-usa. org/pubs/fb_teen_sex.html#20a (accessed September 21, 2005).

108. Maternal and Child Health Bureau, Sexually Transmitted Diseases, *Child Health USA 2002*, p. 37.

109. Maternal and Child Health Bureau, Adolescent HIV Infection, *Child Health USA 2002*, p. 38. Also see Hader SL and others, HIV Infection in Women in the United States: Status at the Millennium, *Journal of the American Medical Association* 285 (2001):1186–92.

110. Evers IM, deValk HW, and Visser GHA, Risk of Complications of Pregnancy in Women with Type I Diabetes: Nationwide Prospective Study in the Netherlands, *British Medical Journal* 328 (2004):915, available at http://bmj.bmjjournals.com/cgi/ content/full/328/7445/915 (accessed April 3, 2006).

111. Evers IM and others, Pregnancy in Women with Diabetes Mellitus Type I: Maternal and Perinatal Complications in Spite of Good Glucose Control, *Ned Tijdschr Geneedskd* 144 (2000):804–9. Also see Gunton JE and others, Outcome of Pregnancies Complicated by Pregestational Diabetes, *Australia–New Zealand Journal of Obstetrics and Gynaecology* 40 (2000):38–43.

112. Levy HL, Historical Background for the Maternal PKU Syndrome, *Pediatrics* 112 (2003):1516–18.

113. With the increasing survivorship of young women with congenital anomalies and chronic illness conditions, obstetricians are facing new questions. They are delivering babies from mothers on medications that were not used ten or twenty years ago and with physical conditions that put the mothers on the margin. The risks of childbirth have rarely been faced, for instance, by young women with corrected congenital heart defects.

114. Smedley BD, Stith AY, and Nelson AR, *Unequal Treatment: Confronting Racial and Ethnic Disparities in Health Care* (Washington, D.C.: National Academy Press, 2003).

115.   Aligne CA and others, Risk Factors for Pediatric Asthma: Contributions of Poverty, Race, and Urban Environment, *American Journal of Respiratory and Critical Care Medicine* 162 (2000):873–77. See also Goodman E, The Role of Socioeconomic Status Gradients in Explaining Differences in US Adolescents' Health, *American Journal of Public Health* 89 (1999):1522–28.

116.   Leung R, Asthma and Migration, *Respirology* 1 (1996):123–26.

117.   Malveaux and Fletcher-Vincent, Environmental Risk Factors of Childhood Asthma in Urban Centers.

118.   Deal LW and others, Unintentional Injuries in Childhood: Analysis and Recommendations, *Future of the Child* 10 (2000):4–22. See also National Public Service Research Institute and National SAFE KIDS Campaign, Childhood Injury: Cost and Prevention Facts, available at www.usa.safekids.org/content_documents/Trends_facts.pdf (accessed September 21, 2005).

119.   The CDC offers an interactive website where families can determine whether their area is at high risk for lead by entering their city name and zip code at www2.cdc .gov/nceh/lead/census90/house11/house11.htm (accessed September 21, 2005).

120.   Brenner RA and others, Where Children Drown, United States, 1995, *Pediatrics* 108 (2001):85–89. The region of the United States with the most drownings is the South. The group at greatest risk for drowning are black males (perhaps because many have not had the opportunity to learn how to swim).

121.   National Committee for Childhood Agricultural Injury Prevention, *Children and Agriculture: Opportunities for Safety and Health* (Marshfield, Wis.: Marshfield Clinic, 1996).

122.   See www.odl.state.ok.us/kids/factbook/ruralkidscount2004/ (accessed September 21, 2005).

123.   Burgdorfer W, Lyme Borreliosis: Ten Years after the Discovery of the Etiologic Agent, Borreloa Burgdorferi, *Infection* 19 (1991):257–62.

124.   The spread of the AIDS epidemic in the United States was from the coasts inward. Internationally, much of the spread is along truck routes. See for instance Gibney L, Saquib N, and Metzger J, Behavioral Risk Factors for STD/HIV Transmission in Bangladesh's Trucking Industry, *Social Science Medicine* 56 (2003):1411–24.

125.   Enserink M, Breakthrough of the Year: SARS, a Pandemic Prevented, *Science* 302 (2003):2045.

126.   Geng E and others, Changes in the Transmission of Tuberculosis in New York City from 1990 to 1999, *New England Journal of Medicine* 346 (2002):1453–58. See also Bloom B, Tuberculosis: The Global View, *New England Journal of Medicine* 346 (2002):1434–35.

127.   Whitney CG and others, Increasing Prevalence of Multidrug-Resistant Streptococcus Pneumoniae in the United States, *New England Journal of Medicine* 343 (2000):1961–63.

128.   Geographic information software (GIS) allows investigators to map geographic areas based on demographic information such as the infant mortality or teen pregnancy rate or the number of cases of cancer or lead poisoning. It also allows the mapping of resources such as the number of health clinics, schools, faith-based centers, and so on.

129.   Nicholas SW and others, Reducing Childhood Asthma through Community-Based Service Delivery, New York City, 2001–2004, *Morbidity and Mortality Weekly Report*, January 14, 2005, pp. 11–14.

130.   The problem of teen substance abuse rose to such high rates in South Boston that a community alliance was formed (under the auspices of the Gavin Foundation) to address the problem. See also the response of Representative Stephen Lynch at www .house.gov/lynch/Newsroom/2004_12/pr_041220_substancetreatment.htm (accessed September 21, 2005).

131.   Perrin JM and others, Variations in Rates of Hospitalization of Children in Three Urban Communities, *New England Journal of Medicine* 320 (1989):1183–87.

132.   Forum, *America's Children: Key National Indicators of Well-Being;* information on

food security is available at www.childstats.gov/americaschildren/eco4.asp (accessed September 21 and October 2, 2005).

133. Nelson DW, The High Cost of Being Poor, in *Kids Count Data Book, 2003* (Baltimore: Annie E. Casey Foundation, 2003), p. 20.

134. Nothnagle M and others, Risk Factors for Late or No Prenatal Care Following Medicaid Expansions in California, *Maternal and Child Health Journal* 4 (2000):251–59.

135. Pollack H and others, Substance Use among Welfare Recipients: Trends and Policy Responses, available at www.jcpr.org/wp/WPprofile.cfm?ID=316 (accessed September 21, 2005). Women poor enough to be on welfare reported being on drugs twice as often as women not eligible for welfare. See also http://endabuse.org/resources/facts/Welfare.pdf (accessed September 21, 2005) for information on the two-way street of domestic violence. Women in poverty are at greater risk of domestic violence, and women who have been victimized either sacrifice financial support for safety or fall into poverty if they leave.

136. Brooks-Gunn J and Duncan G, The Effects of Poverty on Children, *Child Trends* 7 (1997):55–71.

137. See Centers for Disease Control, *Vital and Health Statistics*, July 2003, table 6: 42.4 percent of the poor report excellent health, 29.2 percent very good health; 48.5 percent of the near-poor report excellent health, 29.4 percent very good health; 63.4 percent of the not-poor report excellent health, 26.1 percent very good health.

138. Forum, *America's Children: Key National Indicators of Well-Being*, table HEALTH2, available at www.childstats.gov/americaschildren/hea.asp (accessed October 29, 2005).

139. Rodewald J and others, Immunization Coverage Levels among 19- to 35-Month-Old Children in 4 Medically Underserved Areas of the United States, *Pediatrics* 113 (2003):296–302; Centers for Disease Control, *CDC Fact Book 2000/2001*, p. 14.

140. Starfield B and Newacheck P, Children's Health Status, Health Risks, and Use of Health Services, in Schlesinger MJ and Eisenberg L, eds., *Children in a Changing Health System* (Baltimore: Johns Hopkins University Press, 1990); Shi L and others, Income Inequality, Primary Care, and Health Indicators, *Journal of Family Practice* 48 (1999):275–84.

141. National Health Interview Survey, *Vital and Health Statistics*, July 2003, tables 15, 16, 18.

142. Maternal and Child Health Bureau, Health Insurance Coverage 2000, *Child Health USA 2002*, table 1. In 2000 among children under 18 years of age, 70.6 percent had private insurance, 23.3 percent had public coverage, and 11.6 percent had no insurance coverage. The percentages add up to more than a 100 because of children with double coverage. See www.census.gov/prod/2003pubs/p60-223.pdf (accessed September 20, 2005).

143. Rosenbaum S, Racial and Ethnic Disparities in Health Care: Issues in the Design, Structure, and Administration of Federal Health Care Financing Programs Supported through Direct Public Financing, in Institute of Medicine, *Unequal Treatment* (Washington, D.C.: National Academy Press, 2003).

144. Sipe WE and others, Barriers to Access: A Transportation Survey in an Urban Pediatric Practice, poster at the annual meeting of the Pediatric Academic Society, San Francisco, 2004.

145. Chang R and Halfon N, Geographic Distribution of Pediatricians in the United States: An Analysis of the Fifty States and Washington, D.C., *Pediatrics* 100 (1997):172–79.

146. The National Health and Examination Survey shows that 71.6 percent of children at or above poverty have had otitis media, as contrasted with 61.5 percent for children below poverty. However, 69.0 percent of children with a regular source of care have otitis media, versus 53.7 percent of those without such care, so the story may well be one of underrecognition and underdiagnosing among the poorer children rather than the likelihood of more cases among the wealthier children. See Auinger P and others, Trends in Otitis Media, *Pediatrics* 112 (2003):514–20.

147. National Cancer Institute, *Acute Lymphoblastic Leukemia,* SEER Pediatric Monograph, table 1.5. A number of studies show higher rates in high socioeconomic groups; the hypothesis is that this may be related to the higher age of exposure to infectious agents. See McWhirter W, The Relationship of the Incidence of Childhood Lympho-blastic Leukemia to Social Class, *British Journal of Cancer* 46 (1982):640–45.

148. Wise PH and others, Racial and Socioeconomic Disparities in Childhood Mortality in Boston, *New England Journal of Medicine* 313 (1985):360–66. Most injuries oc-cur at greater frequency among poor children. Automobile occupant injuries are the one exception—these are more likely to occur among wealthier individuals, probably because of greater access to personal automobiles. This finding is also documented in Marcin JP and others, A Population-Based Analysis of Socioeconomic Status and Insurance Status and Their Relationship with Pediatric Trauma Hospitalization and Mortality Rates, *American Journal of Public Health 93* (2003):461–66.

149. Patel DR and Luckstead EF, Sport Participation, Risk Taking, and High-Risk Behav-iors, *Adolescent Medicine* 11 (2000):141–55.

150. Kitzrow MA, The Mental Health Needs of Today's College Students: Challenges and Recommendations, *NASPA Journal* 41 (2000):1–15; Levine A and Cureton S, *When Hope and Fear Collide: A Portrait of Today's College Student* (San Francisco: Jossey Bass, 1998).

151. Warheit GJ and others, Prevalence of Bulimic Behaviors and Bulimia among a Sample of the General Population, *American Journal of Epidemiology* 137 (1993):569–76.

152. National Sudden Infant Syndrome/Infant Death Resource Center, *SIDS Deaths by Race and Ethnicity, 1995–2001* (Health Resources and Services Administration, 2004). The Back to Sleep Campaign has been successful in reducing the rate of SIDS for all races from 87.2 per 100,000 live births in 1995 to 55.5 per 100,000 live births in 2001 (a 36% improvement). Blacks have paralleled improvements for whites, but disparity remains: the black rate in 2001 was 113.5 per 100,000, while the white rate was 45.6 per 100,000.

153. Infant Mortality and Low Birth Weight among Black and White Infants, United States, 1980–2000, *Morbidity and Mortality Weekly Report,* July 12, 2002, pp. 589–92.

154. The protection in the Hispanic group has been attributed to better nutrition and less smoking. Also, women of child-bearing age who migrate may possibly be healthier to begin with, that is, may exhibit the "healthy migrant effect." See discussion on the American Public Health Association website, www.apha.org/ppp/red/LatinAmeric .htm (accessed August 1, 2004).

155. Molina C, Zambrabe RE, and Aquirre-Molina M, The Influence of Culture, Class, and Environment on Health Care, in Molina C and Aquirre-Molina M, eds., *Latino Health in the US: A Growing Challenge* (Washington, D.C.: American Public Health Associa-tion, 1994); Hayes-Batista DE, The Latino Health Research Agenda for the Twenty-First Century, in Suárez-Orozco M and Páez M, eds., *Latinos: Remaking America* (Berkeley: University of California Press, 2002).

156. The Pew Hispanic Center, *Hispanic Health: Divergent and Changing* (University of Southern California, 2002). Most Hispanic families have infant mortality rates as low as or lower than non-Hispanic whites. However, differences can be discerned among Hispanic subgroups. For instance, the Puerto Rican infant mortality rate in 1998 was 8.0 per 1,000, compared with 5.5 per 1,000 for Cuban babies.

157. Maternal and Child Health Bureau, Adolescent Birth Rates, by Age and Race of the Mother, 2001, *Child Health USA 2002,* p. 35. Low pregnancy rates among Asians (20.5 per 1,000) may hold hints for teen pregnancy prevention.

158. Nearly 1 million teenagers become pregnant each year. Those who are unsupported are at high risk for dropping out of school, falling into abuse situations, and ending up in a downward psychosocial spiral. See Alan Guttmacher Institute website, www .agi-usa.org (accessed April 13, 2005).

159. Maternal and Child Health Bureau, Breast-Feeding for the Year 2000, *Child Health USA 2002,* p. 18.

160. Some controversy about the relationship between breast-feeding and later obesity remains. However, studies like Grummer-Strawn LM and Mei Z, Does Breast-Feeding Protect against Pediatric Overweight? Analysis of Longitudinal Data from the CDC and Prevention Pediatric Nutrition Surveillance System, *Pediatrics* 113 (2004):81–86, offer suggestive evidence that prolonged breast-feeding may be protective among certain groups of children. Their study shows a clear relationship among non-Hispanic whites but not among Hispanics or blacks.

161. Aye T and Levitsky LL, Type 2 Diabetes: An Epidemic Disease in Childhood, *Current Opinions in Pediatrics* 15 (2003):411–15; American Diabetes Association, Type 2 Diabetes in Children and Adolescents, *Diabetes Care* 23 (2000):381–89; McConnaughey J, Lifestyle Puts 1 in 3 Kids at Diabetes Risk, speech at the American Diabetes Association annual meeting, New Orleans, June 14, 2003, available at www.drwoolard.com/peinnews/warning_4_children.htm (accessed September 21, 2005).

162. Galtier-Dereure F, Boegner C, and Bringer F, Obesity and Pregnancy: Complications and Cost, *American Journal of Clinical Nutrition* 71 (2000):1242–48; Colman-Brochu S, Deep Vein Thrombosis in Pregnancy, *American Journal of Maternal Child Nursing* 29 (2004):186–92; Kral JG, Preventing and Treating Obesity in Girls and Young Women to Curb the Epidemic, *Obesity Research* 12 (2004):1539–46.

163. Centers for Disease Control, Division of HIV/AIDS Prevention, Young People at Risk: HIV/AIDS among American Youth, available at www.cdc.gov/hiv/pubs/facts/youth.htm (accessed September 21, 2005).

164. HIV/AIDS affects African Americans and African American women in increasing proportions. African American women were diagnosed with AIDS at twenty-five times the rate of white women in 2003. Although African American and Hispanic women together represent less than one-fourth of all U.S. women, they account for 85 percent of AIDS diagnoses reported in 2003. See www.cdc.gov/hiv/pubs/facts/women.htm (accessed September 21, 2005).

165. From July 2000 through June 2001, 128 pediatric AIDS cases were reported for black non-Hispanic children, compared with 28 such cases for white non-Hispanic children. See Centers for Disease Control, *HIV/AIDS Surveillance Report 2001* 13 (2001):22, table 15, available at www.cdc.gov/hiv/stats/hasr1301/table15.htm (accessed September 21, 2005). See also *Pediatric AIDS Facts* at www.cdc.gov/hiv/pubs/facts/perinatl.htm (accessed September 15, 2005).

166. Data on firearm injuries and racial disparities are available at www.childstats.gov/americaschildren/hea8.asp (accessed September 21, 2005). See also www.childtrendsdatabank.org/PDF/Violence.pdf (accessed September 21, 2005).

167. Child Trends Data Bank, Estimated Life Expectancy of Newborns by Year of Birth, Race, and Gender, Selected Years 1970–2001, available at www.childtrendsdatabank.org/figures/78-Figure-2.gif (accessed September 21, 2005).

168. Kawasaki disease rates for children under the age of 5 are 120–50 per 100,000 in Japan, 4–15 per 100,000 among U.S. Caucasians, and 3–8 per 100,000 among Europeans. Falcini F, Calabri GB, and Vierucci SA, Kawasaki Disease in the Third Millenium: A Syndrome Still at Risk to Be Unrecognized or Underdiagnosed, available at www.pedrheumonlinejournal.org/April/PDF/kawasaki.pdf (accessed July 12, 2004).

169. Asthma Mortality and Hospitalization among Children and Young Adults, United States, 1980–1993, *Morbidity and Mortality Weekly Report,* May 3, 1996, pp. 350–53. Among children aged 5–14 years, the asthma death rate nearly doubled from 1980 to 1993 (from 1.7 to 3.2 per million population). In 1993, among children 5–14 years, blacks were 4.0 times more likely than whites to die from asthma, and boys were 1.3 times more likely than girls.

170. White children are more likely to be diagnosed with acute lymphoblastic leukemia, but black children have lower five-year survival rates (64% vs. 78%). See figure I.8, ALL 5-Year Survival Rates by Sex, Race, Age, and Time Period, SEER (9 areas), 1975–84 and 1985–94, in National Cancer Institute, SEER Pediatric Monograph, *Acute Lymphoblastic Leukemia,* p. 27.

171.   Racial Disparities in Median Age at Death of Persons with Down Syndrome, United States, 1968–1997, *Morbidity and Mortality Weekly Report*, June 8, 2001, pp. 463–65.

172.   Institute of Medicine, *Unequal Treatment* (Washington, D.C.: National Academy Press, 2003). Also see www.cdc.gov/nchs/data/hus/hus04trend.pdf#hi (accessed September 21, 2005), which reports that in 2002 blacks were twice as likely as whites to use the hospital emergency room.

173.   Centers for Disease Control, *CDC Fact Book 2000/2001*, p. 23.

174.   Boudreaux ED and others, Multicenter Airway Research Collaboration Investigators Race: Ethnicity and Asthma among Children Presenting to the Emergency Department: Differences in Disease Severity and Management, *Pediatrics* 111 (2003):615–21; Finkelstein JA and others, Quality of Care for Preschool Children with Asthma: The Role of Social Factors and Practice Setting, *Pediatrics* 95 (1995):389–94.

175.   Fadima A, *The Spirit Catches You and You Fall Down* (New York: Farrar, Strauss, and Giroux, 1997).

176.   Vivarelli C, L.E.A.R.N. the 4 T's: Helpful Hints for Culturally Effective Health Care Practice, program presented at Children's Hospital of Philadelphia, Spring 2003.

177.   Gonzalez P and Stoll B, The Color of Medicine: Strategies for Increasing the Diversity of the US Physician Workforce, *Community Catalyst* (Boston, 2002), available at www.communitycatalyst.org (accessed September 21, 2005); Hayes-Bautista DE and others, Latino Physician Supply: Sources, Locations, and Projections, *Academic Medicine* 75 (2000):727–36; Stoddard JJ, Back MR, and Brotherton SE, The Respective Racial and Ethnic Diversity of US Pediatricians and American Children, *Pediatrics* 105 (2000):27–31.

Chapter Four. Clinical Advocacy

1.   Marmot MG and Wilkinson RG, eds., *Social Determinants of Health* (New York: Oxford University Press, 1999); Spencer N, Social, Economic, and Political Determinants of Child Health, *Pediatrics* 112 (2003):704–6; Brooks-Gunn J and Greg Duncan G, The Effects of Poverty on Children, *The Future of Children* 7 (1997):55–71. See also Palfrey JS, *Community Child Health: An Action Plan for Today* (Hartford, Conn.: Praeger, 1994).

2.   World Health Organization, *Alma Ata Declaration on Primary Care* (Geneva, 1978), available at www.who.int/hpr/NPH/docs/declaration_almaata.pdf (accessed November 14, 2004). The Alma Ata Convention introduced the "4A" methodology.

3.   See www.dol.gov/esa/regs/statutes/ofccp/ada.htm (accessed May 5, 2005).

4.   Bartels P and others, *Your New Baby/Su Nuevo Bebe* (Boston: Children's Hospital, 1993).

5.   See www.mcedservices.com/feeding.html (accessed January 19, 2005).

6.   American Public Health Association, Understanding the Health Culture of Recent Immigrants to the United States: A Cross-Cultural Maternal Health Information Catalog, available at www.apha.org/ppp/red/summary.htm. Also see Management Science for Health, available at http://erc.msh.org/mainpage.cfm?file=5.3.0f.htm&module=provider&language=English. A comprehensive bibliography on cultural sensitivity is offered at www.sunyit.edu/library/html/culturedmed/bib/puerto/. All three websites accessed January 19, 2005.

7.   Foster GM, *Hippocrates' Latin American Legacy: Humoral Medicine in the New World* (Langhorne, Pa.: Gordon and Breach, 1994), available at http://sunsite.berkeley.edu/Anthro/foster/pub/reviews/fo25.html (accessed October 4, 2005).

8.   See Maternal and Child Health Policy Research Center, www.mchpolicy.org/publications/medicaid.html (accessed May 8, 2005).

9.   Palfrey JS and others, Patterns of Family Response to Raising a Child with Chronic Disabilities: An Assessment in Five Metropolitan School Districts, *American Journal of Orthopsychiatry* 59 (1989):94–98.

10.   Silva TJ, Sofis LA, and Palfrey JS, *Practicing Comprehensive Care: A Physician's Opera-

tions Manual for Implementing a Medical Home for Children with Special Health Care Needs (Boston: Massachusetts Institute for Community Inclusion, 2000), available at www.ici.org.

11.   See www.aap.org/commpeds/cpti/cptihistory.htm (accessed April 9, 2006) for a description of the programs participating in the initiative. Also see Richmond JB, Patient Reaction to the Teaching and Research Situation, *Journal of Medical Education* 36 (1961):347–52, for a discussion of teaching residents about respect.

12.   Geographic information software can provide a picture of the clinic population. In addition, most cities issue health reports or report cards by neighborhood. Clinic directors who are made aware of a particular health problem in the neighborhood they serve can focus on that problem.

13.   Bethell CD and others, Identifying Children with Special Health Care Needs: Development and Evaluation of a Short Screening Instrument, *Ambulatory Pediatrics* 2 (2002):38–47.

14.   Strine TW and others, Vaccination Coverage of Foreign-Born Children 19 to 35 Months of Age: Findings from the National Immunization Survey, 1999–2000, *Pediatrics* 110 (2002):e15; Ackerman LK, Health Problems of Refugees, *Journal of Family Practice* 10 (1997):337–48; Au L, Tso A, and Chin K, Asian-American Adolescent Immigrants: The New York City Schools Experience, *Journal of School Health* 67 (1997):277–79.

15.   Anand V and others, Child Health Improvement through Computer Automation: The CHICA System, *Medinformation* 11 (2004):187–91.

16.   Liu GC and others, A Spatial Analysis of Obesogenic Environments for Children, *Proceedings of the American Medical Informatics Association, 2002*, pp. 459–63.

17.   Ebert RH, The Role of the Medical School in Planning the Health Care System, *Journal of Medical Education* 42 (1967):481–88; Ebert RH, The New Health Era, *Health Matrix* 4 (1986–87):3–6.

18.   Ferris TG and others, Changes in the Daily Practice of Primary Care for Children, *Archives of Pediatrics and Adolescent Medicine* 152 (1998):227–33.

19.   Kogan MD and others, Routine Assessment of Family and Community Health Risks: Parent Views and What They Receive, *Pediatrics* 113 supp. (2004):1934–43; Wissow LS, Roter D, and Wilson MEH, Pediatrician Interview Style and Mothers' Disclosure of Psychosocial Issues, *Pediatrics* 93 (1994):289–95; Roter DL and others, Communication Patterns of Primary Care Physicians, *Journal of the American Medical Association* 277 (1997):350–56.

20.   See www.nichq.org (accessed April 8, 2005).

21.   Injury-Free Coalition for Kids, www.injuryfree.org (accessed October 4, 2005).

22.   Alanon and Alateen offer comprehensive supports for the spouses and children of people affected by alcoholism.

23.   The pink triangle indicates a safe zone for the discussion of bisexual, gay, lesbian, and questioning issues. Colored triangular symbols were originally used by the Nazis to label Jews, homosexuals, and others who were being persecuted.

24.   Knight JR and others, Validity of the CRAFFT Substance Abuse Screening Test among Adolescent Clinic Patients, *Archives of Pediatrics and Adolescent Medicine* 156 (2002):607–14. Also see www.ceasar-boston.org/ (accessed March 9, 2005).

25.   Goldenring J and Cohen E, Getting into Adolescents Heads, *Community Pediatrics*, July 1988, pp. 75–80. For substance abuse screening in adolescents, the CRAFFT has proved reliable. Glascoe F and Shapiro H provide an overview of instruments for developmental screening at www.dbpeds.org/articles/detail.cfm?TextID=5 (accessed March 9, 2005). The Bright Futures Mental Health Toolbook also includes useful screening and assessment tools.

26.   Satcher D, keynote address, Anne E. Dyson Annual Symposium, Rochester, New York, 2000.

Notes to Pages 101–114 263

27. *Bright Futures in Practice: Physical Activity* (Washington, D.C.: National Center for Education in Maternal and Child Health, 2005). See for instance www.bikesnotbombs.org/youth-prog.htm (accessed April 4, 2005).

28. Tom Tonniges, Michael Shannon, and Bron Anders, personal communication with author.

29. Kaczorowski J and Shipley LJ, presentation at the Anne E. Dyson Annual Symposium Rochester, New York, 2000.

30. Kagan J and Swidman N, *The Long Shadow of Temperament* (Cambridge, Mass.: Harvard University Press, 2004).

31. Kim Wilson, personal communication with author. See also Farmer P, *Pathologies of Power* (Berkeley: University of California Press, 2003).

32. See www.projecthealth.org. Also see discussion in chapters 2 and 5.

33. The notion of one-stop shopping is also promoted in elder health care, women's care, and substance abuse care. It is the ability to bring health, public health, and other human services together under one roof.

34. See www.aap.org/commpeds/cpti/cptihistory.htm (accessed April 9 2006).

35. See www.foodlinkny.org/Initiatives.html#Kidscafe (accessed April 13, 2005).

36. Schainker E, *Grand Rounds Presentation* (Boston: Children's Hospital, 2000).

37. See www.kidsource.com/kidsource/content4/promote.phyed.html; www.ahrq.gov/ppip/activity.htm#HHS96; www.ahrq.gov (all accessed April 9, 2005).

38. Margaret Heagarty, personal communication with author.

39. Li R and others, Prevalence of Breast-Feeding in the United States: The 2001 National Immunization Survey, *Pediatrics* 111 (2000):1198–1201.

40. DeGraw C and others, New Opportunities to Serve Young Children, P.L. 99-457, *Journal of Pediatrics* 113 (1988):971–74.

41. Richmond JB, Stipek DJ, and Zigler E, A Decade of Head Start, in Zigler E and Valentine J, eds., *Project Head Start: A Legacy of the War on Poverty* (New York: Free Press, 1979).

42. Smith PJ and others, Educating Children with Disabilities: How Pediatricians Can Help, *Contemporary Pediatrics* 19 (2002):102–6.

43. See www.injuryfree.org; http://corporate.burlingtoncoatfactory.com/corpinfo/releases/safensound.shtml.

44. Benson PL, Mobilizing Communities to Promote Developmental Assets: A Promising Strategy for the Prevention of High-Risk Behaviors, *Family Science Review* 11(1988):220–38; Scales PC and Leffert N, *Developmental Assets: A Synthesis of the Scientific Research on Adolescent Development*, 2d ed. (Minneapolis: Search Institute, 2004).

45. Porter S, Freeman L, and Griffin LR, *Transition Planning for Adolescents with Special Health Care Needs and Disabilities* (Boston: Massachusetts Department of Public Health, 2000).

46. The history of Mid-City in San Diego is found in part at www.midcitycan.org/pages/history.html.

47. Olds DL and others, Long-Term Effects of Home Visitation on Maternal Life Course and Child Abuse and Neglect: Fifteen-Year Follow-Up of a Randomized Trial, *Journal of the American Medical Association* 278 (1997):637–43.

48. See www.agi-usa.org/pubs/archives/nr_340502.html (accessed July 1, 2004): "Declines in abortion rates were especially steep among adolescents, particularly 15–17-year-olds. The rate for this group fell to 15 abortions per 1,000 women in 2000 from 24 abortions per 1,000 women in 1994, a decline of 39%. Both abortion rates and birth rates for adolescents have been declining since the early 1990s, reflecting that fewer teens are becoming pregnant. However, the proportion of adolescent pregnancies ending in abortion remained stable from 1994 to 2000. An Alan Gutmacher Institute

analysis examining reasons for declining teen pregnancy rates between 1988 and 1995 found that three-quarters of the decrease was due to improved contraceptive use, while one-quarter was due to delayed sexual activity."

49. See Spiegel CN and Lindaman FC, Children Can't Fly: A Program to Prevent Childhood Morbidity and Mortality from Window Falls, *American Journal of Public Health* 67 (1977):1143–47, for an evaluation of the original New York City program. The program in Boston had similar results, which were reported by Sig Kharasch from the Boston Medical Center Emergency Department.

50. Palfrey JS and others, Educating the Next Generation of Pediatricians in Urban Health Care: The Anne E. Dyson Community Pediatrics Training Initiative, *Academy of Medicine* 79 (2004):1184–91.

51. Nicholas SW and others, Reducing Childhood Asthma through Community-Based Service Delivery, New York City, 2001–2004, *Morbidity and Mortality Weekly Report,* January 14, 2005, pp. 11–14.

52. Tonniges TF, Palfrey JS, and Mitchell M, Introduction to the Medical Home, *Pediatrics* 113 supp. (2004):1472. Also see www.medicalhomeinfo.org/about/cshcn.html (accessed October 4, 2005).

53. American Academy of Pediatrics, The Medical Home, *Pediatrics* 110 (2002):184–86.

Chapter Five. Group Advocacy

1. Vintn-Johansen P, *Cholera, Chloroform, and the Science of Medicine* (Oxford, UK: Oxford University Press, 2003).

2. Schmidt WM, *Martha May Eliot: Social Pediatrician, Children's Bureau Chief, 1981– 1978,* available at www.harvardsquarelibrary.org/unitarians/eliot_m.html (accessed September 21, 2005).

3. Dietz WH and Gortmaker SL, Do We Fatten Our Children at the Television Set? Obesity and Television Viewing in Children and Adolescents, *Pediatrics* 75 (1985):807–12.

4. Glied S and Litt SE, The Uninsured and the Benefits of Medical Progress, *Health Affairs* 22 (2003):210–19.

5. Amartya Sen quotation from lecture, The Idea of Identity, Pardee Lectureship, Boston University, November 27, 2001.

6. In the description of the Chinese boy, there are assumptions about gender interests. See Krieger N, Genders, Sexes, and Health: What Are the Connections and Why Does It Matter? *International Journal of Epidemiology* 32 (2003):652–57.

7. Community organizers argue that reaching a consensus among community groups is critical; see Alinsky S, *Rules for Radicals* (New York: Random House, 1971).

8. Bethell CD and others, Identifying Children with Special Health Care Needs: Development and Evaluation of a Short Screening Instrument, *Ambulatory Pediatrics* 2 (2002):38–47.

9. Jellinek MS and others, Use of the Pediatric Symptom Checklist to Screen for Psychosocial Problems in Pediatric Primary Care: A National Feasibility Study, *Archives of Pediatrics and Adolescent Medicine* 153 (1999):254–60.

10. See www.cdc.gov/nip/casa/c_casa.htm (accessed September 21, 2005).

11. Glascoe FP, Developmental Screening, in Parker S. and Zuckerman B., eds., *Behavioral and Developmental Pediatrics: A Handbook for Primary Care* (Boston: Little, Brown, 1995).

12. Knight JR and others, Validity of the CRAFFT Substance Abuse Screening Test among Adolescent Clinic Patients, *Archive of Pediatrics and Adolescent Medicine* 156 (2002):607–14.

13. The Family Violence Prevention Fund, *Preventing Domestic Violence: Clinical Guidelines on Routine Screening,* available at http://endabuse.org/programs/healthcare/files/screpol.pdf (accessed September 21, 2005).

14. Folkins J, The Language Used to Describe Individuals with Disabilities: Resource on

Person-First Language, available at /www.asha.org/about/publications/ journal-abstracts/submissions/person_first.htm (accessed September 29, 2005).

15. Barnett WS, Long-Term Effects of Early Childhood Programs on Cognitive and School Outcomes, *The Future of Children* 5 (1995):25–50; Schweinhart LJ, Barnes HV, and Weikart DP, *Significant Benefits: The High/Scope Perry Preschool Study through Age 27* (Ypsilanti, Mich.: High/Scope Press, 1993); Campbell FA and others, Early Childhood Education: Young Adult Outcomes from the Abecedarian Project, *Applied Developmental Science* 6 (2002):42–57; Palfrey JS and others, The 25-Year Follow-Up of the Brookline Early Education Project, *Pediatrics* 116 (2005):144–52.

16. Brazelton TB, *To Listen to a Child: Understanding the Normal Problems of Growing Up* (Boston: Addison-Wesley, 1992); Brazelton TB, *Touchpoints: Your Child's Emotional and Behavioral Development* (Cambridge, Mass.: Perseus, 2002).

17. Erikson E, Eight Stages of Man, in *Childhood and Society*, 2d ed. (New York: W.W. Norton, 1963).

18. Buka S and Earls F, Early Determinants of Delinquency and Violence, *Health Affairs* (Millwood) 12 (1993):46–64.

19. Shonkoff J and Phillips DA, eds., *From Neurons to Neighborhoods* (Washington, D.C.: National Academy Press, 2001).

20. Hubel D and Wiesel T, *Brain and Visual Perception: The Story of a 25-Year Collaboration* (Oxford, UK: Oxford University Press, 2004).

21. Hack H, Klein NK, and Taylor HG, Long-Term Developmental Outcomes of Low Birth Weight Infants, *Future of Children* 5 (1995):176–96; McCormick MC, Long-Term Follow-Up of Infants Discharged from Neonatal Intensive Care Units, *Journal of the American Medical Association* 261 (1989):1767–72; McCormick MC, The Infant Health and Development Program: Enhancing the Outcomes of Low Birth Weight and Premature Infants, *Journal of the American Medical Association* 263 (1990):3035–42.

22. Teplin SW and others, Neurodevelopmental, Health, and Growth Status at Age Six of Children with Birth Weights Less than 1,001 Grams, *Journal of Pediatrics* 118 (1991):768–77.

23. Bhushan V, Paneth N, and Kiely JL, Impact of Improved Survival of Very Low Birth Weight Infants on the Recent Secular Trends in the Prevalence of Cerebral Palsy, *Pediatrics* 91 (1993):1094–1100. Also see McCormick MC and others, The Health and Developmental Status of Very-Low-Birth-Weight Children at School Age, *Journal of the American Medical Association* 267 (1992):2204–8.

24. Hack M and others, The Effect of Very Low Birth Weight and Social Risk on Neurocognitive Abilities at School Age, *Journal of Developmental and Behavioral Pediatrics* 13 (1992):412–20; Taylor HG, Klein N, and Hack M, Academic Functioning in <750-gm Birth Weight Children and Their Peers: Evidence for Specific Learning Disabilities, *Pediatric Research* 35 (1994):289A.

25. Szatmari P and others, Psychiatric Disorders at Five Years among Children with Birth Weights <1,000 Grams: A Regional Perspective, *Developmental Medicine and Child Neurology* 32 (1990):954–62.

26. Cox J, The Young Parents Program, *Ambulatory Pediatric Association Newsletter*, May 2005, pp. 5–6; Woods ER and others, The Parenting Project for Teen Mothers: The Impact of a Nurturing Curriculum on Adolescent Parenting Skills and Life Hassles, *Ambulatory Pediatrics* 3 (2003):240–45.

27. See www.highscope.org (accessed September 21, 2005).

28. Garofalo R and others, Association between Sexual Orientation and Health Risk Behaviors among a School-Based Sample of Adolescents, *Pediatrics* 101 (1998):895–902.

29. See www.jri.org/jrhealth.htm#sidney; www.howardbrown.org; www.youth.org/loco/ personproject/alerts/states/hawaii/conference.html (all accessed April 3, 2006).

30. Leslie LK and others, Comprehensive Assessments for Children Entering Foster Care: A National Perspective, *Pediatrics* 112 (2003):134–42.

31.   Anne E. Dyson Community Pediatrics Training Initiative, Annual Report, *Caring Altogether* (Boston: 2004), p. 12.

32.   See www.sanfranciscochinatown.com/attractions/chinesehospital.html (accessed September 15, 2005) for the history of how the Chinese were segregated into one section of the city when the bubonic plague was spreading in San Francisco. Currently, the Chinese Hospital is the hub of a large managed care company, the Chinese Community Health Plan, that insures more than 8,000 members and oversees the health care of 7,000 members of Medi-Cal.

33.   The National Institute of Allergy and Infectious Diseases, HIV/AIDS Statistics, NIAID Facts and Figures, available at www.niaid.nih.gov/Factsheets/aidsstat.htm; www .advocatesforyouth.org/publications/factsheet/fshivaid.htm (both accessed September 21, 2005); AAP, Committee on Pediatric AIDS, Planning for Children Whose Parents Are Dying of HIV/AIDS, *Pediatrics* 103 (1999):509–11.

34.   Havens PL and others, Structure of a Primary Care Support System to Coordinate Comprehensive Care for Children and Families Infected/Affected by Human Immunodeficiency Virus in a Managed Care Environment, *Pediatric Infectious Disease Journal* 16 (1997):211–16.

35.   Blumberg SJ, Comparing States Using Survey Data on Health Care Services for Children with Special Health Care Needs (CSHCN), available at www.cdc.gov/nchs/data/ slaits/Comparing_States_CSHCNA.pdf (accessed February 1, 2004).

36.   Palfrey JS and others, Pediatric Alliance for Coordinated Care: Evaluation of a Medical Home Model, *Pediatrics* 113 supp. (2004):1507–16.

Chapter Six. Legislative Advocacy

1.   See www.strategiesforchildren.org/eea/EEA1_staff.htm (accessed April 3, 2006).

2.   For a comprehensive review of the issues around gun control, see entire issue of *Future of Children* 12 (2002), titled Child, Youth, and Gun Violence. See also www .helpnetwork.org (accessed September 22, 2005).

3.   Osterling J and Dawson G, Early Recognition of Children with Autism: A Study of First-Birthday Home Visit Tapes, *Journal of Autism and Developmental Disorders* 24 (1994):247–57. The authors reviewed home birthday party videotapes of eleven children with autism and compared them to similar tapes of eleven typically developing children. They identified differences in three areas: social interaction, joint attention, and autism-like symptoms.

4.   Torrey EF and Knabe MB, Scientologists, Antipsychiatrists, and "Consumer Survivors," in *Surviving Manic Depression: A Manual on Bipolar Disorder for Patients, Families, and Providers* (New York: Basic Books, 2002).

5.   Richmond JB, The Hull House Era: Vintage Years for Children, *American Journal of Orthopsychiatry* 65 (1995):10–20.

6.   See Strain J, Agenda for Change in the U.S. Child Health Care System, *Health Matrix* 4 (1994):107, in which James Strain, the former executive director of the AAP, reviews the formation of the Children's Bureau and the Shepard-Towner Act; also see Hutchins VL, MCHB: Roots, *Pediatrics* 94 (1994):695–99, which reviews the tensions in the founding and launching of the Children's Bureau. The Children's Bureau work on child labor faced enormous criticism as well. Provisions against child labor drew fire from all sides, including employers and even parents. No sooner had legislation against child labor been passed than a case made its way to the Supreme Court, where the provisions were struck down as unconstitutional. See also Markel H and Golden J, Successes and Missed Opportunities in Protecting Our Children's Health: Critical Junctures in the History of Children's Health Policy in the United States, *Pediatrics* 115 supp. (2005):1129–33.

7.   The project depended on 3,000 volunteer women, who walked door to door to register births. For a description of the campaign, see www.webguild.com/sentinel/ women_infants.htm (accessed September 21, 2005).

8.   Mankiller W and others, eds., *Readers Companion to U.S. Women's History* (Boston: Houghton Mifflin, 1998).

9.   Hutchins, MCHB: Roots. Will Rogers's quote is on p. 696.

10.   Louis Pasteur's famous statement, "Chance favors the prepared mind," is one of the favorite aphorisms of many child health advocates, including Julius Richmond. While there is no way to know whether it was one of Martha May Eliot's favorites, she certainly acted as if it were.

11.   Vince Hutchins reports on the funding for the Children's Bureau under Title V in his article MCHB: Roots. The initial funding was $1.6 million for maternal and child health, $1.2 million for services for crippled children. In 1939, at the request of the AAP, $1.0 million was added for services for children with rheumatic heart disease. These sums certainly gave the Children's Bureau more resources than the original appropriation of $26,640, which was intended to pay for fifteen positions plus that of the chief.

12.   Gittler JG, Title V of the Social Security Act and State Programs for Children with Special Health Care Needs Legislative History, in *Implementing Title V CSHCN Programs: A Reference Manual for State Programs* (U.S. Department of Health and Human Services, 1998), p. 5.

13.   See www.amchp.org/policy/stateprofiles.htm as (accessed October 22, 2005).

14.   See www.cnn.com/SPECIALS/1999/century/episodes/05/currents/ (accessed October 22, 2005).

15.   McPherson M and others, A New Definition of Children with Special Health Care Needs, *Pediatrics* 102 (1998):137–40.

16.   Blumberg SJ, Comparing States Using Survey Data on Health Care Services for Children with Special Health Care Needs, available at www.cdc.gov/nchs/data/slaits/Comparing_States_CSHCNA.pdf (accessed September 21, 2005).

17.   Beers NS, Kemeny A, Sherritt L, and Palfrey JS, Variations in State-Level Definitions: Children with Special Health Care Needs, *Public Health Report* 118 (2003): 434–47.

18.   *Olmstead v L.C. ex. Rel. Zimring (Olmstead).*

19.   See www.hhs.gov/newfreedom/ (accessed October 22, 2005).

20.   For trends over time and comparisons of expenditures for adults and disabled individuals, see www.cms.hhs.gov/charts/medicaid/InfoMedicaid_schip.pdf (accessed September 21, 2005).

21.   Fein R, *Medical Care, Medical Costs* (Cambridge, Mass.: Harvard University Press, 1986).

22.   See www.cdc.gov/nchs/hus/hus04trend.pdf#hi (accessed September 21, 2005), table 129.

23.   It probably goes without saying that only the Pilgrims were afforded health benefits. The most substantial codification of these benefits came with the GI Bill of Rights, passed in 1944 for the veterans of World War II.

24.   See Wegman ME, The American Pediatric Society, the AAP, and the Children's Bureau: 1944–1945, in Pearson HA, ed., *The Centennial History of the American Pediatric Society 1888–1988* (New Haven, Conn.: American Pediatric Society, 1988). The case that Eliot made for the importance of child health was, in part, that 50 percent of young men had been rejected for military service because of poor health; see www.ssa.gov/history/pdf/child2.pdf.url (accessed spring 2005).

25.   Lyndon Johnson's Great Society speech was give at the University of Michigan graduation ceremony in May 1964. For the full text, see www.cnn.com/SPECIALS/cold.war/episodes/13/documents/lbj/ (accessed September 22, 2005).

26.   Fein, *Medical Care, Medical Costs.*

27.   The Centers for Medicare and Medicaid Services (CMS) administer Medicare, Medicaid, and S-CHIP. For information on eligibility and benefits, see www.cms.hhs.gov/default.asp (accessed September 22, 2005). Eligibility criteria for Medicaid are

at www.cms.hhs.gov/medicaid/eligibility/criteria.asp (accessed September 22, 2005). Finding this information is time-consuming, emblematic of the hoops that Medicaid recipients must jump through. There is also the problem of "churning": as many as 50–70 percent of Medicaid enrollees are taken off the rolls at least once a year, particularly in those states that subcontract their Medicaid business to managed care organizations (Jim Hunt, president of the Massachusetts League of Neighborhood Health Centers, personal communication with author).

28. The GAO report commissioned by Senator Diane Feinstein is available at www.gao.gov/new.items/d03620.pdf (accessed September 22, 2005); it shows that the per capita income figure used for the Medicaid formula puts states with large populations in poverty at a disadvantage and favors states with small poverty populations. The provision that the federal match can be no lower than 50 percent means that some states that could afford to put more state funds into Medicaid still receive the federal financing assistance.

29. Maryland Medicaid Fact Sheet (courtesy Karen Hendricks, AAP Washington office). The fact sheet urges the state to maintain coverage for children's care and reminds legislators that every state dollar voted for Medicaid leverages matching funds from the federal government.

30. Tang SS, Olson L, and Yudkowsky BK, Uninsured Children: How We Count Matters, *Pediatrics* 112 (2003):168–73, discusses the problem of partial-year coverage. In 1999, "although 6.6 million children (8.4%) were uninsured throughout 1999, an additional 11.4 million (14.4%) were uninsured for part of the year" (p. 168). Also see a discussion of underinsurance at www.kaisernetwork.org/health_cast/uploaded_files/4060.pdf (accessed September 22, 2005).

31. Ku L and Nimalendran S, Improving Children's Health: A Chartbook about the Roles of Medicaid and SCHIP (Center on Budget and Policy Priorities, January 2004), available at www.cbpp.org/1-15-04health.pdf (accessed September 22, 2005). The authors argue that in some cases Medicaid benefits are superior to those offered by private insurance plans. The paper also reports positive health outcomes for Medicaid recipients. See also Palfrey JS and others, Health Care Reform: What's in It for Children with Chronic Illness and Disability? *Journal of School Health* 64 (1995):234–37.

32. See www.mchpolicy.org/publications/medicaid.html (accessed April 8, 2005). See also www.allhealth.org/recent/audio_09-09-05/Medicaid%20Benefits%20for%20Children%20and%20Adults.pdf (accessed September 22, 2005).

33. For a description of the benefits covered under EPSDT, see www.cms.hhs.gov/medicaid/epsdt/default.asp (accessed September 22, 2005).

34. AAP Statement to the National Governor's Association, 2005. In it, the AAP declares concerns about proposed changes in the Medicaid benefit package, cost-sharing, and continued inadequate reimbursement; urges improving the quality of monitoring, home and community-based care, chronic care management, and prescription drugs; and AAP argues that Medicaid must stand as a safety net program protected by federal Medicaid law (statement courtesy of Karen Hendricks, AAP Washington office, Summer, 2005).

35. See www.cms.hhs.gov/medicaid/epsdt/default.asp (accessed September 22, 2005).

36. The CMS website www.cms.hhs.gov/default.asp? (accessed September 22, 2005) describes SCHIP: "The Balanced Budget Act of 1997 created a new children's health insurance program under Title XXI of the Social Security Act called the State Children's Health Insurance Program (SCHIP).... The statute set broad outlines of the program's structure, and established a partnership between Federal and State governments. States were given broad flexibility in tailoring the programs to meet their own circumstances. States could create or expand their own separate insurance programs, expand Medicaid, or combine both approaches. States can choose among several benchmark benefit packages, develop a benefit package that is actuarially equivalent to or better than one of the benchmark plans, or use the Medicaid benefit. States also have the opportunity to set eligibility criteria regarding age, income, resources, residency, and duration of coverage within broad Federal guidelines."

37.   See www.cms.hhs.gov/default.asp? (accessed September 22, 2005).

38.   Alabama, Colorado, Florida, Maryland, Montana, and Utah also "capped" or "froze"
      SCHIP enrollment in the 2003–4 period; see Ku and Nimalendran, Improving Chil-
      dren's Health.

39.   The number and percentage of children without health insurance remained steady
      during 2001 and 2002: 8.5 million children, or 11.5 percent of the population under
      18 years of age; see www.census.gov/prod/2003pubs/p60-223.pdf (accessed Septem-
      ber 20, 2005).

40.   The highly publicized investigations of the conditions at Willowbrook exposed the
      poor practices of institutional care to public scrutiny.

41.   Arc parents elicited the support of scholars, including Grover Power, Seymour Sara-
      son, and Thomas Gladwin. They also provided grants and seed money to young re-
      searchers to stimulate the study of mental retardation. For a chronological review, see
      www.thearc.org/history/resprevhis.htm (accessed September 22, 2005).

42.   Ibid. Also see Crocker AC, The Causes of Mental Retardation, *Pediatric Annals* 18
      (1989):623–36; Mental Retardation, a Handbook for the Primary Physician, *Journal of
      the American Medical Association* 191 (1965):117–56. Again, Julius Richmond was at
      the frontier, chairing the committee and writing the report on the physician's role in
      the early identification of and early intervention for mental retardation.

43.   Stossell S, *Sarge: The Life and Times of Sargent Shriver* (Washington, D.C.: Smith-
      sonian Books, 2004).

44.   Palfrey JS and Rodman J, Legislation for the Education of Children with Disabilities:
      Families and Professionals Working Together, in Levine MD, Carey WB, and Crocker
      AC, eds., *Developmental-Behavioral Pediatrics*, 3d ed. (Philadelphia: W.B. Saunders,
      1999).

45.   Smith PJ and others, Educating Children with Disabilities: How Pediatricians Can
      Help, *Contemporary Pediatrics* 19 (2002):102–6.

46.   DeGraw C and others, New Opportunities to Serve Young Children, P.L. 99-457,
      Journal of Pediatrics 113 (1988):971–74.

47.   For a full description of IDEA 2004, see www.wrightslaw.com-idea-idea.2004.all.pdf
      (accessed September 22, 2005).

48.   For a discussion of the testing requirements under IDEA 2004, see www.ld.org/
      NCLB/MakingNCLBwork.pdf (accessed September 22, 2005).

49.   See www.ld.org (accessed September 22, 2005).

50.   The story of Terrence Bell's unfortunate trip to the chambers of Congress was re-
      ported in the AAP, Reprieve for P.L. 94-142, *Government Activities Report* (Evanston,
      Ill.: AAP, 1982).

Chapter Seven. Professional Advocacy

1.   The Ethics and Human Rights Committee of the American College of Physicians,
      American Society of Internal Medicine, published two articles: Coyle SL, Physi-
      cian-Industry Relations, pt. 1, Individual Physicians, *Annals Internal Medicine* 136
      (2000):396–402; Coyle SL, Physician-Industry Relations, pt. 2, Organizational Issues,
      Annals Internal Medicine 136 (2000):403–6.

2.   Smedley BD, Stith AY, and Nelson AR, *Unequal Treatment: Confronting Racial and
      Ethnic Disparities in Health Care* (Washington, D.C.: National Academy Press, 2003);
      Satcher D, Closing the Gap, September 16, 2003, available at www.healthgap.omhrc.
      gov (accessed March 6, 2004).

3.   U.S. Bureau of the Census, *Population Projections of the United States by Age, Race, and
      Hispanic Origin: 1995–2050;* Flores G, Culture and the Patient-Physician Relationship:
      Achieving Cultural Competency in Health Care, *Journal of Pediatrics* 136 (2000):14–
      23; Agency for Healthcare Research and Quality, *National Healthcare Disparities Re-
      port* (Rockville, Md.: U.S. Department of Health and Human Services, 2003); Ross

Roundtable, *Child Health in the Multicultural Environment* (Abbott Park, Ill.: Ross Products Division, 2000).

4. See Gonzalez P and Stoll B, *The Color of Medicine: Strategies for Increasing the Diversity of the US Physician Workforce* (Boston: Community Catalyst, 2002), available at www.communitycatalyst.org (accessed September 22, 2005).

5. For the cost-saving argument for prenatal care, see Huntington J and Connell FA, For Every Dollar Spent: The Cost Saving Argument for Prenatal Care, *New England Journal of Medicine* 331 (1994):1303–7; Postma MJ and others, Cost Effectiveness of Periconceptual Supplementation of Folic Acid, *Pharm World Sci* 24 (2002):8–11.

6. Thomas L, The Technology of Medicine, in *Lives of a Cell* (New York: Bantam Books, 1975).

7. The Judith M. Power Clinic in Cleveland provides a full range of services for patients on dialysis and emphasizes the care of the "complete child." See program descriptions at http://cms.clevelandclinic.org/childrenshospital/?id=74 (accessed July 13, 2005).

8. HIPAA, the Health Insurance Portability and Assurances Act of 1996, stipulates the privacy of health information. The Office of Civil Rights oversees this protection. See www.cms.hhs.gov/hipaa/hipaa1/content/cons.asp (accessed September 22, 2005).

9. Szilagy P and others, *Interventions Aimed at Improving Immunization Rates*, CD003941, Cochrane Database of Systematic Reviews 2002.

10. Office of Surgeon General, *Closing the Gap: A National Blueprint to Improve the Health of Persons with Mental Retardation*, Report of the Surgeon General's Conference on Health Disparities and Mental Retardation, available at www.surgeongeneral.gov/topics/mentalretardation/retardation.pdf (accessed September 22, 2005).

11. I am most grateful to Katie Plax for spurring an exploration of this topic.

12. Haggerty F, Beyond Curricular Reform: Confronting Medicine's Hidden Curriculum, *Academic Medicine* 73 (1998)):403–7.

13. For more on the medical model, see Palfrey JS, *Community Child Health: An Action Plan for Today* (Westport, Conn.: Praeger, 1994), pp. 48–49.

14. Mandela N, *Long Walk to Freedom: The Autobiography of Nelson Mandela* (New York: Little, Brown, 1994). Mandela describes his concept of leadership as being like that of a shepherd who steers his flock from behind, always allowing them to set the original direction but being there to gently keep them from obvious dangers.

15. Palfrey JS and others, Evaluation of the Medical Home for Children with Special Health Care Needs: How Feasible Is the Model? *Pediatrics* 113 supp. (2004):1507–16. See also Hirsch AT, The Economic Survival of Pediatric Practice, *Pediatrics* 96 (1995):825–29, discussion at 829–31; Antonelli RC and Antonelli DM, Providing a Medical Home: The Cost of Care Coordination Services in a Community-Based, General Pediatric Practice, *Pediatrics* 113 supp. (2004):1522–28; AAP Committee on Pediatric Emergency Medicine, Overcrowding Crisis in Our Nation's Emergency Departments: Is Our Safety Net Unraveling? *Pediatrics* 114 (2004):878–88.

16. Berwick DM, Disseminating Innovations in Health Care, *Journal of the American Medical Association* 289 (2003):1969–75. See also Vastag B, Interview with Donald M. Berwick, MD, MPP: Advocate for Evidence-Based Health System Reform, *Journal of the American Medical Association* 291 (2004):1945–47.

17. See www.nichq.org/ (accessed September 22, 2005) for descriptions of the quality assurance programs on immunization delivery, asthma care, care for children with special health care needs, and children with ADHD.

18. One of the most effective quality improvement tools is the P-D-S-A (plan, do, study, act cycle). Instructions and supports for using quality improvement methodology are available at the Institute for Health Care Improvement website, www.ihi.org/IHI/Topics/Improvement/ImprovementMethods/HowToImprove/ (accessed September 22, 2005).

19. Since the late 1990s the Agency for Health Care Quality has sponsored the collection and analysis of data on child health care utilization and expenditure. The findings are startling, elucidating, and helpful. Even while health care expenditures in general are

skyrocketing and the youth population is expanding, children's health care expenses have been held essentially in check. See Simpson L and others, Health Care for Children and Youth in the United States: 2000 Report on Trends in Access, Utilization, Quality, and Expenditures, *Ambulatory Pediatrics* 4 (2004): 131–53.

20. Fischman W and others, *Making Good: How Young People Cope with Moral Dilemma at Work* (Howard University Press); Howard Gardner, talk on good work, Apthorp House, October 2004.

21. Gonzalez and Stoll, *The Color of Medicine.*

22. Angela Diaz, speech, Open Society, Soros Foundation, New York, 2003.

23. The federal government now has a number of generous loan repayment programs especially for physicians from underrepresented minorities. At many universities special offices of minority affairs provide career guidance to trainees and junior faculty. Joan Reede at Harvard Medical School offers programs for junior high and high school students who aspire to a career in science and medicine and has developed a large cadre of mentors in the Medical School who offer everything from one-time advice to summer job placement.

24. The Partnership in Boston was started by a group of professionals from underrepresented minority backgrounds as a support for young people starting out in the city to give them access to a network of successful individuals they could call on throughout their careers. Each year a number of fellows are chosen from the area's large institutions, including the hospitals.

Chapter Eight. Political Will

1. John Mayer, chief of pediatric cardiac surgery, Children's Hospital, Boston, personal communication with author. To get proper recompense for surgical procedures for newborns with congenital heart disease, the pediatric cardiac surgeons had to wage a campaign for several years to convince the payors of the technical complexities of anesthetizing and operating on small infants (some of whom were even premature and low birth weight).

2. The federal government leaves most issues related to families in the hands of the states. See Morgan LW, The Federalization of Child Support, a Shift in the Ruling Paradigm: Child Support as Outside the Contours of Family Law, *Journal of American Academy of Matrimonial Law* 16 (1999):195–221.

3. See www.unicef.org/crc/crc.htm (accessed September 22, 2005) for a description of the convention; for the Implementation Handbook, see www.unicef.org/publications/index_5598.html. One of the impediments to the U.S. signature has been the language in the document prohibiting capital punishment for minors. The Supreme Court decision *Roper v. Simmons* of March 1, 2005, made the U.S. stance on this decision more compatible with the convention statements.

4. The UNICEF comment on the U.S. refusal to sign the convention is also found at www.unicef.org/crc/crc.htm (accessed September 22, 2005).

5. Ross Roundtable, *Environmental Health* (Abbott Park, Ill.: Ross Products Division, 1996); Needleman HL and Landrigan PJ, *Raising Children Toxic Free* (New York: Farrar, Strauss, and Giroux, 1994).

6. Lombardi J, Starting Right, *American Prospect,* November 2004, pp. 14–15; Meyers M and Gornick JC, The European Model, *American Prospect,* November 2004, pp. 21–22.

7. The birth rate (births per 1,000 women ages 15–44) has varied over the century. At the beginning of the twentieth century the rate was 120; during the Depression and the years of World War II, the rate was 76; in the postwar years it was again in the 120 range. See www.cdc.gov/nchs/data/nvsr/nvsr51/nvsr51_04.pdf; also see U.S. Department of Commerce, *Historical Statistics of the United States, Colonial Times to 1970,* pt. 1, series B–10, p. 49 (Government Printing Office, 1975).

8. U.S. Census 2000, *Demographic Trends in the 20th Century,* particularly table 15, Households by Type, by Presence of Own Children under 18, and by Age of Householder, 1950–2000. In 2000, 52 percent of households had no children under the

age of 18, while in the 1960s the share was 43 percent. Also see table 13, Households by Size,1900–2000: in 1940 one-person households accounted for only 8 percent of households; in 2000 this share was 26 percent.

9. The overall good health and the longer life expectancy of American society has dramatically affected U.S. age-group distributions. Two shifts have occurred for children and youth. First, children and youth ages birth to 19 years have become a smaller proportion of the overall population (U.S. Census 2000, *Demographic Trends in the 20th Century*, particularly figure 2-2). Second, at the age of 19, youth do not become independent adults but instead enter a kind of waiting period, not fully dependent on their families but rarely independent, either. Young people looking for work find that there are few jobs, especially for the inexperienced. They are encouraged to continue their education, get a degree, take out educational loans, and put off entering the world of work. At the same time, they are lured into adulthood at ever-younger ages: good nutrition has changed their growth patterns, with a secular downward trend in the age of menarche. (The average age of menarche in the 1840s is said to have been 16.5; in 1988 it was 12.5 years; see www.infoforhealth.org/pr/j41/j41chap1 _2.shtml#top [accessed September 22, 2005]). Further, children are treated increasingly like little adults, with television, the Internet, the movies, and the commercial markets conceiving of them as consumers. In 1997, children's direct influences on parental purchases was estimated at $188 billion. See www.globalissues.org/ traderelated/consumption/children.asp (accessed April 9, 2006).

10. Barnett WS, *Lives in the Balance: Age 27 Benefit-Cost Analysis of the High/Scope Perry Preschool Program* (Ypsilanti, Mich.: High/Scope Press, 1997), p. xi: "In 1992 constant dollars discounted at 3% annually, the program cost $12,356 per participant to operate ($7,252 per child per school year, with 13 children attending 1 year and 45 attending 2 years). Offsetting this investment were the following per participant returns to the taxpayers: a $6,287 return due to the participant's decreased overall schooling costs, an $8,847 return from increased taxes paid on the participant's higher earnings, a $2,918 return due to reduced cost of welfare assistance to the participant, a $12,796 return due to decreased justice-system costs, and a $57,585 return due to decreased crime-victim costs. Thus the $12,356 investment per participant provided a total return to taxpayers of $88,433, which is $7.16 for every dollar invested."

11. See www.saintjamescathedral.org/sandwich_sunday.asp.

12. See http//blogs.law.harvard.edu/palfrey.

13. March of Dimes comments on the proposed rule to redefine child under SCHIP are available at www.marchofdimes.com/aboutus/855_1946.asp (accessed September 22, 2005). Along with the American College of Obstetricians and Gynecologists and the American Academy of Pediatrics, the March of Dimes points out that the Bush plan to cover only unborn children would lead to disparities in prenatal care for poor mothers: "The proposed rule does not meet the well-established and clinically based standards of care for pregnancy developed and approved by the AAP and ACOG and published in Guideline for Perinatal Care."

14. Johnson KA and Kafer K, Why More Money Will Not Solve America's Education Crisis, at www. heritage.org/Research/Education/BG1448.cfm (accessed June 29, 2005).

15. Montana's smaller schools outperform larger schools; see www.mrea-mt.org/rsctfile2 .html (accessed June 29, 2005).

16. The National Institute for Child Health and Development and the Centers for Disease Control have proposed a major children's study to assess the effects of the environment and community on the health and development of a cohort of 100,000 children; see http://nationalchildrensstudy.gov/ (accessed September 22, 2005).

17. The Boston Miracle, or Operation Ceasefire, was the combined effort of the Boston Police Department and the Ten-Point Coalition of religious leaders to counter youth violence. In the late 1990s the program had very promising results, with a 60–70 percent decrease in youth homicide; see http://ojjdp.ncjrs.org/pubs/gun_violence/ profile21.html (accessed June 29, 2005). Also see Prothrow-Stith D and Spivak HR,

Murder Is No Accident: Understanding and Preventing Youth Violence in America (New York: John Wiley and Sons, 2004).

18. Robert Blendon uses polling techniques to determine public opinion about health topics; see Blendon R and others, America's Views on Children's Health *Journal of the American Medical Association* 280 (1998):2122–27, available at www.edbriefs.com/usa97-98/usa12.15.97.html.

19. The Children's Charter was drawn up at the 1930 White House Conference on Child Health and Protection; see Markel H and Golden J, Successes and Missed Opportunities in Protecting Our Children's Health: Critical Junctures in the History of Children's Health Policy in the United States, *Pediatrics* 115 supp. (2005):1129–33.

20. Clinton HR, *It Takes a Village* (New York: Simon and Schuster, 1996).

21. Marian Wright Edelman speaks of the cooption of the Children's Defense Fund phrase, "Leave No Child Behind," by the Bush administration as the act of a "deceptive weasel." See CDF Action Council, *A Nation and a Century Defining Time: Where Is America Going?* (Washington, D.C.: CDF, 2004). See www.cdfactioncouncil.org (accessed June 29, 2005) for a discussion of the Dodd-Miller "Act to Leave No Child Behind."

22. See http://nces.ed.gov/programs/digest/d03/tables/dt166.asp (accessed June 29, 2005).

23. See http://nces.ed.gov/surveys/pisa/PISA2003Highlights.asp (accessed June 29, 2005).

24. U.S. Department of Education, Ten Facts about K–12 Education Funding, available at www.ed.gov/about/overview/fed/10facts/index.html#chart7 (accessed June 29, 2005).

25. Urban Health Initiative; see www.urbanhealth.org/ (accessed June 29, 2005).

26. See www.cdfactioncouncil.org (accessed June 29, 2005).

27. Edelman M, Stand Up for Children Now, at www.cdfactioncouncil.org/stand_up_for_children_now.pdf (accessed April 9, 2006).

28. See www.usatoday.com/money/companies/2004-03-22-fortune-500-list_x.htm.

29. Edelman, Stand Up For Children Now.

Index

geographic information software (GIS),
72–73
geography, and health, 71–74
Gingrich, Newt, 181
Ginsberg, Ruth Bader, 166
globalization, 60
global warming, 213
gonorrhea, 69
Great Society, 168
group advocacy, 12, 121–143; age groupings,
128–135; clinical conditions groupings,
140–143; gay and lesbian youth, 134–135;
grouping systems, 128–143; guidelines,
125–127; national/ethnic/cultural attri-
butes groupings, 138–139; problems of
grouping, 122–124; social factors groupings, 135–138

Hack, Maureen, 131–132
Haggerty, Robert, 30–31, 33, 43
Hamilton, Alice, 20–24
happiness, pursuit of, 4, 239
Harlem Children's Zone, 73, 117
Harlem Children's Zone Asthma Initiative,
118
Harlem Hospital, 117
Harlem Injury Prevention program, 38
Hatch, Orrin, 174
Hawaii Healthy Start, 43
Head Start, 35, 108–110, 138
Head Start Alumni Parents, 115
Heagarty, Margaret, 38–40
health, defined, 1
health and health care disparities, 70–84;
family income and health, 74–77; geography and health, 71–74; race/ethnicity and
health, 77–84
health care: accessibility, 90–91; affordability,
91–92; appropriateness, 95; availability,
4–5, 75, 92–95; information sheets, 93–94;
reform, 173
Health Care Committee, 147
health care industry, 183
health insurance, 74–76, 162, 166–176; availability, 91–92; racial disparities and, 82;
State Child Health Insurance Program,
172–176; uninsured and underinsured
children, 91, 136–138
Health Insurance Portability and Assurances
Act (HIPAA), 190
Health Services and Centers Act of 1978, 36
Healthy Child Car America, 45
Healthy Children 2010, 164–165
Healthy People, 9, 36, 164–165, 202
Healthy Tomorrows, 45
Hearn, Ruby, 44, 229
Hein, Karen, 219

Helmholz, Henry, 167
HELP (Handgun Epidemic Lowering Plan),
155
Help Desks, 104, 116
Heritage Foundation, 222
Herrera, Vicki, 192
Herrick, James B., 28
HiB vaccine, 58
high-risk sports, 76
high school graduation rates, 54
HighScope, 133
Hippocratic oath, 184
Hispanic children, infant mortality and, 78
HIV/AIDS: black youth and, 80; education
and counseling, 162; epidemic, 63–64, 72,
140–142, 163; geography and, 72; HIV in-
fection, 57, 62, 69; prevention services, 111
Hole in the Wall Gang, 47
holistic care, 188
homeless children, 3, 138
Homer, Charles, 74, 98, 197
homicide, 57, 86
Hoover, Herbert, 225
HOPE Clinic, 138
housing, 3, 239
Howard Hughes Institute, 204–205
Hubel, David, 131
Hull House, 20–22, 24
Humphrey, Hubert, 178
Hunt, James, 228
Hutchins, Vince, 159, 161
hypoplastic left heart syndrome, 61

illness, causes of, 58–70; acute illness, 58–70;
chronic illness, 61–70; globalization and,
60
illness, vaccines and, 59
immigrants: health care benefits and, 91,
176; understanding culture of, 103
immigration trends, U.S., 52
immunizations, 60; poverty and, 75; tracking, 190
income: for child health advocates, 191–193;
family, 3, 239
Indian Health Service, 200
individualized health plan (IHP), 62, 93, 143,
165, 178
Individuals with Disabilities Education Act
(IDEA), 66, 176–181, 227
industrial development, children and, 213
industrial disease, 22
infant car seats, 101
infant mortality rate, 78, 159
infection: geographic areas and, 72; infectious disease patterns, 60; stress and, 31
injury: as cause of death, 57, 71; injury prevention initiative, 110